KU-467-499

SYSTEMS OF THE BODY

The Cardiovascular System

BASIC SCIENCE AND CLINICAL CONDITIONS

SECOND EDITION

Alan Noble BSc PhD
Visiting Lecturer in Physiology
School of Medicine
University of Southampton
Southampton, UK

Alan Thomas MA PhD MIBiol
Lecturer in Physiology
School of Biological Sciences
University of Southampton
Southampton, UK

Robert Johnson BA BM MRCP
Consultant in Paediatric Cardiology
Alder Hey Children's NHS Foundation Trust
Liverpool, UK

Paul Bass BSc MD FRCPath
Consultant Histopathologist and Honorary
Senior Clinical Lecturer
Department of Histopathology
Southampton University Hospitals
Southampton, UK

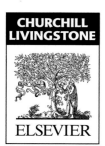

CHURCHILL LIVINGSTONE

ELSEVIER

EDINBURGH LONDON NEW YORK OXFORD PHILADELPHIA ST LOUIS SYDNEY TORONTO 2010

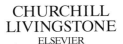

CHURCHILL LIVINGSTONE
ELSEVIER

First Edition 2005, Elsevier Limited.
Second Edition © 2010, Elsevier Limited. All rights reserved.

No part of this publication may be reproduced or transmitted in any form or by any means, electronic or mechanical, including photocopying, recording, or any information storage and retrieval system, without permission in writing from the publisher. Permissions may be sought directly from Elsevier's Rights Department: phone: (+1) 215 239 3804 (US) or (+44) 1865 843830 (UK); fax: (+44) 1865 853333; e-mail: healthpermissions@elsevier.com. You may also complete your request online via the Elsevier website at http://www.elsevier.com/permissions.

ISBN: 978-0-7020-3374-2

British Library Cataloguing in Publication Data
A catalogue record for this book is available from the British Library

Library of Congress Cataloging in Publication Data
A catalog record for this book is available from the Library of Congress

Notice
Knowledge and best practice in this field are constantly changing. As new research and experience broaden our knowledge, changes in practice, treatment and drug therapy may become necessary or appropriate. Readers are advised to check the most current information provided (i) on procedures featured or (ii) by the manufacturer of each product to be administered, to verify the recommended dose or formula, the method and duration of administration, and contraindications. It is the responsibility of the practitioner, relying on their own experience and knowledge of the patient, to make diagnoses, to determine dosages and the best treatment for each individual patient, and to take all appropriate safety precautions. To the fullest extent of the law, neither the Publisher nor the Authors assume any liability for any injury and/or damage to persons or property arising out of or related to any use of the material contained in this book.

The Publisher

ELSEVIER your source for books, journals and multimedia in the health sciences

www.elsevierhealth.com

Printed in China

Working together to grow libraries in developing countries

www.elsevier.com | www.bookaid.org | www.sabre.org

ELSEVIER   **BOOK AID** International   **Sabre Foundation**

The Publisher's policy is to use **paper manufactured from sustainable forests**

When we set about planning the First Edition of this book we were very conscious of the fact that medical education, in many centres, has moved on from traditional discipline-based curricula. The Systems of the Body series of books was conceived at Elsevier as being particularly suitable for integrated system-based or problem-based learning courses. In order to try to assist with this form of learning, our book on the cardiovascular system therefore includes relevant aspects of anatomy, physiology, pharmacology and pathology, all introduced in a 'whole-body' clinical context. We have included illustrative case histories which we hope will help to provide a framework for understanding the main content of each chapter.

In updating the book for the Second Edition we have included a series of "interesting facts" boxes which are scattered through the text. Some of these contributions identify particularly important concepts, some provide a historical context to the material in the Chapter concerned and others identify a more offbeat aspect of the topics discussed. A section of the book which demanded substantial modification was that concerned with the techniques currently in use to assess aspects of cardiac function. This reflects the remarkable technological advances which have been made in the only four year period between producing the two editions of this book.

All four of the co-authors of this book have been associated, in varying ways, with medical education programmes in the University of Southampton. In 1971 the Medical School was established with a systems-course basis and so it was a very early example of this type of course. The course has evolved steadily since its inception and the original educational concepts have been retained and developed.

A fundamental aspect of studying anything is to develop an understanding of the language that is used. In order to try to help with this, we have included a glossary of commonly used terms at the end of the book.

We do hope that you find this book useful and that you enjoy reading it.

ACKNOWLEDGEMENTS

We particularly wish to acknowledge the contribution of Sue Noble to the production of this book. She has been a major source of help and enthusiasm for both editions. Lynn Watt, the Project Development Manager at the publishers, Elsevier, was exceptionally helpful in producing the First Edition of this book and for the Second Edition Lulu Stader has been similarly outstanding.

Our colleague, Professor Geraldine Clough, provided very helpful and constructive criticism of a draft of Chapter 11: Capillary function and the lymphatic system.

Paul Bass acknowledges the patience and encouragement of his family, Paulina, Aaron, David and Abraham and Alan Noble would similarly like to acknowledge Sue, Kate, Liz and Han.

A DESIGN SPECIFICATION FOR THE CARDIOVASCULAR SYSTEM

1

Chapter objectives

After studying this chapter you should be able to:

1. Explain the necessity for our enormously profuse circulatory system.

2. Describe the limitations posed by diffusion as a way of delivering oxygen to tissues and removing carbon dioxide.

3. Outline the mechanisms whereby the pH of body fluids is kept within narrow limits.

4. Briefly outline the characteristic changes in cell structure and function associated with cell death.

5. Describe the gross structure and function of the major types of blood vessel within the circulation.

6. Define angiogenesis and outline its role in the mature cardiovascular system.

7. Explain the pattern of presentation of cardiovascular disease with peaks in the very young and in older members of society.

The gross structure and function of the cardiovascular system is dictated firstly by the need to deliver oxygen continuously to the 100 000 000 000 000 (10^{14}) cells which make up the 'textbook person'. Oxygen is used by cells to generate ATP, the metabolic energy source for all the functions of the body. Oxygen is not particularly soluble in water and will only diffuse quickly over short distances. Moreover, oxidative metabolism generates acidic products, particularly CO_2, and continuous removal of these sources of H^+ is essential for the maintenance of life. Marginal failure of either oxygen delivery or hydrogen ion removal will result in illness and tissue damage but total failure of either will end in death within a few minutes. For example, cessation of oxygen supply to the brain leads to a loss of consciousness in 8–10 seconds and permanent brain damage in 5–10 minutes.

As a consequence of these performance requirements we have evolved with a circulatory system which in the textbook person, if stretched out end to end, would measure 60 000 miles or 96 000 km. This is enough to encircle the world three times. This book is about the organization and control of this circulatory system, the causes and effects of failure and the basis for treatment regimens aimed at avoiding or minimizing the effects of circulatory failure. An example of a clinical history of a patient with developing circulatory problems is introduced in Case 1.1:1.

Some fundamental concepts in relation to these opening paragraphs need further explanation.

Textbook person

Textbooks of basic biomedical sciences are inherently sexist, ageist and do not recognize either relatively small or large individuals. They are written primarily about male, 70 kg subjects in the age range 20–25 years. Textbooks contain statements such as 'cardiac output is 5 L/min'. This is a figure which may well apply to the textbook person at rest, but there are wide variations which all represent perfectly normal values for a given individual within the population at large.

Oxygen consumption

Our textbook subject at rest consumes about 250 mL O_2/min and generates 200 mL CO_2/min. This gives rise to the concept of a respiratory quotient (RQ):

$$\text{Respiratory quotient (RQ)} = \frac{CO_2 \text{ produced}}{O_2 \text{ consumed}}$$

The precise value for RQ in any individual will reflect the composition of their diet but for a typical person consuming a mixed diet of carbohydrate, fat and protein the RQ would be about 0.8. This means that we normally consume more oxygen than we produce carbon dioxide. During exercise oxygen consumption may increase to

---

Case 1.1   A design specification for the cardiovascular system: 1

A young man with a history of insulin-dependent diabetes mellitus

Calvin was first diagnosed with diabetes when he was 10 years old. He had initially responded well to the need to comply with his treatment regimen of dietary control and regular doses of insulin given by self-injection. He was familiar with these problems as both his father and grandfather also had diabetes.

However, by the time Calvin reached 18 years old his diabetes did not fit well with his own self-image. He wanted to be out enjoying life with his friends and did not like to feel he was 'an invalid'. This led to him becoming lax with his medication and his blood glucose control became less rigorous.

There were a number of occasions on which Calvin felt unwell and over a period of 5 years there was a series of eight emergency hospital admissions. On one such occasion he had been drinking more water than usual (polydipsia) and had been producing greater than normal amounts of urine (polyuria) for about 3 weeks. He had become drowsy and lethargic and, for the 3 days prior to the hospital admission, he had been vomiting.

The doctor in the emergency room noted that he was underweight for his age and build. Initial observations included a pulse rate of 142 beats/min, a blood pressure of 100/60 mm Hg and abnormally deep breathing. A venous blood sample provided the following data:

[Glucose] = 37 mmol/L (3.5–5.5 fasting)
[Na^+] = 132 mmol/L (135–145)
[K^+] = 5.5 mmol/L (3.5–5.0)
[Haemoglobin] = 17.5 g/100 mL (13.5–18.0)

Normal reference values are shown in brackets.

A urine dipstick test also showed the presence of glucose and ketones.

This case history raises the following questions:

1. What evidence is there in this history of body fluid volume depletion?
2. What is the link between volume depletion, Calvin's low blood pressure and his fast heart rate?
3. What aspects of this history give immediate cause for concern and form the basis for clinical management strategies?

Aspects of the answers to these questions are discussed in Case 1.1:2 and in the text of this chapter.

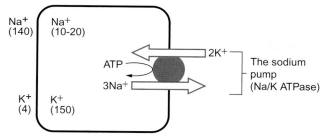

Fig. 1.1 The left hand side of this diagram shows typical concentrations of Na and K inside and outside cells. The right hand side depicts the sodium pump which uses ATP to maintain the ionic gradients across cell walls. Concentration units are mmol/L.

about 10 times the resting value and the RQ may move closer to a value of 1 due to preferential metabolism of carbohydrate.

Interesting facts

30–40% of all the food we consume in our lifetime is used to generate ATP to drive the sodium pump which maintains the sodium and potassium concentration gradients across cell membranes.

Oxygen is used within the mitochondria of cells to generate adenosine triphosphate (ATP). This provides the energy for movement, for the synthesis of macromolecules and to drive the movement of ions, particularly Na^+ ions, across cell membranes against a concentration gradient. The distribution of Na^+ and K^+ inside and outside cells is summarized in Figure 1.1. The ion gradients are maintained by the sodium pump which expels three Na^+ ions and pulls two K^+ ions into the cell each time it operates. As both of these ion movements are against a concentration gradient, an ATP molecule is hydrolysed to provide the energy. For some cells there may be about a million sodium pumps each operating at about thirty times a second. In the body as a whole the sodium pump accounts for about 30% of all of our energy intake over our lifetime. In this way, ionic gradients are maintained which are essential for the continuing function of nerves and muscles, including the heart. Failure to maintain ATP generation in hypoxic tissues leads to osmotic swelling of cells and to a loss of normal cellular function (see p. 7). To serve all the requirements, the quantities of ATP which must be synthesized are quite prodigious and amount to something roughly equivalent to an individual's body weight every day.

Diffusion

Diffusion is the movement of particles from an area of high concentration to an area of low concentration. The concentration of a gas in solution is actually the product of the partial pressure and the solubility coefficient (a constant at a given temperature). Two sets of units are in common usage for gas pressures. The appropriate conversion factors are as follows:

$$1 \, kPa \equiv 7.5 \, mm \, Hg$$

$$1 \, mm \, Hg \equiv 0.133 \, kPa$$

Some important parameters determining rate of diffusion are:

- the diffusive gradient (concentration difference between two points)

- the solubility of the particle in the solvent; if it is not very soluble the concentration will be low

- the size of the solute particle (small particles will diffuse faster than large particles)

- temperature: diffusion is faster at high temperatures than at low temperatures; body temperature is about 37°C in normal human subjects.

Most diffusion in living systems takes place in an environment in which water is the solvent, although molecules such as oxygen and carbon dioxide also have to diffuse through the lipid bilayer which makes up cell membranes. Special provision, in the form of transport proteins and ion channels, is made for ions which carry a charge and are therefore not lipid soluble.

Einstein (1905) showed that the time taken for a molecule to diffuse between two points varies as the square of the distance between the points. In physiological terms, diffusion is fine as a process for moving molecules short distances. A typical cell diameter in the body is about 10 μm and the time taken for an oxygen molecule to diffuse this distance would be a few milliseconds. Diffusion of oxygen over longer distances, however, such as the approximately 10 mm (a thousand times 10 μm) thickness of the ventricular wall of the heart, would take a million times as long, a time measured in hours. This would be inconsistent with maintaining life as, given the composition of the atmosphere, the diffusive gradients of oxygen available to us would be too small. The solution to these problems is to have an amazingly profuse circulatory system which delivers the oxygen and other nutrients very close to the cells where they will be used. Cells in the body are rarely more than 50 μm from a capillary and most are not more than 10–20 μm away.

The diffusive gradients concerned with loading of oxygen into pulmonary capillary blood at the lungs and the delivery of oxygen into the tissues are shown in Figures 1.2 and 1.3. Figure 1.2 shows the events at the interface between an alveolus and a pulmonary capillary. A typical Po_2 in the alveolus is 13.3 kPa (100 mm Hg). Blood returning to the lungs has a Po_2 of about 5.3 kPa (40 mm Hg) and so oxygen diffuses into the pulmonary capillary blood from the alveolus. The diffusive gradient for unloading CO_2 at the lungs is much smaller than for O_2. Mixed venous blood Pco_2 is about 6.1 kPa (46 mm Hg) whilst alveolar Pco_2 is typically 5.3 kPa (40 mm Hg).

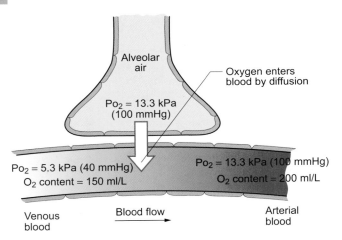

Fig. 1.2 Loading of oxygen by diffusion from the alveolae into pulmonary capillaries.

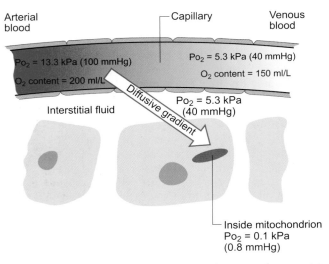

Fig. 1.3 Diffusive gradient. Diffusive gradient for oxygen from arterial blood to the mitochondrion of a cell where the oxygen is used. The interstitial fluid outside the cell is part of the way down this diffusive gradient. When blood leaves the tissue as venous blood it has equilibrated with the interstitial fluid.

The diffusive gradient for CO_2 (0.8 kPa) is 10% of the diffusive gradient for O_2 (8 kPa). Both diffuse at about the same rate because CO_2 is 20 times as soluble in water as O_2. The transit time for red blood cells through pulmonary capillaries at rest is about 1 second but the diffusive exchange of O_2 and CO_2 is normally complete in about 0.25 seconds.

Delivery of O_2 into the tissues (Fig. 1.3) starts with the arterial blood which has picked up O_2 in the lungs (P_{O_2} = 13.3 kPa; 100 mm Hg). Oxygen is used inside the mitochondria and the P_{O_2} here is of the order of 0.1 kPa (about 1 mm Hg). The interstitial fluid outside a cell is part of the way down a continuous diffusive gradient between

the arterial blood and the inside of a mitochondrion. A typical P_{O_2} in the interstitial fluid is 5.3 kPa (40 mm Hg). Blood leaving a capillary has equilibrated with this fluid and so venous P_{O_2} is the same as in the interstitial fluid.

Interesting facts

Under normal circumstances, the lungs have spare capacity for several of their functions. For example, completion of the exchange of oxygen and carbon dioxide at the pulmonary capillary: alveolus interface only takes about a quarter of the approximately 1 second available for gas exchange. These safety factors mean that some degree of malfunction of the heart and lungs can be tolerated.

Carriage of oxygen in blood

A further consequence of the poor solubility of oxygen in water is that we have evolved with an oxygen-carrying pigment, haemoglobin (Hb). The oxygen-binding characteristics of haemoglobin are such that it is nearly fully saturated with oxygen at the partial pressure of oxygen normally present in the alveoli of the lungs. Figure 1.4 shows the oxyhaemoglobin dissociation curve. At a P_{O_2} of 13.3 kPa (100 mm Hg), a typical figure for the alveolus, Hb is 97–98% saturated with O_2. This information can be used to calculate the amount of oxygen carried bound to haemoglobin as follows:

Amount O_2 carried bound to Hb = [Hb] × 1.34
× % saturation Hb with O_2 (mLO$_2$/L blood).

Typical values for [Hb] are 120 g/L (women), 140 g/L (men). The figure 1.34 mL/g is the volume (mL) of oxygen bound to 1 g Hb when it is fully saturated. These figures mean that arterial blood contains about 200 mL O_2 bound to Hb per litre blood. A small amount (0.3 mL/L) is carried as dissolved O_2

Reference to the oxyhaemoglobin dissociation curve (Fig. 1.4) shows that venous blood is about 75% saturated with O_2 at P_{O_2} = 5.3 kPa (40 mm Hg) and therefore about one quarter of the O_2 carried in arterial blood has moved into the tissues. One quarter of the 200 mL O_2/L present in arterial blood is 50 mL. If 50 mL of O_2 is typically deposited in the tissues from each litre of arterial blood, and the textbook person's cardiac output (volume of blood pumped per minute from each side of the heart—see Chapter 4) is 5 L/min, then 250 mL O_2/min is delivered to the tissues. This is the amount of oxygen identified previously as a figure for O_2 consumption rate for the textbook person at rest.

All tissues do not have the same oxygen consumption rate relative to blood flow. The figure quoted above, that 'venous blood is typically 75% saturated with oxygen', refers to 'mixed venous blood', i.e. the blood in the right side of the heart which is a mixture of all the venous drainages for the whole body. Venous blood from the kidneys, which have a high flow rate but relatively low O_2 consumption, has an oxygen saturation of about 90%. By contrast, the blood in the venous drainage from the

Calvin's acute circulatory problems

Calvin's fundamental problem was a lack of insulin, a hormone which moves glucose from the circulation into cells particularly in the liver and skeletal muscle. In addition, in the absence of insulin gluconeogenesis, the conversion of amino acids from the breakdown of protein into glucose is promoted. The high blood [glucose] leads to an osmotic diuresis, excessive urine production and hence body fluid volume depletion. Responses to volume depletion in the form of blood loss (haemorrhage) are discussed in Chapter 14.

The diuresis is the cause of a high [haemoglobin] due to loss of fluid from the extracellular compartment. An appropriate clinical test for volume depletion is to compare standing and lying arterial blood pressure measurements. Normally there will be no substantial difference but in the volume-depleted patient there is a drop in pressure (postural drop) on standing.

In Chapter 4 of this book the links between blood volume and cardiac output (the volume of blood pumped by the heart per minute) are discussed. Basically, the fall in blood volume (a decreased preload on the heart) leads to a decrease in cardiac output and, as a consequence, a fall in arterial blood pressure. The baroreceptor reflex (see Chapter 10) reacts to a fall in blood pressure with an increase in heart rate and constriction of peripheral blood vessels.

Body fluid replacement with a combination of 0.9% saline and 5% glucose is the first priority in order to avoid circulatory collapse. The apparent anomaly of giving extra glucose to a patient with an already high blood [glucose] is explained as follows.

The textbook person contains about 42 L of water. The factors which determine the distribution of this volume between different compartments are described in detail in Chapter 11. Basically, about 14 L is in the extracellular compartment, which includes blood plasma and 28 L is in the intracellular compartment. An increase in the osmotic strength of body fluids, due to high blood [glucose] combined with a decrease in capillary blood pressure associated with volume depletion, means that there is movement of water from the intracellular compartment to the extracellular compartment. As a consequence Calvin suffers both intracellular and extracellular volume depletion. There is a high [Na^+] in extracellular fluid and a low [Na^+] in the intracellular fluid. Infusion of saline into a patient will therefore selectively expand the extracellular compartment. Administration of 5% glucose solution initially does not substantially change the osmotic strength of body fluids but, once the glucose has become distributed around the body, insulin supplements will drive the glucose into cells where it can be metabolized to CO_2 and water. Giving 5% glucose is therefore equivalent to an infusion of pure water and will initially dilute the extracellular compartment. The osmotic gradient created will move water into the intracellular compartment. Infusion of 5% glucose will therefore expand both the intracellular and extracellular compartments. These ideas are explained in more detail in Chapters 11 and 14.

A further potential cause for concern is the increase in plasma [K^+]. This is likely to be a result of a ketoacidosis, a form of metabolic acidosis. At a level of 5.5 mmol/L this is not a significant problem, but further increases in potassium as a result of acidosis-induced movement of K^+ from inside to outside cells can lead to the development of cardiac arrhythmias and potentially cardiac arrest (see Chapters 2 and 7). Despite a raised plasma [K^+] there may be whole body depletion of K^+ as most of the K^+ is in the intracellular compartment.

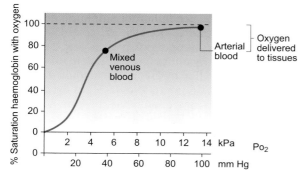

Fig. 1.4 Oxygen–haemoglobin dissociation curve.

Interesting facts

The task of working out the three-dimensional structure of haemoglobin was undertaken by Max Perutz in Cambridge. It took him 23 years but the answer taught us a huge amount about how the oxygen carriage mechanism works. He was awarded the Nobel Prize in 1962.

The shape and position of the oxyhaemoglobin dissociation curve (Fig. 1.4) shows one of the safety factors in relation to lung function. The top of the curve is nearly flat from 13 kPa (100 mm Hg), normal arterial Po_2, down to about 10 kPa (75 mm Hg). This means that a decrease in Po_2 within this range makes little difference to the % saturation of haemoglobin with oxygen, that is little change to the total amount of oxygen carried in arterial blood. Put another way, we can afford to have a certain degree of lung malfunction before it makes any significant difference to oxygen delivery to the tissues.

heart is only 25% saturated with O_2. This is an important concept in relation to physiological control mechanisms and to the pathological consequences of disturbances of coronary blood flow (see Chapter 5).

Cyanosis

Cyanosis is an important clinical sign. It refers to the blue colouration of the skin and mucous membranes produced by the presence of excessive amounts of deoxygenated haemoglobin in arterial blood. It is fundamentally classified into central and peripheral cyanosis.

Central cyanosis is often observed on the lips particularly but is conveniently looked for in a warm environment, the inside of the mouth. It represents a failure of the heart and lungs to ensure adequate oxygenation of the blood during passage through the lungs. There is no agreed quantitative standard for central cyanosis but the presence of 50 g of deoxygenated haemoglobin in 1 L of arterial blood is a commonly used definition. In some laboratories lower levels down to 20 g deoxygenated Hb in 1 L of blood are used to define central cyanosis. In a patient with 150 g Hb in 1 L of blood, 50 g/L as deoxygenated Hb is one third of the total, i.e. a % saturation of 67%. In anaemic patients, despite poor oxygenation of their tissues, a point is reached at which it would be impossible for them to become cyanosed. A patient with 70 g Hb in 1 L blood (about half normal) which is normally saturated with oxygen (97–98%) has enough oxygen delivery to the tissues to support life. However if 50 g Hb/L out of 70 g Hb/L in arterial blood was deoxygenated the patient would be dead not cyanosed.

Peripheral cyanosis which is visible in extremities such as fingers and ears is caused by impaired local blood flow and excessive local extraction of oxygen from the available blood supply. This occurs for example in cold environments (hence the expression 'blue with the cold') or in peripheral vascular diseases such as Raynaud's disease (see Chapter 9).

Interesting facts

Polymorphisms of the haemoglobin molecule are thought to be the most numerous naturally occurring genetically determined variations of any protein in the body.

The battle against the hydrogen ion: acid–base balance

Proteins play many important roles in the body, as structural proteins, membrane ion channels and transporters and as enzymes.

The amino acids which make up proteins have a number of side groups which can bind or release H^+ ions. These include carboxylic acid groups ($-COO^- + H^+ \rightleftarrows COOH$), amino groups ($-NH_2 + H^+ \rightleftarrows NH_3^+$) and the imidazole side group of histidine which can be protonated. Increasing $[H^+]$ will make it more likely that these sites bind an H^+ ion and, conversely, decreasing $[H^+]$ will make it more likely that H^+ ions are released. These anionic and cationic sites are involved in forming ionic bonds which stabilize the three-dimensional structure of proteins and therefore changes in $[H^+]$ will alter the shape of proteins and will modify their functional characteristics. For example, altering the shape of ion channels will alter ion permeability and hence bring about changes in the membrane potential of the conducting system of the heart (see Chapter 2), and in the nervous system, which can be lethal. Close regulation of extracellular and intracellular $[H^+]$ is therefore crucially important.

Under normal conditions extracellular fluid pH is maintained within the narrow range of 7.36–7.44. A pH of 7.4 corresponds to a $[H^+]$ of 40 nmol/L (40×10^{-9} M). This is a very low concentration, especially compared to the other constituents of body fluids. Typical $[Na^+]$ in plasma, for example, is 140 mmol/L, over three million times the free $[H^+]$, yet it is commonly changes in $[H^+]$ which ultimately lead to death. The extremes of pH which are compatible with human life are thought to be pH 6.8–7.8 ($[H^+] = 160$ to 16 nmol/L). It must be stressed however that these extremes could only be tolerated for a very short period of time and, clinically, very much smaller deviations from the normal range are a cause for concern.

Although we need to maintain $[H^+]$ in body fluids at a very low level, oxidative metabolism generates large quantities of H^+. The major source of this H^+ is carbon dioxide.

The textbook person generates about 14 moles of CO_2 per day. Failure of the circulation (as the transport system) and the lungs (as the site of excretion) to adequately get rid of this CO_2 leads to respiratory acidosis, a common feature of lung disease. Acutely, complete failure to excrete CO_2 for only a few minutes would lead to a rapid fall in pH and death. Overvigorous excretion of CO_2 (i.e. hyperventilation) leads to respiratory alkalosis, a pH above the normal range. Clinically, alkalosis is much less common than acidosis but is still potentially dangerous when it does occur.

The second form of acid to be excreted comes from the oxidative metabolism of dietary constituents. Complete metabolism of sulphur-containing amino acids, for example, will lead to the generation of sulphuric acid which must be excreted via the kidneys. The total load of such 'metabolic acid' for the textbook person is of the order of 50–100 mmol/day. Quantitatively this is a smaller challenge than the excretion of CO_2 but nevertheless it is very significant considering the low $[H^+]$ in body fluids. Failure to excrete H^+ adequately via the kidneys leads to metabolic acidosis. Examples of this are renal failure or the overproduction of keto acids which occurs in poorly controlled diabetes mellitus, as in the case history of Calvin described in this chapter. Depletion of metabolic acid, as in vomiting, leads to a metabolic alkalosis.

The roles of the circulatory system in relation to acid–base balance can be summarized as buffering and transport. Buffering of H^+ is essential to prevent substantial fluctuations in pH during the transport of H^+ from the site of generation in the cells to the site of excretion in the lungs or kidneys. The most important buffering systems in blood are proteins, especially haemoglobin, and the bicarbonate

Case 1.1 — A design specification for the cardiovascular system: 3

Arterial blood gas measurements

Calvin provided an arterial blood sample for blood gas analysis, which gave the following results:

P_{CO_2} = 1.4 kPa (4.7–6.0) = 10.5 mm Hg (35–45)
P_{O_2} = 15.9 kPa (11–13) = 119 mm Hg (80–100)
pH = 7.15 (7.35–7.45)
$[HCO_3^-]$ = 3.5 mmol/L (24–30)
Base excess = −22 mmol/L (−2 to +2)
Normal reference values are shown in brackets.

Calvin has a ketoacidosis, a form of metabolic acidosis. This is shown by the large negative base excess. He is hyperventilating as a response to H^+ ions detected by his peripheral chemoreceptors. The CO_2 produced in his tissues is being diluted into a volume of alveolar gas about three to four times the normal volume and hence P_{CO_2} is a quarter to a third of normal values. The P_{O_2} is high as a result of the hyperventilation and there is no indication of lung malfunction. An increase in P_{O_2} at this level does not significantly increase the volume of oxygen carried in the blood as haemoglobin is already 97–98% saturated at normal arterial P_{O_2} (Fig. 1.4).

Base excess is a quantitative assessment of the metabolic component of the acid–base disorder. Thus in this case each litre of body fluids has been depleted of bicarbonate (HCO_3^-) by 22 mmol/L. This can be viewed as the result of bicarbonate

binding to hydrogen ions and being excreted at the lungs as CO_2.

$$H^+ + HCO_3^- \rightleftarrows H_2CO_3 \rightleftarrows H_2O + CO_2$$

Clinical management of the acidosis may involve infusion of sodium bicarbonate but it will often be corrected just by administration of insulin. This will end the ketoacid production and hence help to normalize acid–base status. A danger in the management of the acidosis is the attendant fluctuations in plasma $[K^+]$. During an acidosis there is effectively an exchange of H^+ and K^+ across cell membranes such that acidosis results in hyperkalaemia. This may itself become life-threatening (see Case 1.1:2). Treatment of the acidosis however brings its own problems. K^+ ions re-enter cells when the acidosis is corrected but also one of the physiological roles of insulin is to move K^+ into cells. This happens normally for example after the intake of a K^+ load, such as a banana, chocolate or orange juice. The combination of a reversal of the acidosis and the effects of insulin administration may cause plasma $[K^+]$ to fall to dangerously low levels with consequent effects on the membrane potential of pacemaker cells in the heart (see Chapter 2).

buffer. Haemoglobin acts as a buffer because the protein component, globin, can absorb or release H^+ as described earlier. The bicarbonate buffer relies on the generation of HCO^-_3 by the kidneys each time a hydrogen ion is excreted into the urine. The transport function of the circulatory system is crucial in maintaining acid–base balance. It is essential to have a very profuse circulatory system with a blood capillary close to every cell in the body so that H^+ ions can be removed immediately they leave the cells where they are generated. Local circulatory failure will lead to local tissue acidosis. This concept is further discussed in relation to shock mechanisms in Chapter 14 of this book.

Apart from its general role as a nutrient delivery and waste collection system in the body, the circulatory system has other functions in relation to the immune system (see Chapter 11) and in thermoregulation (see Chapter 9).

Cell injury and cell death

Cell injury

Cell injury may be reversible or irreversible. Often a cell/group of cells will initially adapt to a given stimulus and there may be no cellular signs of injury. An example is the cardiac muscle cell in mild hypertension. However, if the stimulus persists or increases in amount/frequency as in severe, long-term hypertension, reversible and ultimately

irreversible injury leading to apoptosis or necrosis may occur.

Causes of cell injury

There are numerous causes of cell injury. These include: hypoxia (lack of oxygen), infection (bacteria, viruses, fungi), physical agents (hot or cold temperatures, ultraviolet radiation), chemicals (acids, alkalis), and immunological stimuli such as autoantibodies against, for example, thyroid epithelium.

Cell injury occurs because a cell has to function outside its normal homeostatic capabilities. Thus, if acid is slowly added to the environment of a cell, initial adaptation may occur, but eventually a point of no return will be reached when the adaptive response can no longer protect the cell and cell death occurs.

Mechanisms of cell injury include:

- cell membrane damage such as that caused by complement pathway-related membrane attack complex or free radicals

- mitochondrial damage as seen in hypoxia and cyanide poisoning

- ribosomal damage as in the effect of alcohol on hepatocytes

- nuclear damage caused by radiation or viruses.

Although a particular agent may preferentially target one part of the cell, there is always a wide-ranging cascade of events. Thus, once the cell membrane is damaged, cell pumps such as the sodium pump described earlier will be compromised, also the cytoplasmic composition will change and this will affect mitochondria, the nucleus and other cell organelles.

The response to injurious agents will depend on both the type of cells involved and the type of agent.

Highly specialized cells with a cytoplasm rich in sensitive organelles, such as cardiac muscle cells or renal proximal tubular epithelial cells, may be more prone to cell injury from factors such as hypoxia or drugs than more simple cells such as fibroblasts. In addition, cells which are already compromised, by hypoxia for example, may be more prone to new or further injury than normal cells. The response of a cell population to injury is also dependent on the ability of the cells to divide. In this respect, the cells of the body can be categorized into three groups designated labile, stable and permanent.

- Labile cells divide continuously as they are maintained in the cell cycle (Fig. 1.5). They are often stem cells or precursor cells in a cell population such as basal epidermal or gut lining cells and bone marrow cells. A reduction in labile cell number can, potentially, be quickly reversed.

- Stable cells are usually excluded from the cell cycle and are found in G_0. They can be driven into the cell cycle, at G_1, by an appropriate stimulus. This usually involves growth factor production by the surviving similar or neighbouring different cells. Once in the cell cycle, they can divide and restore cell numbers. Examples of this include renal tubular epithelial cells after acute tubular necrosis or hepatocytes after viral hepatitis.

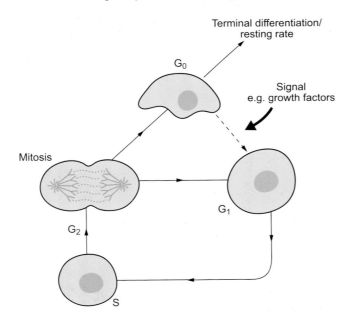

Fig. 1.5 The cell cycle. G_0, non-dividing (resting) state; G_1 and G_2, gap/preparation phases; S, replication of DNA. Source: Bass et al., 2009.

In both labile and stable cell populations there is a large potential 'reserve' for restoring cell numbers and therefore tissue/organ function. This replenishment of a cell population by exactly similar cells is known as 'regeneration'.

- Permanent cells have no ability to divide and are excluded from the cell cycle. The classic examples are neurones and cardiac myocytes. Thus, after the brain and heart have been fully formed in utero, no new neurones or cardiac muscle cells will appear. These cells cannot replicate when cells are lost as, for example, after significant hypoxia. The body therefore has an alternative strategy. 'Scarring' known as gliosis in the brain and fibrosis in the heart, occurs and the dead cells are replaced by inert, non-specialized, fibrous tissue composed mainly of collagen. This is laid down by myofibroblasts found in granulation tissue. The process whereby the cells of a tissue are replaced by scar tissue is known as 'repair'.

The type of agent causing the injury will also be important. Some cells, such as cardiac myocytes, are more prone to hypoxia than for example fibroblasts. The length of time cells are exposed to the injurious agent is also important, and after a significant time period even fibroblasts will be injured by hypoxia. A further critical variable is the severity of the exposure. Cardiac myocytes are more prone to injury in anoxic (no oxygen) conditions than mild hypoxic (relative lack of oxygen) conditions.

Cell death: apoptosis and necrosis

It is now well established that cell death is actually a spectrum of cellular events and changes. At one end of this spectrum is 'apoptosis', a recognized normal physiological event, and at the other is the pathological process of 'necrosis'.

Apoptosis occurs when cell populations need to be fine-tuned. Although essentially a physiological event, it can occur as part of pathological processes. Physiologically, during fetal development, the digits of the hands and feet develop from solid 'bars' of tissue and the interdigital webs are removed by apoptosis. Similarly, the lumen in many hollow viscera is produced by apoptosis of the central cells. Autoreactive T lymphocyte cells are deleted from the young thymus by apoptosis. During the apoptotic process, the cell itself switches on genes which code for new proteins and some of these proteins cause the cell to die. Hence the term 'cell suicide' is used to describe apoptosis. Endonucleases cause DNA fragmentation and caspases destroy proteins. The cell is effectively killed from within. Cell membrane pumps may remain viable until the very end of the process. Morphologically, the cell shrinks, the nuclear chromatin condenses and the cell breaks up into a number of apoptotic bodies, which are cleared up (phagocytosed) by macrophages or neighbouring cells. The apoptotic cells are recognized by novel surface signal molecules. The apoptotic process is extremely quick, lasting a few minutes. It often only affects a relatively small number of cells and causes no lasting tissue damage.

At the other end of the cell death spectrum is necrosis. Necrosis is the sum of the morphological changes that result from cell death in a living tissue. Necrosis is pathological, involves large numbers of cells and, importantly, evokes a potentially damaging, inflammatory response. Table 1.1 shows a comparison between apoptosis and necrosis. There are five main types of necrosis and these are outlined in Table 1.2.

Overall, therefore, cell death usually results in cessation of function of a tissue or organ. In necrosis, the dead cells rupture and there is spillage of cell contents. Amongst the extruded material there may be enzymes/proteins from the cytoplasm or specific organelles that enter the blood stream. These enzymes/proteins can be used as clinical 'markers' to assess which cells are damaged, the extent of the damage and even the timing/duration of the process. Examples of this include enzymes released following myocardial necrosis (see Chapter 5).

Overall functional structure of the cardiovascular system

The gross structure of the cardiovascular system is that we have two populations of blood vessels, the systemic and pulmonary circulations, which are perfused by two pumps mounted in series (Fig. 1.6). The fact that the two pumps are joined together in the heart with a common control system is convenient but is not theoretically essential.

The relatively high pressure developed in the systemic arterial system, a result of the left ventricle pumping against the resistance to blood flowing through the rest of the systemic circulation, provides the driving force to perfuse all the tissues of the body with blood except the lungs (see Chapter 10). A series of arterial vessels branching from the aorta distribute the blood to the tissues of the body. Within these tissues, distribution of blood flow is primarily controlled at the level of the arterioles and pre-capillary sphincters but exchange of nutrients and waste

Table 1.1 Comparison of apoptosis and necrosis

Feature	Apoptosis	Necrosis
Type of process	Programmed cell death usually physiological	Pathological cell death
Purpose of process	Process used to 'fine tune' cell populations—individual cells/groups of cells involved (e.g. finger webs in embryogenesis)	Pathological event, often causing massive tissue destruction with numerous cells dying (e.g. myocardial infarction)
Progression of process	Complex 'triggered' series of intracellular biochemical events involving enzyme production and activation (DNA switched on)	Pathological insult tips cells out of limits of adaptability and irreversible cell death occurs
Rate of process	Very rapid	Usually slow
Final result	Ultimately cell shrinks, nucleus condenses and cell fragments into apoptotic bodies which are phagocytosed. No inflammation occurs	Ultimately the cells swell, burst and the intracellular contents often provoke intense inflammation

Table 1.2 Types of necrosis

Type	Aetiopathogenesis	Morphology	Example
Coagulative	Denaturation of intracellular proteins	Firm tissue. Cell 'ghosts' seen	Heart Kidney
Liquefaction (colliquative)	Enzymatic tissue dissolution (lysomes in neurones)	Soft semi-fluid tissue. Destroyed architecture	Brain
Fat	Damage to adipocytes (enzymatic or traumatic)	Firm yellowy tissue. Dead adipocytes seen±inflammation with giant cells	Pancreas Breast
Gangrenous	Coagulative necrosis and putrefaction as a result of infection particularly with clostridia	Black foul-smelling tissue	Limb Bowel
Caseous	Intracellular infection with *Mycobacterium tuberculosis*	Soft, white tissue. No cell 'ghosts' seen	Tuberculosis

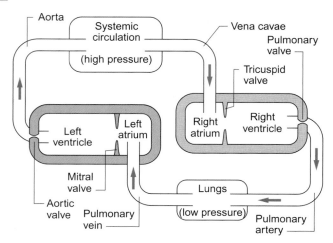

Fig. 1.6 Gross structure of the circulation. The arrows indicate the direction of blood flow.

products takes place in the capillaries (see Chapter 11). Blood then drains through venules into small veins and eventually the great veins (superior and inferior vena cavae) to return to the right side of the heart. The structures and functions of each of these types of blood vessel will be described later in this chapter.

The output from the right side of the heart serves the relatively low pressure pulmonary circuit (Fig. 1.6). Blood leaves the right ventricle in the pulmonary artery and gas exchange between blood and the alveoli of the lungs occurs in the pulmonary capillaries. Carbon dioxide diffuses from the blood into the alveoli and oxygen diffuses in the reverse direction. Blood returns to the left side of the heart in the pulmonary veins.

Blood pressure in the circulation

The systemic loop is a relatively high-pressure circuit. The peak (systolic) pressure generated in the aorta when the left ventricle contracts is typically 120 mm Hg and the trough (diastolic) pressure reached when the ventricle is refilling is typically 80 mm Hg. Mean pressure is 93 mm Hg (see Chapter 10). After passage of blood through a series of resistances, small arteries, arterioles, capillaries, venules and veins, the blood returns to the right atrium where the mean pressure is typically 0–5 mm Hg. There is a continuous drop in pressure going round each of the loop circulations. This is of course essential for blood to flow from one point to the next, that is downhill in pressure terms.

The pulmonary blood supply is a relatively low-pressure loop. The systolic pressure generated in the pulmonary artery is typically 20–25 mm Hg and the diastolic pressure 8–12 mm Hg. Pulmonary capillary blood pressure is about 8–11 mm Hg and any significant increase in this value leads to excessive movement of water out of the pulmonary capillaries and a major clinical problem, pulmonary oedema (see Chapter 11). Pressure in the pulmonary vein and the left atrium is normally about 5–8 mm Hg.

Case 1.1 — A design specification for the cardiovascular system: 4

Calvin's cardiovascular problems later in life

By the time Calvin was 40 he had developed hypertension. His GP told him that this was more common in diabetic than non-diabetic subjects and this was especially true for people of Afro-Caribbean descent such as Calvin. Hypertension affects over half of all people with diabetes. The regulation of arterial blood pressure and the development of hypertension are discussed in Chapter 10. The GP explained to Calvin that he was concerned because the combination of his still poorly controlled diabetes and his hypertension posed a considerable risk of a future heart attack or stroke. These problems are often secondary to the development of atheroma (see Chapters 5 and 8).

The risk of myocardial infarction or angina is between two and four times greater in diabetic patients than in the general population. Cardiovascular disease is the major cause of death in diabetes.

Now 48 years old Calvin began to notice a new set of problems. His feet lost their sensitivity to touch and pain. This meant that his feet were frequently damaged because he bumped into things or cut them. He could not tell whether shoes fitted correctly or not. The damaged area would ulcerate and become infected. The process of healing was very slow and eventually the ends of two of his toes on his right foot became necrotic (gangrenous) and had to be amputated. The loss of sensation in Calvin's foot is called a neuropathy. It arises because of the altered metabolic state in diabetes and particularly affects the sensory nerve endings in the hands or feet ('glove' and 'stocking').

Calvin had been referred to a hospital clinic where the team had been monitoring his kidney function regularly. Previously a regular series of urine dipstick tests for albumin conducted in the surgery had failed to show any positive results, although urine samples sent to the local hospital laboratory had provided evidence of microalbuminuria (a raised level of protein in the urine but still below the sensitivity of a dipstick test). He was prescribed an angiotensin converting enzyme inhibitor (ACE I) drug. It was hoped that this would help, in combination with other drugs, to control his raised blood pressure but also would slow the progression of renal failure by attenuating fibrotic mechanisms (see Chapter 9). The situation changed and now the albumin in Calvin's urine did become detectable by dipstick.

Some of Calvin's new problems were the result of diabetes-induced vascular damage. The background to this is outlined in Case 4.1:5.

Note: pressures in the circulatory system are measured relative to atmospheric pressure. Thus a pressure of 0 mm Hg in the right atrium means that it is the same as atmospheric pressure. Factors determining arterial blood pressure are described in Chapter 10.

Circulation time

The blood volume of an individual can be estimated to be between 7 and 8% of total body weight. For the textbook person weighing 70 kg, therefore, blood volume would be between 4.9 and 5.6 L. For a lean person, the figure of 8% is more appropriate, whereas 7% would apply to those more generously provided with adipose tissue.

Resting cardiac output for the textbook subject is about 5 L/min (see Chapter 4). This means that, at rest, the average red blood cell is doing a complete circuit of the double loop circulation described above every minute. During exercise (see Chapter 13) cardiac output may increase about fivefold. As blood volume is still the same, the average red cell is now completing the double circuit in 12 seconds.

Structure and function of blood vessels

The entire circulation consists of a tube of endothelial cells surrounded by varying amounts of the other tissue types which make up the blood vessel wall. The properties of endothelial cells as sources of vasoactive mediators (see Chapter 9) and their role in determining the functional properties of capillaries (see Chapter 11) are discussed later in this book.

The blood volume of the textbook person is about 5 L and its distribution among the various types of blood vessel is illustrated in Figure 1.7.

Structure of the blood vessel walls

With the exception of capillaries, blood vessel walls each consist of three layers, tunica intima (inner layer), tunica media (middle layer) and tunica adventitia (outer layer) (Fig. 1.8).

The tunica intima consists of the endothelial cells. The endothelial cells provide a physical barrier between the blood and the rest of the blood vessel wall. Disruption of this barrier is an important step in the development of atheroma (see Chapter 5).

The tunica media has two layers of elastic tissue, the internal and external elastic laminae, sandwiching a layer of smooth muscle. The media layer is a source of mechanical strength for the blood vessel and, as it contains smooth muscle, the means by which the diameter of the vessel can be altered.

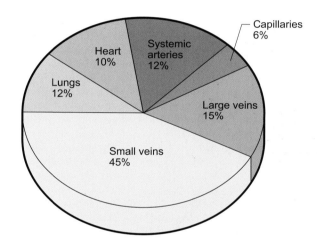

Fig. 1.7 Distribution of blood volume in a subject at rest. (Data taken from Davies A, Blakeley AGM, Kidd C Human physiology. London: Churchill Livingstone; 2001.)

	Aorta	Small artery	Arteriole	Capillary	Venule	Vein	Vena cava
Lumen diameter (typical size)	25 mm	4 mm	30 μm	5 μm	20 μm	5 mm	30 mm
Wall thickness	2 mm	1 mm	8 μm	0.5 μm	1 μm	0.5 mm	1.5 mm
Endothelium	✓	✓	✓	✓	✓	✓	✓
Elastic tissue	✓✓✓	✓✓✓	✓✓			✓	✓✓
Smooth muscle	✓	✓✓✓	✓✓✓		✓	✓	✓✓
Fibrous tissue	✓✓✓	✓✓	✓✓		✓	✓✓	✓✓✓

Fig. 1.8 Comparison of the size and typical wall composition of the major types of blood vessel. The relative amounts of the component tissues within each type of blood vessel are shown, not the absolute amount compared to other vessels.

The tunica adventitia is a layer of connective tissue containing fibrous tissue which serves to hold the blood vessel in place. The small blood vessels which supply the wall of large blood vessels with nutrients, the vasa vasorum, run through the adventitia connective tissue.

Arteries

Artery is a collective term which covers vessels with varying structures and varying functions. They exist on the high pressure side of the circulation and have an external diameter larger than about $100\,\mu m$. Arteries contain about 12% of the total blood volume (Fig. 1.7). They are conveniently divided into elastic and muscular arteries on the basis of their functions.

Large arteries (elastic arteries)

The adult human aorta has an internal diameter of the order of 25 mm and, at about 2 mm, the thickest walls in the peripheral circulation. The large arteries, the aorta and its major branches, are distensible and are referred to as 'elastic arteries'. The walls contain substantial amounts of both fibrous tissue and elastic tissue. Fibrous tissue is rich in collagen, which provides strength to the large arteries. The abundant elastic tissue in the walls of large arteries means that they can be inflated by the entry of additional blood each time the heart muscle contracts (systole). During the cardiac refilling phase, diastole, when blood is no longer entering the arteries from the heart, the large arteries recoil against the blood and help to maintain peripheral tissue perfusion. This is sometimes called the 'Windkessel effect' and the arteries concerned are referred to as 'Windkessel vessels'.

The amount of collagen and how firmly it is anchored in the wall of large arteries, increases with age and therefore the elasticity of the vessel is reduced. As a consequence, pulse pressure (systolic pressure minus diastolic pressure) also increases with age. Measurements of arterial wall stiffness are being developed as a non-invasive way of assessing the structural and functional integrity of arterial walls.

The walls of very large arteries, such as the aorta, do contain smooth muscle but, in relative terms, not as much as in smaller arteries. Large arteries play little role in the regulation of the peripheral circulation.

Small arteries (muscular arteries)

Vessels classified as small arteries have an internal diameter of 0.1–10 mm and typical examples would include the radial artery in the wrist and the cerebral and coronary arteries. The walls have a substantial amount of elastic tissue but a smaller fibrous tissue component compared to large arteries. These small arteries have relatively more smooth muscle than large arteries and, as a consequence, have some involvement in circulatory control mechanisms, especially in relation to the cerebral circulation. By the time blood has reached the end of the small artery segment of the circulation, mean arterial pressure has fallen from about 93 mm Hg (aorta) to 55 mm Hg, showing that this segment of the circulation poses a considerable, but not the greatest, resistance to blood flow.

Arterioles

Arterioles typically have a lumen diameter of about $30\,\mu m$ and a wall thickness of about $6\,\mu m$. Smooth muscle is a major component of the vessel wall and contraction is regulated by a range of mechanisms (see Chapter 9). The arterioles, together with some small arteries, are referred to as 'resistance vessels' and are the major site for regulation of the distribution of blood flow and for arterial blood pressure regulation (see Chapter 10). During passage through the arterioles blood pressure drops from about 55 mm Hg to 25 mm Hg at the entrance to the capillary segment. In the resistance vessels the pulsatile blood flow is smoothed out to a constant vessel pressure.

Figure 1.9 is a diagram of the 'microcirculatory unit', the arrangement of arterioles, pre-capillary sphincters, capillaries and venules inside a tissue. At the entrance to a capillary bed from an arteriole there is a small cuff of smooth muscle which acts as a pre-capillary sphincter. Closure of the sphincter means that the capillary is not perfused with blood. In resting muscle tissue, of the order of 90% of sphincters may be shut at any one time but will open during exercise (see Chapter 13). The sphincters have no nerve supply but are regulated by local metabolite concentrations.

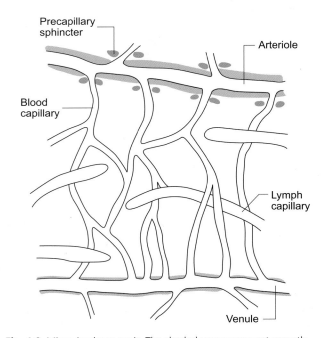

Fig. 1.9 Microcirculatory unit. The shaded areas represent smooth muscle.

Capillaries

Capillary walls have a single layer of endothelial cells about 0.5 μm thick with a surrounding, non-cellular, basement membrane. Capillary walls do not have smooth muscle but contractile elements within endothelial cells allow them to change shape in response to chemical mediators. This occurs, for example, as part of inflammatory reactions. The cells are not uniform in either structure or function throughout the body and this is discussed in more detail at the start of Chapter 11. Capillaries are the site of exchange of nutrients and waste products between the circulation and the interstitial fluid surrounding cells in the body. This is aided by the low velocity of flow through capillaries. They are the smallest blood vessels and make by far the largest contribution to the 60 000 miles of tubing which comprise the entire circulation. Despite this, only about 6% of total blood volume is flowing through capillaries at any one time (Fig. 1.7).

The capillaries, because they are so profuse, present an enormous cross-sectional area and therefore have a relatively small resistance to blood flow, especially compared to the arterioles. Pressure drop across a typical capillary bed is from 25 mm Hg at the arteriolar end to 15 mm Hg at the venule end.

Venules

These vessels have an internal diameter of the order of 30 μm and a wall about 3 μm thick. The wall comprises an endothelial cell lining together with small amounts of fibrous tissue and an often incomplete layer of smooth muscle. In common with capillaries, venule walls are an important site for the movement of water and nutrients between the circulation and the interstitial fluid (see Chapter 11).

Veins

Small veins typically have an internal diameter of the order of 5 mm and a wall thickness of about 0.5 mm. The walls of veins do contain both elastic and fibrous tissues and also smooth muscle but all of these are in smaller quantities than equivalent-sized arteries.

Veins are very distensible, in other words, if pressure increases inside a vein it will expand easily. Small veins accommodate a high percentage of total blood volume (about 45%) (Fig. 1.7) and have an effective venoconstrictor sympathetic nerve supply. This is important to avoid venous pooling of blood in the lower half of the body, especially during changes in posture (see Chapter 9). Small veins in the lower half of the body have valves which are an important aspect of the venous return mechanisms which move blood against the force of gravity from the legs back to the heart (see Chapter 4).

Pressure drop from the end of the venules (15 mm Hg) through the small veins and vena cava to the right atrium

Box 1.1 Microvascular and macrovascular disease in diabetes

Diabetes increases the risk of both microvascular and macrovascular complications. This will be made worse by the coexistence of other risk factors such as hypertension, cigarette smoking and hypercholesterolaemia (see Chapter 5).

Poorly controlled diabetes is associated with an increased risk of microvascular complications. Capillary basement membranes become thickened with consequent alterations in their permeability and structural integrity (see Chapter 11). The capillaries of the retina and the kidney are particularly susceptible. Damage to the blood vessels of the retina makes diabetes the commonest cause of blindness in people aged 30–69, a 20-fold increase in risk compared to non-diabetic patients.

In the kidney, glomerular basement membrane changes lead to an increasing permeability to plasma proteins and the entry of increasing amounts of albumin into the nephron. Normally, the small amounts of protein filtered in normal subjects are reabsorbed in the proximal tubule but eventually this mechanism is overwhelmed resulting in proteinuria. This may lead on to the development of oedema (see Chapter 11) and eventually to end-stage renal failure which must be managed by either dialysis or transplantation.

Microvascular problems in diabetes are not however the major cause of cardiovascular death in diabetic patients. Macrovascular complications are 70 times more likely to be fatal. Ischaemic heart disease and peripheral vascular disorders affecting large arterial blood vessels in the legs for example are usually secondary to the development of atheroma (see Chapter 5). About 85% of strokes are atherothrombotic and the risk of this is two to three times higher in patients with diabetes. The remaining 15% of strokes follow an intracranial haemorrhage and the incidence is similar in diabetic and non-diabetic subjects.

(0–5 mm Hg) is sufficient to ensure flow of blood back to the heart but the small gradient illustrates the fact that these vessels do not pose a major resistance to blood flow.

Vena cavae and other large veins

The inferior and superior vena cavae are sometimes referred to as the great veins. The inferior vena cava has an internal diameter of about 30 mm, larger than the aorta, but a wall thickness (1.5 mm) which is less than the aorta. The walls of the vena cavae contain quite a lot of fibrous tissue together with some elastic tissue and smooth muscle. These large veins contain about 15% of total blood volume (Fig. 1.7).

The fibrous tissue in the wall of the vena cava provides strength. This is necessary because wall tension in this large vessel is significant. This can be illustrated by reference to the law of Laplace. This law applies to any distensible structure and links wall tension (T), radius (R)

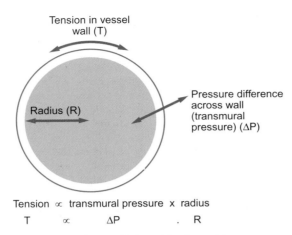

Tension in vessel wall (T)

Radius (R)

Pressure difference across wall (transmural pressure) (ΔP)

Tension ∝ transmural pressure × radius

$$T \quad \propto \quad \Delta P \quad . \quad R$$

Fig. 1.10 Law of Laplace applied to a blood vessel.

and the pressure difference (ΔP) across the wall of the vessel, the transmural pressure (Fig. 1.10):

$$T \alpha \Delta P \times R$$

Although pressure inside the vena cavae is low, the radius is large and so a significant wall tension is developed. Application of this principle to capillaries, which have a very small radius, reveals that capillaries have very low wall tension and so do not tend to burst despite having a wall only one cell thick and containing blood at a higher pressure than the veins.

Angiogenesis

Most of the cells which make up blood vessel walls have a very long turnover time which is measurable in terms of months or years. In the brain capillary turnover time is particularly long.

In certain circumstances, such as in wound repair and in replacing the endometrium of the uterus every 28 days in menstruating women, there is a need for the formation of new blood vessels—angiogenesis. Excessive unwanted angiogenesis also occurs to support tumour growth and in chronic conditions such as psoriasis and rheumatoid arthritis. Conversely, insufficient angiogenesis is thought to be a feature of some aspects of heart disease, strokes and other pathological states.

New blood vessels form as branches (sprouts) from existing capillary blood vessels. The first stage involves the proteolytic digestion of a portion of the basement membrane followed by endothelial cell proliferation. This occurs close to the parent blood vessel and allows the immature blood vessel to grow towards a chemical stimulus generated by, for example, a hypoxic site or developing tumour cells. The migrating endothelial cells have eventually to form a tube and link up with another set of migrating cells before blood circulation can occur.

There are a host of cytokine agents implicated in both promoting and inhibiting angiogenesis. There is much research interest in their role in disease mechanisms and

in exercise physiology. The potential therapeutic use of drugs which could, for instance, suppress the development of the new blood vessels which allow tumours to increase in size is widely recognized.

From cradle to grave—the presentation of heart disease

Heart disease may present at any age though there are two clear peaks—the very young and the old. However the range of pathologies is quite distinct. Most children with cardiac problems are born with their heart disease whereas most adults acquire theirs. The Barker hypothesis suggests that in fact we are born with the potential for the acquired forms.

Babies with major heart problems may be diagnosed before birth and antenatal screening methods are improving all the time. The majority of major defects will present within a few hours of birth with symptoms such as breathlessness and poor feeding and signs such as cyanosis and murmurs (see Chapter 12). Incidental findings subsequently become the major route by which cardiac defects are identified, usually when children present to their GP or hospital with other illness which may be exacerbated by underlying heart disease.

An increasing number of conditions are found through screening children where there is a family history of genetically transmitted pathology, such as hypertrophic obstructive cardiomyopathy or long QT syndrome. Some cardiac illnesses are acquired during childhood. The commonest of these is Kawasaki's disease, an acute vasculitis which may lead to involvement of the coronary arteries with dilatation and stenosis. In the developing world rheumatic heart disease is a common cause of acquired heart disease in childhood triggered by streptococcal infection.

Between the ages of 5 and 40 the incidence of new cardiac disease reaches its nadir. There is a steady trickle through GP's surgeries and hospital clinics of chest pain, palpitations and exercise intolerance—all associated in the public and physician's mind with cardiac disease but seldom demonstrating any convincing pathology in this age group. Some will be musculoskeletal in origin, some atypical asthma, the majority nothing at all. Sadly, one of the major presentations of heart disease in this age group is sudden death for which a cardiac cause may be identified. This may trigger the screening of other family members in order to identify those at risk. An important group of patients is those in whom a familial dyslipidaemia is the underlying cause of accelerated atheromatous coronary disease. A carefully taken history looking at the incidence of sudden death or cardiac disease in young people will provide important clues to the likelihood of underlying pathology.

Slowly the classical features of coronary artery disease will begin to dominate the population as it ages. Symptoms such as swollen ankles (see Chapter 11), chest pain (see Chapter 6) or dyspnoea with exertion (see Chapter 5)

Case 1.1 — A design specification for the cardiovascular system: 5

Calvin's macrovascular complications

Calvin is now aged 62. His diabetes is reasonably well controlled but his compliance with the drugs he has been prescribed to reduce his blood pressure is not good. The problems with his feet and the toe amputations have reduced his mobility and this contributes to his being overweight and to a generally depressed approach to life.

Three months ago he started to experience crushing chest pains and to become more breathless. A coronary angiogram showed significant narrowing of his coronary arteries. Further tests are planned but Calvin feels he is just waiting for a heart attack to happen. Coronary blood flow regulation and myocardial infarction are discussed in Chapter 5.

---

herald the long-term decline related to progressive obstruction of the coronary arteries. The prevalence of cardiovascular disease rises steadily from the fourth decade. The initial evidence may come in the first acute myocardial infarction or even sudden death (the more common presentation in women over the age of 50). Various risk factors are recognized as increasing the progression of this condition; lifestyle factors such as smoking, obesity, inactivity and alcohol intake; medical problems such as diabetes, hypertension; genetic factors leading to familial predisposition. All must be assessed and factored in to the risk assessment and management of the individual.

Increasingly the detection of coronary heart disease occurs in screening programmes. So called 'Well Person Clinics' check for risk factors. The importance of this type of screening is increasing as it becomes more obvious that risk factors may be modified by interventions such as lifestyle changes and pharmacological therapy including cholesterol-lowering and antihypertensive drugs.

Further reading

Aaronson, P.I., Ward, J.P.T., 2007. The Cardiovascular System at a Glance. Blackwell Publishing, Oxford.

Abelow, B., 1998. Understanding Acid–Base. Williams and Wilkins, Baltimore.

Bass, P., Burroughs, S., Carr, N., Way, C., 2009. Master Medicine: General and Systematic Pathology, third ed. Churchill Livingstone, Edinburgh.

Davies, A., Moore, C., 2009. The Respiratory System, second ed. Churchill Livingstone, Edinburgh.

Donnelly, R., Emslie-Smith, A.M., Gardner, I.D., Morris, A.D., 2000. Vascular complications of diabetes. In: Donnelly, R., London, N.J.M. (Eds.), ABC of Arterial and Venous Disease. BMJ Books, London.

Folkman, J., 2006. Angiogenesis. Ann. Rev. Med. 57, 1–18.

Levick, J.R., 2009. An introduction to Cardiovascular Physiology, fifth ed. Arnold, London.

CARDIAC MUSCLE STRUCTURE AND FUNCTION

2

Chapter objectives

After studying this chapter you should be able to:

1. Describe the structural characteristics of cardiac muscle cells.

2. Discuss the role played by calcium ions in the regulation of cardiac muscle function.

3. Explain the ionic basis for the resting potential of the ventricular muscle cells.

4. List the characteristics of the pacemaker potential in sinoatrial and atrioventricular node tissue.

5. Explain the importance of the shape and duration of the cardiac muscle action potential in avoiding the development of a sustained tetanic contraction in the heart.

6. Explain the role of the bundles of His and the Purkinje fibres in distributing a wave of excitation to the ventricular muscle.

7. Describe the basis for some major arrhythmias of the heart and the actions of drugs which combat arrhythmias.

Cardiac muscle

The heart's role in producing the pressure gradient by which the body's tissues are perfused with blood means that cardiac muscle is active from about the fourth week of fetal life until death. The muscle which forms the contractile elements of the atria and ventricles is highly specialized. It shares many of its properties with skeletal (or voluntary) muscles although its action is not of course under conscious control. It also has properties which are more typical of involuntary or smooth muscle but the contractile mechanism is most like that in skeletal muscle. One of the main requirements of cardiac muscle is that it must contract in a rhythmic and coordinated fashion but it must not under any circumstance enter into a state of maintained, tetanic contraction. This requirement for a rhythmic pumping action is met by the electrical-charge-sensitive properties of the ion channels in the muscle cells. These properties result in a prolonged action potential which outlasts the mechanical twitch it produces and prevents sequential contractions from fusing into a single tetanic contraction. (Note: a 'tetanic' contraction means that if the frequency of stimulation of a muscle is increased, eventually a point is reached where the separate individual contractions become fused into a single sustained contraction.)

In skeletal muscle, fibres can be activated individually or in groups to vary the strength of the contraction. In the heart, the coordinated contraction resulting from the spread of activity across the atria and the ventricles requires that the cardiac muscle cells are electrically connected through gap junctions. In skeletal muscle the strength of contraction of individual fibres can be varied by changing the frequency of action potentials, but this is not an option for the heart where rhythmic contractions involve all of the cardiac muscle cells. Instead, the strength of contraction of cardiac muscle is regulated, as in smooth muscle, by varying the intracellular calcium concentration during activation of the cells. This provides a target site for drugs which affect the strength of cardiac contraction and hence cardiac output. The actions of these 'inotrope' drugs are discussed in Chapter 4.

Structure of cardiac muscle

The fundamental contractile unit in both skeletal and cardiac muscle is the sarcomere (Fig. 2.1). These units are about $2\,\mu m$ long and are defined at each end by the Z line which is formed from the protein α-actinin. Attached to the Z lines are the thin filaments made from F-actin which in turn consist of G-actin monomers joined together, in a structure sometimes said to resemble a helical string of beads, to form the thin filament (Fig. 2.2). These actin thin filaments are arranged in a parallel sandwich structure with the protein myosin (thick filament). Under polarized light microscopy the arrangement of the actin and myosin protein creates a striated (striped)

appearance in which the A band is generated by the myosin filaments and the I band is composed mainly of actin (Fig. 2.1).

Parallel bundles of sarcomeres are joined end to end to make up a myofibril. The myocytes primarily contain bundles of myofibrils together with mitochondria and the cell nucleus, which is displaced to one side of the cell. Unlike skeletal muscle the myocytes of the atria and ventricles are not attached to specific skeletal insertion points by tendons but instead they are joined together in a branched meshwork to form a muscular bag in which the cells contract against their attachment to adjacent cells. Each individual myocyte in the adult human heart is about $50–100\,\mu m$ in

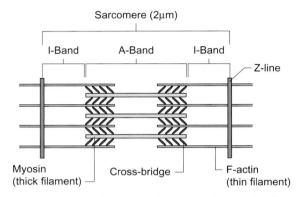

Fig. 2.1 Arrangement of actin (thin filament) and myosin (thick filament) within the contractile unit of cardiac muscle, the sarcomere. Cross-bridges, which can shorten, are formed between the myosin head and binding sites on the actin filament.

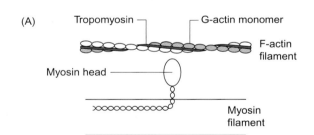

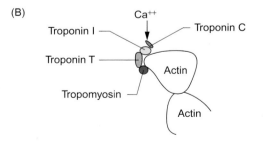

Fig. 2.2 (A) Cross-bridge between myosin and actin filaments in the resting state. Each actin filament (F-actin) is composed of two chains of G-actin monomers twisted around each other. (B) Ca^{++} binds to troponin C and this results in a rearrangement of the troponin complex, followed by movement of the tropomyosin filament and exposure of the myosin binding site on actin.

length and about 10–20 µm in diameter. In order to work as an effective contractile unit and to permit electrical activity to spread across heart muscle the individual muscle cells must be both physically joined together and electrically connected. This is achieved by the presence of 'intercalated discs'—sites of apposition and thickening of the sarcolemma of adjacent cells. The intercalated discs contain both high conductance gap junctions (connexons) which provide for electrical continuity and desmosomes containing the protein cadherin to form a junction with adequate physical strength.

Contractile mechanism in cardiac muscle

An increase in intracellular [Ca^{++}] causes contraction of the myocardial cell by a sliding filament mechanism similar to that in skeletal muscle. The actin and myosin filaments pass over each other as a result of the breaking and reforming of cross-bridges between the filaments (Fig. 2.2). The cross-bridges are formed between the heads of the myosin-filaments and the actin filaments. When the [Ca^{++}_i] (the intracellular calcium ion concentration) rises the calcium ions bind to troponin C, a part of the three protein troponin complex. Troponin C is attached to tropomyosin, a protein which in the resting state shields a specific myosin binding region on the actin filament. The resulting 'cross-bridge' between myosin and actin undergoes a structural change which moves the actin filament over the myosin filament producing a small contraction. The myosin head then disengages and the process is repeated causing the actin to 'walk' down the myosin filament. The force of contraction depends on the number of cross-bridges formed, a parameter which in turn depends on the [Ca^{++}] inside the muscle cell. Under resting conditions only a relatively small proportion of the potential total cross-bridge formation actually occurs. This means that physiological stimulation, via sympathetic nervous system activation, and drugs which increase intracellular [Ca^{++}] can generate a more forceful cardiac muscle contraction than occurs at resting levels.

Each cycle of cross-bridge formation involves the hydrolysis of an ATP molecule to alter the configuration of the myosin head as part of the contraction process. Cardiac muscle cells are continually contracting and require substantial amounts of energy. Metabolically they are similar to 'slow' skeletal muscle fibres in that they derive their energy from ATP generated by oxidative phosphorylation and the myocytes thus contain large numbers of mitochondria. It must be appreciated that, like any muscle, the contraction of cardiac muscle, particularly in the left ventricle, impedes the flow of blood through the coronary blood vessels and thus the heart muscle is only effectively perfused during its relaxation (diastolic) phase (see Chapter 5). A period of powerful cardiac contractions at a rapid rate such as might occur during exercise may result in the oxygen supply to the myocardium being insufficient to meet the metabolic demand. Responses to exercise are discussed in Chapter 13.

Regulation of intracellular [Ca^{++}] in cardiac muscle

As previously noted, the force of cardiac muscle contraction depends on the intracellular [Ca^{++}]. Opposite each Z line there is a tubular structure, the T tubule, running at right angles to the plasma membrane of the cell (Fig. 2.3). The T tubules help to spread electrical excitation rapidly into the cell and they run close to the sarcoplasmic reticulum (SR) in which Ca^{++} ions are stored. Ca^{++} is pumped into the stores by using Ca^{++} ATPase pumps which are regulated by the inhibitory protein phospholamban. The Ca^{++} used to trigger contraction of cardiac muscle therefore comes from two sources, the SR (about 75% of the total) and also transmembrane flux of Ca^{++} from the extracellular fluid (about 25% of the total). This is in contrast to skeletal muscle which only uses SR stores of Ca^{++} for contraction.

Interesting facts

Contraction of all three types of muscle, skeletal, cardiac and smooth muscle is triggered by a rise in intracellular [Ca^{++}]. The source of Ca^{++} for the contractile mechanism is different in the three muscle types.

The resting intracellular [Ca^{++}] is about 0.1 µmol/L and when an action potential (see p. 21) occurs in a cardiac muscle cell it triggers an initial increase in the intracellular calcium ion [Ca^{++}_i] concentration. The action potential results in an inward flow of calcium from the extracellular fluid where the ionized calcium concentration is about 1.2 mmol/L. This takes place through L-type calcium channels located in the T tubules and in the plasma membrane. The initial small increase in [Ca^{++}_i] causes the release of further calcium ions from the SR stores—the so-called calcium-induced calcium release. This is mediated by a Ca^{++} binding site on the SR which is part of a calcium channel protein often referred to as a 'ryanodine-sensitive receptor' or as a 'foot protein' (Fig. 2.3). As a result of calcium release from the SR the [Ca^{++}_i] increases, normally to about 0.5–2 µmol/L. In heart failure (see Chapter 6) there are significant alterations in how myocyte [Ca^{++}] is regulated.

During relaxation some Ca^{++} has to be exported back out of the cell and some replaced into the SR. Ca^{++} is predominantly expelled from the myocyte via a $3Na^+ - Ca^{++}$ exchanger which uses the inward 'downhill' movement of the $3Na^+$ to move Ca^{++} out of the cell (Fig. 2.3). This mechanism per se does not consume ATP although the Na^+/K^+-ATPase actively expels Na^+ across the plasma membrane in order to maintain the electrochemical gradient for Na^+. A portion of the Ca^{++} is actively expelled from the cell across the plasma membrane by Ca ATPases. ATP is also used to pump Ca^{++} back into the SR stores. Within the SR much of the calcium is stored as ionized Ca^{++}. However some is attached to calcium binding proteins of which calsequestrin is one of the most important.

Physiological stimulation of sympathetic nerves to the heart results in an increased force of contraction (see

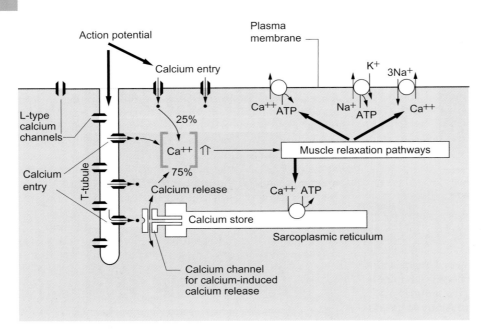

Fig. 2.3 Regulation of intracellular [Ca^{++}] in cardiac muscle. The increase in [Ca^{++}] which produces contraction follows the arrival of an action potential. This opens L-type calcium channels in the plasma membrane and T-tubule system and promotes Ca^{++} entry from the extracellular fluid. Ca^{++} ions entering via the T-tubule trigger further Ca^{++} release from the sarcoplasmic reticulum stores. For muscle relaxation to occur Ca^{++} must either be pumped back into the sarcoplasmic reticulum or expelled across the plasma membrane. The 3Na^{+}–Ca^{++} exchanger is driven by the [Na^{+}] gradient across the plasma membrane which in turn is maintained by the Na^{+}/K^{+}-ATPase.

Chapter 4). The β_1-adrenoceptor activation leads to a rise in intracellular cyclic AMP (see Fig. 4.6), a second messenger which activates several protein kinases. Subsequent phosphorylation of the protein phospholamban accelerates transport of Ca^{++} into the SR thus favouring retention of Ca^{++} in the SR at the expense of efflux back across the plasma membrane. Contractility of the heart is therefore increased by raising the amount of Ca^{++} stored in the SR. The rate of relaxation of cardiac muscle is also increased as the Ca^{++} re-enters the SR more quickly. The effects of cAMP in these events can be manipulated by drugs such as milrinone and caffeine which act as phosphodiesterase inhibitors and hence prolong the half-life of cAMP.

Interesting facts

Before the mid-1980s, dilated cardiomyopathy was a common disease in domestic cats. In most cases this was secondary to taurine deficiency. The problem has now largely been overcome by changes in diet formulation.

Cardiac electrical activity

Resting potential of ventricular muscle cells

The resting potential of a cardiac muscle cell is about −85 mV and, as in other excitable cells, this occurs as a result of the ionic concentration gradients maintained by the action of the Na^{+}/K^{+}-ATPase (see Chapter 1). The intracellular [K$^{+}_i$] is about 140 mmol/L whilst the extracellular [K$^{+}_o$] is about 4 mmol/L. We can consider a theoretical cell with such a concentration gradient for K^{+} and, initially, an equal number of positive and negative charges inside the cell. There is a diffusion gradient for positively charged potassium ions to move out of this theoretical cell and thus create a charge imbalance (potential difference) across the cell membrane with the inside of the cell negatively charged. The negative charge inside cells is mainly in the form of organic phosphates and ionizable groups on proteins, molecules which are too large to follow the K^{+} across the cell membrane. Eventually a situation is reached where the tendency for K^{+} ions to move out of the cell down the concentration gradient is balanced by the electrical gradient which will tend to move K^{+} ions back into the cell. This concept of the balance between the diffusive gradient and the electrical gradient is the basis for the derivation of the Nernst equation.

The work which would have to be done to move a mole of K^{+} ions against an electrical gradient of E volts is:

$$EZF \text{ Joules}$$

where E = the potential difference in volts, Z = the valency of the ion (i.e. 1, in the case of Na^{+} and K^{+}) and F = the number of charges in one mole of ions (the Faraday).

The work which would have to be done to move a mole of K^{+} ions against a chemical concentration gradient is:

$$RT \log_e (K_o/K_i) \text{ Joules}$$

where R = the gas constant, T = temperature in degrees Kelvin, K_o = potassium concentration outside the cell and K_i = potassium concentration inside the cell.

At equilibrium:

$$E_K \, ZF = RT \log_e (K_o/K_i)$$

or

$$E_K = \frac{RT}{ZF} \log_e (K_o/K_i) - \text{The Nernst equation}$$

Box 2.1 Goldman equation

The resting potential of nerve and muscle cells is predominantly determined by the concentration gradient and cell permeability for K$^+$ ions. The resting potential is therefore close to the potassium equilibrium potential (E_K) which can be calculated using the Nernst equation (see text). However the resting potential is also affected by other ions. If the impact of ions such as Na$^+$ and Cl$^-$ is taken into account the membrane potential can be calculated using the Goldman equation.

$$\text{Membrane potential} = \frac{RT}{F}\log_e\left[\frac{P_k[K_o^+] + P_{Na}[Na_o^+] + P_{Cl}[Cl_i^-]}{P_k[K_i^+] + P_{Na}[Na_i^+] + P_{Cl}[Cl_o^-]}\right]$$

where P_K, P_{Na}, P_{Cl} refer to the permeability to each ion, R is the universal gas constant, T is the temperature in degrees Kelvin, F is the Faraday constant.

A more complex form of the equation can be used to take account of other ions. The concentration gradient for negatively charged ions is reversed (compared to the cations).

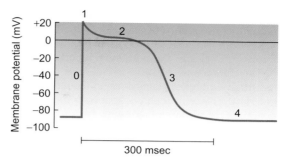

Fig. 2.4 Ventricular muscle action potential. The ionic fluxes associated with the five phases are described in the text.

For a monovalent cation such as K$^+$ at a typical body temperature of 37°C (310°K) this equation can be simplified to $E_K = 61.5 \log_{10} (K_o/K_i)$ by multiplying all the constants together and converting from natural logarithms to base 10 logarithms.

E_K is called the equilibrium potential for potassium. This means it is the membrane potential at which the net of flow of potassium ions out of a cell down the diffusive gradient is exactly balanced by their net movement into a cell down the electrical gradient. Implicit in the concept of an equilibrium potential is that only a single ion is considered each time.

The equilibrium potential for K$^+$ in cardiac muscle cells (−94 mV) is a little more negative than the actual resting potential (RP) of the cells which is about −85 mV. This is because the resting potential is also partly determined by the movement of ions other than K$^+$. However because the membrane is relatively permeable to K$^+$ and there is a substantial K$^+$ gradient maintained by the Na$^+$/K$^+$-ATPase, potassium normally has the greatest influence on the magnitude of the resting potential. In practice the membrane is also a little permeable to Na$^+$. It is possible to calculate the true resting potential by combining the concentration gradients of K$^+$, Na$^+$ and other ions weighted according to their relative permeabilities. Negatively charged ions have their concentration gradient reversed. The resulting equation is called the Goldman equation (see Box 2.1 for further explanation).

Cardiac action potential in ventricular muscle

The resting potential in cardiac myocytes is about −85 mV. When, as a result of a wave of excitation generated by pacemaker tissue, the cardiac muscle membrane potential has depolarized to the threshold potential (−60 to −65 mV) the opening of sodium gates in the membrane is triggered. As in other excitable cells, an action potential is then generated.

The ventricular muscle action potential has five phases (Fig. 2.4). In phase 0 the sodium gates open and the permeability to sodium (P_{Na}) increases about a hundred-fold which makes the sodium permeability much greater than that for other ions, including K$^+$. As a result the membrane potential rises to between +20 and +30 mV, that is approaching the equilibrium potential for sodium (E_{Na}) which is about +40 mV. At this point the sodium gates are 'inactivated' by the electric charge distribution across the cell membrane and the sodium permeability falls.

In phase 1 the K$^+$ permeability (P_K) begins to increase and K$^+$ leaves the cell at an increased rate down both a favourable concentration and electrical gradient. However the membrane potential does not immediately fall to E_K because there is a simultaneous opening of L-type voltage-gated Ca^{++} channels and an inward flow of Ca^{++} ions from outside the cell (phase 2). This calcium current results in a plateau phase of the membrane potential which lasts for as long as the calcium current flows. As described earlier, these events cause the release of a larger quantity of Ca^{++} from the sarcoplasmic reticulum which generates myocyte contraction (Fig. 2.3). Eventually the calcium channels are inactivated partly as a direct result of the rise in intracellular [Ca^{++}]. The membrane potential, under the influence of increased K$^+$ channel opening, falls (phase 3) to a value close to the potassium equilibrium potential (E_K). At this stage the cycle recommences from the resting potential (phase 4).

As described, the Na$^+$ channels in the muscle cell close at the peak of the action potential. They clearly have to be returned to a state where they can be stimulated to re-open before another action potential can be produced. The Na$^+$ channels remain closed during the plateau phase of the action potential (Fig. 2.4) and stimulation of the muscle during this phase cannot produce a further action potential. This is the 'absolute refractory' period of the myocytes. During repolarization (phase 3) many, but not all, of the Na$^+$ channels have re-opened by the time the membrane potential reaches −50 mV. Between −50 mV and complete repolarization a further action potential can be generated but this requires a greater than normal stimulation. This is the 'relative refractory period'. This has an important consequence in clinical medicine. Hyperkalaemia, a rise in plasma [K$^+$], is a frequent consequence of acidosis or inadequate excretion of K$^+$ from the body, a process normally regulated by aldosterone effects on the kidney. Hyperkalaemia may become life threatening because it will lead to depolarization of cardiac myocytes, that is a rise in the resting potential towards zero. This will mean that return to a sufficiently low (negative) membrane potential to ensure opening of all populations of Na$^+$ channels will not take place. Cardiac arrest may be the consequence.

The shape of the cardiac action potential is crucial to the functioning of the heart because the long plateau phase in the muscle cells outlasts the mechanical activity. This means that however hard the heart is stimulated individual contractions cannot fuse into a maintained tetanic contraction as happens in skeletal muscle. The heart is thus bound to beat rhythmically.

Pacemaker tissue

Cardiac muscle differs from skeletal muscle and most neurones in that in some areas of the heart the 'resting potential' is particularly unstable. After an action potential in these areas the membrane potential gradually drifts upwards (depolarizes) until a threshold potential is reached where the opening of sodium ion channel gates is triggered and ion permeability rises rapidly producing another action potential. Cardiac muscle therefore has the property of producing rhythmic depolarizations which, in turn, result in rhythmic contractions. The mammalian heart is said to be capable of myogenic activity. This can be seen when a piece of cardiac muscle is removed from a living heart. If it is kept warm and oxygenated in an artificial extracellular fluid environment it will continue to contract and relax spontaneously for some time. The resting and action potentials generated in the sinoatrial node are illustrated in Fig. 2.5.

The ability of a piece of cardiac muscle tissue to undergo spontaneous depolarization and hence generate action potentials is called automaticity. The parts of the heart which display automaticity are the sinoatrial node, the atrioventricular node and the bundle of His together with its Purkinje fibres. Ordinary ventricular muscle cells do not normally have automaticity.

The rate of contraction of any given piece of muscle will depend upon the rate of depolarization of the resting potential in the muscle cells. The part of the heart with the fastest rate of drift of the resting potential will have the fastest intrinsic rhythm. In the human heart this is the sinoatrial node (SAN), which is a band of tissue in the right atrium close to the junction with the superior vena cava (Fig. 2.6). In the SAN the K$^+$ permeability is lower and hence the initial resting potential (-60 mV) is less negative than elsewhere in the heart mainly because of the absence of one type of K$^+$ channel (the 'inward rectifier' potassium channel). The membrane potential drifts upwards (depolarizes) faster than in other parts of the heart and is called a pacemaker potential. The ionic events which contribute to the pacemaker potential are complex and include inward movement of Na$^+$ ions, an outward movement of K$^+$ ions which decays with time and, once the pacemaker potential has depolarized past -55 mV, there is an inward Ca^{++} current. The latter ion movement accelerates the rate of depolarization towards the threshold potential of between -55 mV and -40 mV at which an action potential is triggered (Fig. 2.5). In the normal heart the SAN serves as the cardiac primary pacemaker and determines the rate at which the whole heart beats. The intrinsic rate of the human SAN is about 110–120 beats per minute (bpm) but at rest it is normally under tonic parasympathetic inhibition so that the resting heart rate is typically about 70 bpm.

If, for some reason, the SAN fails to function or becomes electrically isolated from the rest of the heart then the area with the next fastest intrinsic rhythm is the atrioventricular node (AVN) which has an intrinsic rate of about 50 bpm. If the conduction of activity to the

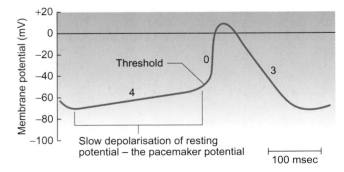

Fig. 2.5 Sinoatrial node potential (pacemaker potential). Increasing the slope of the slow depolarization of the resting potential leads to earlier arrival at the threshold potential and therefore an increase in heart rate.

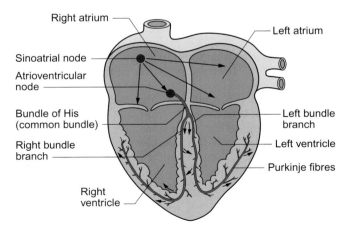

Fig. 2.6 Conduction pathway in the normal heart. Excitation originates in the sinoatrial node, spreads through the atria and is then transmitted to the ventricles via the atrioventricular node. The bundle of His has right and left branches to carry the wave of excitation to both ventricles.

ventricle through the AVN is interrupted ('complete heart block') then the ventricles will beat at their own rate of about 30–40 bpm driven by the intrinsic depolarization rate of the Purkinje fibres.

The control of heart rate is discussed in Chapter 4. Sympathetic nerve stimulation at the SAN increases the rate of phase 4 depolarization and therefore the threshold potential is reached more quickly and heart rate increases. Parasympathetic nerve stimulation via the vagus nerve slows the heart rate by a combination of two mechanisms. The SAN cells are hyperpolarized and the rate of rise of the phase 4 resting potential is also reduced. Both of these effects mean that it takes longer for the resting potential to reach the threshold potential.

An outline of a case history of a child with a disturbance of the cardiac conduction system is described in Case 2.1:1.

<hr>

Interesting facts

Mammalian hearts do not need a nerve supply to make them contract. Because of their intrinsic contractile ability (automaticity) they are described as being myogenic. Other types of animals such as insects, molluscs and crustaceans have neurogenic hearts which only beat in response to nerve stimulation.

<hr>

The transmission of the cardiac action potential

The cardiac action potential normally originates at the SAN because it is the region of the heart with the fastest intrinsic contractile rate. The action potential then spreads across the left and right atria. The atrial action potential is similar in shape to that of the ventricle although the plateau phase is shorter. There is a region of fibrous tissue called the annulus fibrosis, part of the fibrous skeleton of the heart, which effectively provides an area of insulation between the atria and the ventricles so that excitation must normally pass through the AVN in order to reach the ventricles. If there is an electrical 'leak' in the ring of fibrous tissue separating the atria and the ventricles this will be an alternative, direct route for excitation to spread from atria to ventricles. When this occurs it is called the Wolff–Parkinson–White (WPW) or pre-excitation syndrome and it generates a characteristic arrhythmia (see Chapter 7).

The cells within the AVN structurally resemble those of the SAN and the shape of their action potentials is similar except that the initial resting potential is about −80 mV and the depolarization 'overshoot' does not normally exceed +5 to +10 mV. The depolarization drift in phase 4 is slower because of the absence of a population of sodium channels, hence the slower intrinsic rate of firing. The AVN provides a junction between the atria and the ventricles but it also inserts a small delay of approximately 0.1 second (AVN delay) into the onward passage of the action potential. This is reflected in the rather gentle slope of phase 0 of the action potential in these cells and is caused by the small diameter of the nodal cells and their complex morphology. The delay allows time for the contraction of the atria to complete ventricular filling before the ventricles contract and expel blood from the heart.

The depolarization passes from the AVN into the 'bundle of His' (Fig. 2.6) which consists of specialized conducting tissue known as Purkinje fibres. These fibres are modified ventricular muscle cells and are grouped together in left and right bundles. They have a relatively large diameter and they are the largest of all the cells in the heart. This means they have a high conduction velocity. Purkinje fibres, together with the AVN tissue, have the longest refractory period of any cardiac cells. The functional importance of this is that is protects the heart against 're-entry' excitation from adjacent myocytes back into the conducting tissue which could potentially spread

<hr>

Case 2.1 Cardiac muscle structure and function: 1

Unplanned consumption of digoxin

Three-year-old Harry was brought to the hospital emergency department by his mother. She was concerned that Harry was found with a bottle of digoxin tablets prescribed for his grandfather for management of his cardiac failure. The bottle was open and there were many tablets scattered on the floor. It was not clear how many tablets were originally in the bottle nor how many Harry may have swallowed. This problem occurred roughly 2 hours earlier, the delay being because Harry's mother had to leave work in order to take him to the hospital.

The triage nurse immediately recognized the potential for serious poisoning and admitted Harry to the observation area where she applied a cardiac monitor. She also performed a 12-lead ECG and called the duty doctor to review Harry. Harry complained that he felt sick and that his 'tummy hurts'. The triage nurse gave Harry some activated charcoal by mouth.

Harry's ECG showed a rate of 63 bpm. Blood pressure was 76/48 mmHg. The P–R interval on the ECG was 0.21 s (normal 0.1 s). The doctor took some blood for electrolyte measurement and a digoxin concentration. The results showed [Na$^+$] = 137 mmol/L (normal range: 135–145 mmol/L), [K$^+$] = 5.7 mmol/L (normal range: 3.5–5.0 mmol/L). The initial plasma digoxin concentration was 8 μg/L (therapeutic range 0.5–2.0 μg/L).

1. Why is Harry's heart rate low and what information does the P–R interval provide?
2. Why is the plasma [K$^+$] high?

The answers to these questions can be found in the text of this chapter, in Box 2.2 and in Chapter 7.

back to the atria and cause dangerous arrhythmias. Other characteristics of the cells which comprise the conducting system are that although they are modified cardiac myocytes they have few myofibrils and so do not contract significantly when they are depolarized.

The Purkinje fibres conduct excitation quickly down each side of the septum before spreading out over the ventricles. As a result, depolarization of the ventricles occurs in a prescribed sequence starting with the papillary muscles and the septum and then spreading to the endocardial (inner) part of the ventricular muscle and out towards the epicardial (outer) surface. This coordinated spread of the electrical activity through the heart is responsible for the shape of the ECG (see Chapter 7). Repolarization of the muscle proceeds from epicardial to endocardial surface, the opposite direction to depolarization. This is the basis for the fact that the QRS complex (depolarization) and the T wave (repolarization) are both upwards deflections in a normal ECG, opposite polarity currents moving in opposite directions.

Drugs which act on the heart

The conducting pathway of the cardiac impulse and the electrical properties of the cardiac myocytes provide important therapeutic targets for drug actions. There are three main types of drugs which act upon the heart, those which are responsible for modifying heart rate, those which are used to regulate the rhythm of the heart and those which are used to regulate the force of cardiac contractions. The first group which broadly mimic or block the actions of the sympathetic and parasympathetic nerves controlling heart rate and the latter group (positive and negative inotropes) are discussed in Chapter 4.

Arrhythmias

The beating of the heart is normally driven by the spontaneous activity of the SAN and the heart is thus said to be in sinus rhythm. However there are occasions when this is not the case and an arrhythmia (the more scientifically rigorous term dysrhythmia is preferable but sadly it is not in widespread use) may be present. Arrhythmias may result from abnormal depolarization of cardiac tissue such that the cardiac rhythm is not being generated by the SAN or they may occur because cardiac excitation originates at the SAN but its conduction through the heart is abnormal (see Chapter 7).

If a piece of cardiac muscle is damaged and unable to conduct activity then the wave of excitation must go around it much like a crowd of people leaving a football match might move to either side of a tree. If one pathway is much longer than the other then, when the activity rejoins the healthy tissue, it may do so after the impulse which took the shorter route has gone and the cells are past their refractory period and capable of being stimulated again. As a result an action potential will be set up which will be

Normal spread of excitation

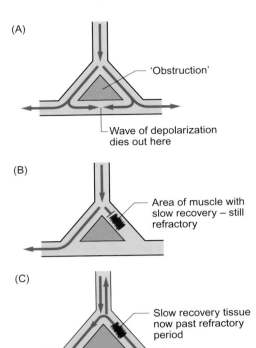

Fig. 2.7 Re-entry or circus mechanism for generation of arrhythmias. (A) Normal passage of a wave of depolarization around a region of non-myocyte tissue such as a blood vessel or fibrosed tissue from a previous infarction. The two waves of excitation meet on the far side of the obstruction and die out. (B) On one of the routes around the obstruction there is an area of tissue which is slow to repolarize, perhaps because of ischaemia. Initially this pathway cannot be excited. (C) The wave of depolarization taking the long route around the obstruction is delayed sufficiently to reach the damaged tissue when it has repolarized and it can now be retrogradely excited. Once past the damaged tissue this wave of depolarization can now carry on to re-excite other normal tissue. This constitutes a self-perpetuating loop or circus.

conducted in the conventional direction but also backwards (retrogradely) along the faster route (Fig. 2.7). This activity may collide with the next impulse passing down the faster route and negate it, or it may carry on around the loop producing what is called a re-entry arrhythmia. In circumstances where the ventricular rate is irregular, not all ventricular contractions may result in sufficient ejection of blood to allow a pulse to be palpated at, for example, the radial or brachial artery. As a result the pulse rate may not be the same as the ventricular rate recorded on an ECG.

On occasions, the ability of the wave of depolarization originating from the SAN to successfully pass through the AVN is impaired and this will result in various degrees of 'heart block'. In first-degree heart block there is a prolongation of the P–R interval of the ECG to greater than 0.2s (see Chapter 7) as transmission through the AVN is slowed. In second-degree heart block one may see a situation where not every wave originating at the

Case 2.1 Cardiac muscle structure and function: 2

Further progress with Harry's digoxin toxicity

Harry was transferred to the regional paediatric cardiology unit for further management. Four hours after his admission Harry became less well. The ECG monitor showed his ventricular rate had become irregular. A rhythm strip on the ECG showed an atrial rate of 155 bpm with second-degree heart block varying between 2:1 and 3:1. Harry's ventricular rate was between 60 and 80 bpm. An ECG showed a P–R interval of 0.24 s. The digoxin concentration was now 15 μg/L.

The National Poisons Unit was contacted for advice. They suggested treatment with lidocaine (lignocaine) (a broad-spectrum membrane stabilizer which acts on sodium channels) and Digibind (a monoclonal Fab antibody specific for digoxin). Over the next 6 hours Harry's heart rate stabilized and he returned to sinus rhythm.

1. Why are the atrial and ventricular rates different?
2. What is the rationale of administering lidocaine and the antibody?

Answers to these questions can be found in the text of this chapter and in Box 2.2.

Box 2.2 Pharmacological and toxic effects of digoxin

Digitalis glycosides are steroid-like compounds which were originally isolated from the foxglove plant and used as a herbal medicine. Digoxin is the most widely used compound among the glycosides which block the Na^+/K^+-ATPase (see Chapter 1) and hence raise the intracellular $[Na^+]$. This reduces the rate of expulsion of Ca^{++} from heart muscle cells via the $3Na^+/Ca^{++}$ co-transporter (Fig. 2.3, and see Fig. 4.7) and produces a positive inotropic action, that is an increase in cardiac muscle contractility (see Chapter 4). This was the therapeutic aim for which Harry's grandfather was prescribed digoxin. Independent of this action digoxin also has actions on the cardiac action potential and its conduction.

Digoxin can generate arrhythmias by increasing the excitability and automaticity of cardiac muscle. There are two mechanisms behind these actions. Blocking the Na^+/K^+-ATPase will lead to depolarization of the muscle cells and hence arrhythmias are more easily initiated. Secondly, digoxin promotes the release of Ca^{++} from the sarcoplasmic reticulum which leads to a transient depolarization of the cardiac muscle cell immediately after an action potential.

Although in the previous paragraph the pro-arrhythmic actions of digoxin are described, the drug also has important clinical actions which oppose the development of arrhythmias. These are mediated by central nervous system actions leading to stimulation of the vagus nerve. This has a modest effect slowing the SAN discharge but digoxin also slows transmission through the AVN. This is the effect seen in Harry with a prolongation of the P–R interval and second-degree heart block.

Digoxin is well absorbed in the gastrointestinal tract and has a long half-life of 1.5 days. This is further lengthened if renal function is impaired although this was not a problem in the case of Harry. Digoxin has a narrow therapeutic index, the difference between therapeutic and toxic doses of the compound. As the drug increases the automaticity of heart muscle toxic effects include the generation of ventricular ectopic beats. Other acute side effects include nausea, vomiting, anorexia, diarrhoea, confusion, malaise, vertigo and yellowed visual disturbances. These side effects are made worse by hypokalaemia. This was also not a problem for Harry.

Treatment of digoxin toxicity may include the use of atropine to block the vagally mediated effects of the drug and the use of monoclonal antibodies to bind and inactivate digoxin. Potassium supplementation may be used if necessary.

SAN is able to pass through the AVN. This usually occurs in a repetitive manner such that perhaps every third or fourth atrial depolarization wave fails to produce ventricular activity. Missed beats are often accompanied by a progressive lengthening of the P–R interval in the two or three preceding beats. Finally, in complete heart block there is no synchronicity between atrial and ventricular activity at all. In patients with complete heart block atrial systole will occasionally coincide with ventricular systole and thus contraction of the right atrium is attempting to move blood against a closed tricuspid valve (see Chapter 3). When this occurs blood from the right atrium flows back up the neck in the jugular vein producing what are known as cannon waves.

The bundle of His has two main branches, right and left. Blockade of conduction through only one branch is called bundle branch block. This is further discussed in Chapter 7 in the context of the characteristic ECG patterns.

Occasionally the phase 4 depolarization in cardiac cells may be more rapid than usual. This is likely to occur in pacemaker cells or in cells where the resting potential is normally stable but their ability to maintain a stable plateau potential is impaired, for example by ischaemia. This may result in the establishment of an ectopic pacemaker in areas of the heart where this does not normally occur. The ability of heart muscle to initiate its own activity, be it at a normal pacemaker site or at an ectopic site, is referred to as 'automaticity'.

Antiarrhythmic drugs

There is a widely used classification of antiarrhythmic drugs—the Vaughan Williams classification.

Class I

These drugs act on phase 0 of the action potential and slow the rate of rise of the action potential by inhibiting fast sodium channels. Class I includes a range of drugs with differing actions on ion channels. They are subdivided into three categories on the basis of their effects on the duration of the action potential: 1a, increases duration (disopyramide, procainamide and quinidine); 1b, decreases duration (lidocaine (lignocaine) and mexiletine); 1c, has no effect on duration (flecainide and propafenone).

Class II

These are β_1-adrenoceptor blocking drugs (beta-blockers). They reduce the rate of depolarization at the SAN and AVN as well as at some other tissues which may be producing an ectopic focus of activity. Conduction of impulses through the AVN is slowed. The most widely used drugs are atenolol and propranolol.

Class III

These drugs inhibit the K^+ channels involved in repolarization thus increasing the duration of the action potential and prolonging the refractory period. Drugs in this category include amiodarone, sotalol and bretylium.

Class IV

Some calcium channel blocking drugs reduce calcium entry and stabilize phase 4 of the action potential in the SAN and especially the AVN thus slowing the heart rate. Verapamil and diltiazem but not the dihydropyridine derivatives such as nifedipine have antiarrhythmic activity.

Digitalis glycosides (see Chapter 4), adenosine (see Chapter 9) and atropine (a muscarinic ACh receptor antagonist) are all used to modify cardiac rhythm disturbances. They do not fit into the Vaughan Williams classification of antiarrhythmic drugs.

Further reading

Bers, D.M., 2006. Altered cardiac myocyte Ca regulation in heart failure. Physiol. 21, 380–387.

DiFrancesco, D., 1993. Pacemaker mechanisms in cardiac tissue. Annu. Rev. Physiol. 55, 451–472.

Irisawa, H., Brown, H.F., Giles, W., 1993. Cardiac pacemaking in the sino atrial node. Physiol. Rev. 73, 197–227.

Katz, A.M., 1992. Physiology of the Heart, second ed. Raven, New York.

Levick, J.R., 2009. An Introduction to Cardiovascular Physiology, fifth ed. Arnold, London.

Noble, D., 1979. The Initiation of the Heart Beat. Clarendon Press, Oxford.

Sanguinetti, M.C., Keating, M.T., 1997. Role of delayed rectifier potassium channels in cardiac repolarization and arrhythmias. News Physiol. Sci. 12, 152–157.

Sommer, I.R., Johnson, E.A., 1979. Ultrastructure of cardiac muscle. In: Berne, R.M. (Ed.), Handbook of Physiology, Cardiovascular System, Vol 1. The Heart. American Physiological Society, Bethesda, pp. 113–186.

Waller, D.G., Renwick, A.G., Hillier, K., 2009. Medical Pharmacology and Therapeutics, third ed. WB Saunders, Edinburgh.

THE HEART AS A PUMP: VALVE FUNCTION AND VALVE DISEASE

3

Chapter objectives

After studying this chapter you should be able to:

1. Describe the gross structure of the heart and its associated valves.

2. Explain the series of events which constitute the cardiac cycle.

3. Describe the basic pathological features of congenital and acquired valve diseases.

4. Outline the key elements of clinical history taking and examination for suspected cardiac disease.

5. Explain the range of investigative methods available for the assessment of cardiac function.

Functional anatomy of the heart

The heart lies obliquely in the thorax within the mediastinum—the space between the lungs which also contains the major blood vessels, oesophagus and trachea. It typically weighs about $325 \pm 75\,g$ in men and $275 \pm 75\,g$ in women. The heart can be described as having three surfaces and an apex. About two thirds of the heart is to the left of the mid-line. The anterior surface of the heart is formed mainly by the right ventricle and is in contact with the ribs and sternum (Fig. 3.1). The inferior surface of the heart is formed mainly by the left ventricle and is in contact with the diaphragm. The posterior surface of the heart is formed mainly by the left atrium. This surface is also known as the base of the heart. The apex which is anterior to the rest of the heart consists only of the left ventricle and forms an important clinical landmark when assessing the size of the heart. The aorta and the pulmonary trunk arise from the left and right ventricles respectively at the superior pole of the heart (Fig. 3.2). The superior and inferior vena cavae open into the upper and lower parts of the right atrium. There are four pulmonary veins which open into the back of the left atrium. The junction between the atria and the ventricles is marked by the atrioventricular groove and the junction between the ventricles both posteriorly and anteriorly is marked by the interventricular grooves.

Interesting facts

About 2500 years ago, Hippocrates, a Greek doctor, recognized that blood vessels were of two different types. He thought that blood travelled from the liver and spleen to be warmed by the heart.

The fibrous skeleton of the heart is a framework of dense collagen around the atrioventricular junction and the arterial outflow. It provides structural support for the heart, particularly by stabilizing the heart valves, and it also prevents the heart from being overstretched (Fig. 3.3). The electrical insulation provided by this fibrous skeleton forms the barrier between the atria and the ventricles and ensures that electrical conduction normally only occurs through the bundle of His (see Chapters 2 and 7).

The heart is surrounded by the pericardium. The fibrous pericardium is a tough sac enclosing the heart and providing attachments to adjacent structures. The serous pericardium has a visceral layer which is attached to the surface of the heart and a parietal layer lining the fibrous pericardium. The smooth layers of the serous

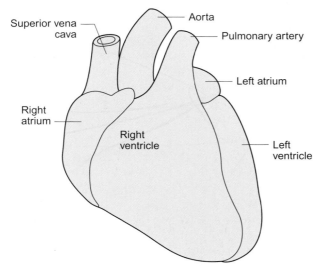

Fig. 3.1 External anatomy of the heart. Frontal (anterior) view of the external anatomy of the heart.

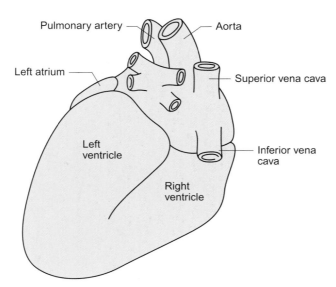

Fig. 3.2 External anatomy of the heart. Posterior-inferior view of the external anatomy of the heart.

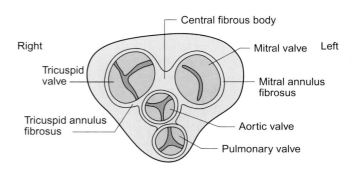

Fig. 3.3 Cross-section of the heart. Cross-section diagram of the heart (anterosuperior aspect) below the level of the atria. The fibrous skeleton of the heart is shown supporting the four valves.

pericardium slide easily over each other and allow the heart to move within the thorax as it beats. The very narrow space between the layers of serous pericardium is filled with pericardial fluid.

The right atrium has only a thin (about 2 mm) wall. There is a rough portion belonging to the auricular appendage and a smooth portion which receives the superior and inferior vena cava and the coronary sinus, the major part of the venous drainage for the heart itself. Blood flows from the right atrium into the right ventricle through an atrioventricular valve which has three cusps—the tricuspid valve (Fig. 3.3). The right ventricle is more muscular (about 4–5 mm thick) than the right atrium. The tricuspid valve is attached to the papillary muscles of the ventricular wall by the chordae tendinae (heart strings) which are made of fibrous tissue and help to stabilize the valve and prevent blood from flowing back into the right atrium when the ventricle contracts.

The left atrium is thin walled (about 3 mm) and, like the right atrium, has a smooth and a roughened portion. The smooth-walled part is formed by the entrance of the four pulmonary veins. The atrioventricular opening in the left side of the heart is guarded by a valve shaped like a bishop's mitre and formed from two cusps—the mitral valve. (In Shaw's play, St Joan declares at her trial that 'Bishops are never in the right'—this may help you to remember that the mitral valve is in the left side of the heart!). The left ventricle has the greatest wall thickness (8–15 mm) of all the cardiac chambers with internal muscular ridges throughout except for a small area at the aortic valve opening. At the tip of the apex the wall of the left ventricle is only about 2 mm thick. The mitral valve is anchored to the left ventricle by papillary muscles and chordae tendinae. The aortic valve has three semilunar cusps. There is a dilatation, the sinus of Valsalva, in the aortic wall just above each cusp. These dilatations allow blood to flow behind the cusps at the very beginning of ventricular relaxation in diastole and thus ensure that the aortic valve shuts and that the cusps are not flattened against the side of the aorta. They also allow blood to freely enter the right and left coronary arteries (see Chapter 5).

The body surface markings of a normal heart extend from the second left and third right costal cartilages down to the fifth left intercostal space and the sixth right costal cartilage. It should be appreciated that these markings will be affected by posture, by breathing (contraction of the diaphragm pulls the heart downwards) and by hypertrophy or dilatation of the ventricles when the apex beat may move from the fifth intercostal space in the mid-clavicular line to the sixth intercostal space in the mid-axillary line. The location of the apex beat is therefore often an important clinical sign.

The arterial blood supply of the heart is via the right and left coronary arteries which originate from the aorta near the aortic valve (see Chapter 5). The left coronary artery branches into the left circumflex and left anterior descending arteries. The right coronary artery branches into the marginal and right posterior descending arteries. The venous drainage of the heart is via a number of veins which drain into the coronary sinus on the inferior surface of the heart in the atrioventricular sulcus. The coronary sinus drains into the right atrium.

The cardiac cycle

The events which comprise the cardiac cycle on the left side of the heart are shown in Figure 3.4. The equivalent values for the right side of the heart are qualitatively similar but the pressures are lower since the pulmonary circulation is a low-resistance circu lation. The onset of ventricular systole is indicated by the first heart sound which is produced by closure of the atrioventricular valves. The end of ventricular systole is indicated by the second heart sound which is produced by closure of the aortic and pulmonary valves.

The sounds produced by valve closure and any murmurs associated with valves are best listened to in four specific areas of the chest:

- aortic valve: second intercostal space, right sternal edge
- pulmonary valve: second intercostal space, left sternal edge
- tricuspid valve: fourth intercostal space, left sternal edge
- mitral valve: at the apex of the heart.

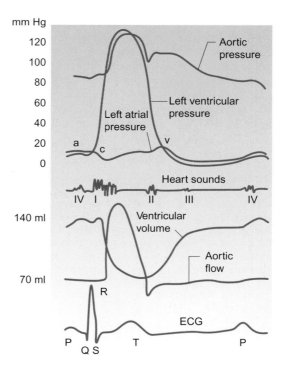

Fig. 3.4 Pressures, volume and flows in the heart. The pressures volumes and flows within the left side of the heart during the cardiac cycle. (Modified from Wiggers 1952 Circulatory dynamics. Grune and Stratton, New York.)

On the ECG the P wave corresponds to atrial depolarization (see Chapter 7) and thus marks the onset of atrial systole. The QRS complex is associated with ventricular depolarization and thus the onset of ventricular systole. The functioning of the heart as an effective pump depends upon the valves between the atria and the ventricles (the tricuspid and mitral valves) and those between the ventricles and the main distributing arteries (the aortic and pulmonary valves) functioning correctly.

In Figure 3.4 the left ventricular pressure wave begins with a small surge of pressure when the left atrium contracts and 'top ups' the ventricle. In some individuals with a hypertrophied left atrium pumping blood into a stiffened left ventricle, as may occur in ischaemic heart disease or hypertension, a sound is generated which is referred to as the fourth heart sound. The increase in ventricular volume associated with atrial systole is very small as most ventricular filling is passive and occurs in the early stage of diastole when blood flows through the relaxed atrium into the relaxed ventricle. With the onset of ventricular contraction ventricular pressure rises and the mitral valve closes. This, along with the normally concurrent closure of the tricuspid valve, causes the first heart sound. If venous return is increased acutely then the closure of the tricuspid valve in the right side of the heart may be slightly delayed and the first heart sound will be 'split', that is closure of the two valves will be heard separately. If either valve fails to close fully then the murmur of mitral or tricuspid regurgitation, an early systolic murmur, will be heard.

In the early phase of ventricular systole all four valves are closed. Ventricular pressure rises and this is called an isovolumic (also called isometric or even isovolumetric) phase of ventricular contraction. When ventricular pressure exceeds aortic pressure the aortic valve will open. If the aortic or pulmonary valves fail to open normally then the early systolic murmur of aortic or pulmonary stenosis will be heard. An aortic stenosis murmur will often radiate up the carotid artery in the neck.

Interesting facts

In 1628 the English physician, William Harvey, published his book 'De motu cordis' in which he proposed that the heart is a pump driving the circulation of blood around the body. Earlier ideas had suggested that blood is continuously produced in the liver. However, Harvey calculated that in one hour, the heart pumped a weight of blood which was three times the weight of a man. Circulation, rather than new synthesis of blood, clearly had to occur.

The ventricle empties the stroke volume of blood into the aorta (see Chapter 4) and ventricular volume typically falls by about 70 mL (Fig. 3.4). Ventricular and aortic pressures follow a similar path as the contraction of the ventricles opposes the elastic recoil of the aorta. Blood flow in the aorta rises substantially at this time. As ventricular relaxation proceeds, ventricular pressure falls and when it is below the pressure in the aorta the aortic valve closes. This is helped by a backflow of blood created by the sinus of Valsalva as described above. Closure of the valve creates a short-lived dip in aortic pressure called the dicrotic notch. The closure of the aortic and pulmonary valves generates the second heart sound. If either the aortic or pulmonary valve fails to close fully then the murmur of aortic or pulmonary regurgitation may be heard. This is an early diastolic murmur. Ventricular pressure continues to fall and eventually the pressure in the ventricle is less than that in the atrium. At this point the mitral valve opens and blood flows into the ventricle (Fig. 3.4). If the mitral or tricuspid valve fails to open properly then the early diastolic murmur of mitral/tricuspid stenosis may be heard. Opening of these valves between the atria and ventricles heralds the period of rapid ventricular filling and may occasionally, especially in individuals with low heart rates and high stroke volumes, produce a third heart sound which is said to be analogous to a 'sail flapping in the wind'. After closure of the aortic valve pressure in the aorta and thus blood flow is maintained by the elastic recoil of the artery wall. The oscillations in aortic pressure are therefore not as large as those seen in the ventricle and aortic flow, although it is pulsatile, is much more uniform than it would otherwise be. This is important to ensure continued perfusion of all the tissues of the body during diastole (see Chapter 10).

The pressure wave in the left atrium is shown in Figure 3.4. The right atrial pulse is qualitatively similar and, since there are no valves at the entrances to the atria, a similar pulse may be seen in the jugular vein if the patient's head and thorax are tilted back at about 45 degrees. The 'a' wave of atrial pressure (7 mm Hg in the left atrium and 5 mm Hg in the right atrium) corresponds to atrial systole, the 'c' wave corresponds to the closure of the atrioventricular valves which bulge back into the atria as they close. The 'v' wave of the jugular or atrial pulse results from atrial filling and immediately precedes the opening of the tricuspid and mitral valves.

The case history of a young girl with a suspected cardiac valve problem is introduced in Case 3.1:1.

Valve pathology

General principles of the pathology of heart valves

Valvular heart disease can be congenital (i.e. the patient is born with the problem) or acquired (the pathology occurs as a result of illness after birth). The spectrum of valvular heart disease, particularly in the developed world, is changing as some diseases such as rheumatic heart disease become much rarer. From a pathologist's viewpoint, disease of a valve can lead to an incompetent valve that allows blood back into the chamber from which it was expelled or a stenotic valve that impedes blood flow from one chamber to the next. A stenotic valve can of course also be incompetent.

<table>
<tr><td>

Case 3.1

The heart as a pump: 1

A young girl with a heart valve problem

Sammy, a 5-year-old girl of Nigerian origin, presented to her GP with a history of breathlessness. Clinical examination showed her to be mildly distressed, tachycardic (heart rate 115 bpm at rest) and tachypnoeic (respiratory rate 33/min). Her apex beat was displaced just lateral to the left mid-clavicular line and was prominent. On ausculation her chest was clear but there was a loud pansystolic murmur, most easily audible at the apex but radiating to the axilla. Sammy's parents gave a history of her having had a sore throat during a visit to relatives in Nigeria 3 weeks before.

The GP was worried that the child showed signs of cardiac disease and referred her urgently to the local paediatric team. An ECG was recorded which showed a prolonged P–R interval (220 ms) and doming ST segment elevation in the lateral chest leads. The paediatric team performed a throat swab and arranged a full blood count. Blood samples were taken for the assessment of Sammy's renal function profile, erythrocyte sedimentation rate (ESR—a crude non-specific test of infection, inflammation and neoplasia), C-reactive protein (CRP—an acute phase protein which increases in inflammatory joint disease), creatine phosphokinase (CK—a non-specific marker for muscle damage which increases in the presence of ischaemic cardiac muscle) and for anti-streptolysin titre (ASOT—a test used for serological diagnosis of β-haemolytic streptococcal disorders). Sammy was referred on to the regional cardiac centre.

The ASOT results came back at twice the upper limit of normal, supporting the diagnosis of a recent streptococcal infection. The CRP result was 93 mg/L (normal <10) and ESR was 42 mm/h (normal <20). CK was normal at 125 IU/L (normal <150). Sammy's throat swab was reported positive for group A streptococci.

At the regional cardiac centre an echocardiogram was performed which showed left ventricular dilatation, mitral valve prolapse and regurgitation and evidence of myocarditis. Sammy was commenced on high-dose aspirin, IV benzylpenicillin and diuretics as acute rheumatic myocarditis was likely. Over a period of 7 days Sammy's symptoms subsided. After 2 weeks in hospital she was discharged with prophylactic penicillin. This clinical history and the management strategy adopted raised the following questions:

1. What is the underlying pathology of the symptoms and signs with which Sammy presented?
2. Why was penicillin used?
3. What was the effect of high-dose aspirin?

Some aspects of the answers to these questions can be found in this chapter but you may need to consult a specialist textbook of pharmacology for a more complete explanation.

</td></tr>
</table>

Congenital heart disease

The common congenital valve diseases are described below.

Bicuspid aortic valve

About 1% of the adult population has a congenital bicuspid aortic valve compared to the tricuspid valve found in the rest of the population. The two cusps may be of the same or different sizes and there may be a median raphe (a fibrous bar) that extends from one cusp to the wall of the aorta. The bicuspid valve is much more prone to calcification (Fig. 3.5) than a normal valve and young patients may present with the symptoms and signs of a heavily calcified valve (aortic stenosis/incompetence) that is then found to be bicuspid.

Aortic valve stenosis

A complete fibrous tissue membrane may be found instead of a normal valve. Occasionally, a unicommissural valve is found—effectively a complete fibrous sheet with a tear towards one side. Subvalvar and supravalvar congenital stenosis can also occur.

Aortic valve incompetence

Aortic valve incompetence may occur because of an intrinsic abnormality of the valve itself or because of dilatation of the aortic root. Aortic root dilatation may be idiopathic, but can be seen in Marfan's syndrome and osteogenesis imperfecta. In both the idiopathic and Marfan's cases, accumulation of mucins occurs in the wall of the aorta.

Mitral valve incompetence

In the condition 'floppy mitral valve' the valve cusps are larger than normal, dome- or parachute-shaped and look

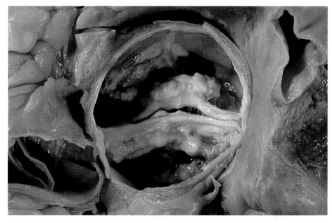

Fig. 3.5 Bicuspid aortic valve which has become calcified. Fibrotic changes in the valve lead to both stenosis and regurgitation. (Source: Stevens & Lowe 2000.)

rather myxoid/mucoidy. The chordae tendinae often also have this appearance and are elongated. Congenital pulmonary valve stenosis (or sub- or supravalvar stenosis) also occurs.

Interesting facts

Rheumatic fever is an inflammatory disease which results from streptococcal infection in children and young adult. Subsequent problems develop in later life with stenosis of mitral and aortic valves frequent outcomes. In developed countries, the incidence of rheumatic fever has decreased markedly since the 1920s. This is mainly associated with improvements in sanitation and the availability of antibiotics.

Infective endocarditis

This is an inflammatory condition affecting the endocardium, particularly on the heart valves. Previously known as bacterial endocarditis, we now know that a large number of other types of microbe can be responsible for the process.

The pathological process leads to the development of friable, often large thrombus-type masses ('vegetations') on the heart valves. Fragments of these thrombi can split off from the main mass and embolize around the bloodstream. They have the potential to impact in distant vessels causing ischaemia/infarction and spread of infection. Classically, infective endocarditis (IE) is divided into acute and subacute forms. It should be understood that this 'temporal' classification is artificial. However, acute forms of the disease tend to be more aggressive and often present more quickly than the subacute forms.

Acute IE most often occurs in the setting of previously normal valves. This form of the disease is usually very destructive and has devastating, often fatal, results. The patient may be feverish and quickly become extremely ill. The classical organism involved is *Staphylococcus aureus*. Intravenous drug users are particularly prone to this disease as they may inject dirty drug solutions. The water used for dissolving the drug may for example be obtained from a toilet bowl. The virulent organisms settle on the valves in the right side of the heart. Large, friable, invasive, thrombus-like masses (Fig. 3.6) occur and embolization is frequent.

Subacute IE is a slow, smouldering disease and the heart valves affected have usually been previously damaged, classically by rheumatic heart disease, or are prosthetic. The damaged valve is more prone to seeding and infection by lower-virulence organisms, typically *Streptococcus viridans*. Subacute IE is usually a more prolonged, non-specific illness with fevers, weight loss and flu-like symptoms. The vegetations in subacute IE are smaller, firmer and embolization is less common.

Infective endocarditis is caused by an interplay between bacteria in the blood and the endocardium of the heart valves. Bacteria in the blood (bacteraemia) is probably a common occurrence in the population at large and in an

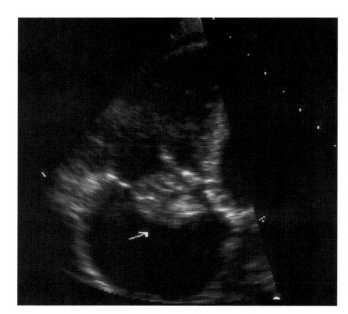

Fig. 3.6 Acute infective endocarditis vegetation on heart. Echocardiograph showing a large vegetation (arrowed) on the tricuspid valve of the heart of an intravenous drug user. (Source: Haslett et al. 2003.)

immunocompetent individual is of no great clinical significance. Bacteria may enter the bloodstream from an infective focus anywhere in the body. Dental work and surgical procedures are particularly likely causes. If the bacteria are especially virulent and/or the heart valves are abnormal, IE may occur. Predisposing cardiac valve abnormalities include congenital or acquired mitral valve prolapse, bicuspid aortic valve and prosthetic valves. Acute IE tends to affect right-sided valves whereas subacute IE tends to affect the left-sided valves (rheumatic heart disease commonly attacks the mitral and aortic valves).

By naked eye, the heart valve vegetations are usually about 0.5–1.0 cm diameter in subacute IE and 1–2 cm in acute IE and look like crumbly nodules. The vegetation may be single or form a confluent, valve-destroying mass. In acute IE, perforation of a valve cusp may be seen or infiltration of the adjacent myocardium/aortic wall may be apparent (with frank abscess formation). The vegetations are usually on the upper (atrial) aspect of the tricuspid and mitral valves and on the ventricular aspect of the pulmonary and aortic valves.

Under the microscope, the vegetations consist of a superficial layer of thrombus-like material with platelets and fibrin with subjacent colonies of bacteria and an inflammatory reaction abutting the heart valve surface. The heart valve itself may show granulation tissue formation and fibrosis.

The common consequences of having infected, friable, vegetations on the heart valve include:

- Embolus formation—the embolus may travel down a coronary artery or enter the systemic circulation typically to the spleen, kidney or brain. At the site of impaction, infection may be set up in the wall of the vessel, leading to a weakened, dilated artery (mycotic aneurysm—see Chapter 8).

- Valve perforation or destruction and/or local spread of infection and inflammation into the myocardium or aorta. This may lead to, or exacerbate, cardiac failure.

- Immune complex tissue injury—immune complexes are generated as a response to continued infection and these may set up local reactions if they settle in the kidneys (glomerulonephritis), skin (vasculitis) or joints (arthralgia).

History taking for cardiac disease

The classical symptoms of cardiac disease are:

- chest pain particularly with exertion
- poor effort tolerance
- dyspnoea (awareness of breathing)
- collapse
- palpitations (awareness of heart beating)
- swelling of the ankles and peripheral oedema.

None of these symptoms is specific to cardiac disease. Chest pain for example may arise from many causes—severe asthma, pneumonia, gastro-oesophageal reflux or musculoskeletal problems. As with any medical assessment the function of history taking is to seek evidence which will support or refute the hypothesis that symptom x is caused by problem y. The wise clinician should always keep an open mind however, as it is easy to be deceived by an atypical presentation of common illness or by classical symptoms for one pathology actually arising from another cause. The clinician should consider the history as a series of important clues. The clues may be reinforced by findings on examination and the results of appropriate tests.

Cardiac pain can broadly be divided into two groups, firstly the pain associated with acute insufficiency of coronary blood flow as a result of coronary vessel obstruction causing either myocardial infarction or unstable angina and secondly the pain related to blood flow insufficiency becoming apparent on exertion which is classical angina pectoris. Cardiac chest pain is typically central, crushing and radiates to the left arm (usually) or both arms or the neck but it is not well localized. Onset of pain during exercise and relief after rest is typical of exertional insufficiency. The resting blood flow may be adequate but the myocardium becomes ischaemic under increased demand. The character of the pain of infarction is similar but more severe. It frequently occurs at rest and is of longer duration. Men frequently describe the pain of infarction as the most severe they have ever known, though this may not be the case for women who have been through childbirth!

In arriving at a diagnosis the associated symptoms and timing may be important. A sharp, stabbing chest pain which is specifically localized may indicate pleuritic pain. A sudden onset of pain accompanied by dyspnoea may suggest a pneumothorax or pulmonary embolism. If the pain is associated with fever and related symptoms then pneumonia may be the underlying cause. A sharp, burning, retrosternal pain linked with eating patterns may point to gastro-oesophageal reflux as the cause.

A careful note of risk factors for cardiac disease should be made:

- smoking
- previous history of vascular disease
- known hypertension
- diabetes
- family history.

The above factors will all be useful in identifying heart failure (see Chapter 6) which in the majority of cases will be preceded by some form of chronic illness. Exercise intolerance and peripheral oedema will point to heart failure as will orthopnoea. This is an inability to breath comfortably when lying flat which causes the individual to prop themselves up with several pillows in order to sleep. Orthopnoea is predominantly a symptom of left heart failure. Sitting up reduces the preload (venous return) on the right side of the heart and hence reduces the output into the pulmonary circuit. Pulmonary engorgement (increased lung stiffness) which generates the sensation of dyspnoea is therefore reduced.

The degree of exercise intolerance as evidenced by the onset of angina may be a useful guide to the level of coronary insufficiency. Chest pain on vigorous exertion such as walking up stairs implies a lower level of insufficiency than chest pain walking on the level. Recording these parameters will allow the progress of disease to be monitored and give a yardstick for benefit from intervention (see Chapters 5 and 13).

Palpitations, simply the awareness of one's own heartbeat, is a common presentation but a rarer symptom of actual cardiac disease. Awareness of an abnormal heart rhythm may precede a collapse, which is usually strong evidence of an arrhythmia compromising cardiac output. However collapse may be the first 'symptom' of a serious arrhythmia. The description by witnesses to a collapse may be crucial, with the major differential diagnosis being neurological events such as seizures. If the individual is aware of the palpitations the key points to elicit in history taking are onset/offset and regularity. The heart cannot be partly in an abnormal rhythm so paroxysmal arrhythmias are typified by sudden onset and offset. Inappropriate sinus tachycardia, the most common cause of palpitations, generally starts and stops gradually. Regularity of palpitations is another important characteristic. Ectopic beats tend to give an occasional irregularity with most beats coming at a normal interval. Bigeminy and trigemini (couplets and triplets) tend to be irregular in a consistent manner. The commonest arrhythmia in clinical practice is atrial fibrillation (see Chapter 7). The chaotic nature of the heart rate means that it is very distinctly 'irregularly irregular'.

Children and young adults may demonstrate sinus arrhythmia, a perfectly normal acceleration and deceleration of the heart rate related to breathing. This usually disappears with advancing age. The author's unquantified guesstimate based on conducting ECG practicals with medical students is that about a third of 18–20 year olds will still show sinus arrhythmia.

Ankle swelling and other signs of peripheral oedema represent evidence of increased right atrial pressure and a resultant increase in hydrostatic pressure in the capillary bed (see Chapter 11). It is particularly a result of right ventricular failure as opposed to the pulmonary oedema of left heart failure (see Chapter 6). Frequently both ventricles will fail together, especially as the commonest cause of right heart failure is left heart failure.

Peripheral oedema will occur in the dependent parts of the body, that is the lowest part with respect to gravity. This is usually the feet and ankles but could also be the sacrum and buttocks in those who are bed bound for most of the time. With mild right heart failure the feet and ankles may swell during the day when an individual is standing for much of the time but go down when they 'put their feet up'. The severity of failure is to some degree evidenced by how far up the legs the oedema can be detected, oedema reaching up to the knee being generally worse than simple swelling of the ankles.

Clinical examination of the cardiovascular system

Detailed discussion of the normal and abnormal features of cardiac disease are beyond the scope of this book and you should refer to a textbook of clinical examination. To summarize the examiner is looking for signs attributable directly to cardiac dysfunction such as an irregular pulse or murmurs and signs which are secondary to cardiovascular dysfunction such as liver distension and oedema. Before performing the examination it is wise to consider the possibilities suggested by the history. Chest pain of itself is unlikely to relate to other physical signs. However ischaemia, either acute or chronic, may leave evidence of heart failure such as a raised jugular venous pressure, peripheral oedema or displacement of the apex beat due to cardiac enlargement.

A thorough examination of the cardiovascular system will encompass at least the following points but may require much more detail;

- examination of the hands for clubbing (Fig. 3.7) and splinter haemorrhages (Fig. 3.8)

- pulse—rate, rhythm, character

- blood pressure

- mucous membranes in the mouth inspected for signs of anaemia

- jugular venous pulse (JVP)

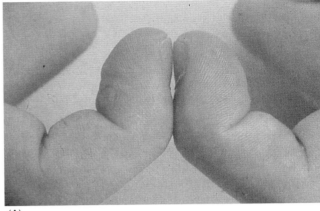

(A)

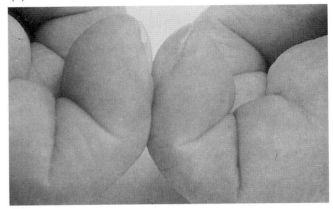

(B)

Fig. 3.7 Finger clubbing. Comparison of (A) normal nail beds and (B) finger clubbing in a patient with infective endocarditis. (Source: Underwood 2004.)

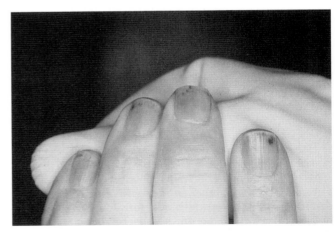

Fig. 3.8 Splinter haemorrhages. Splinter haemorrhages in the nail bed of a patient with infective endocarditis. (Source: Underwood 2004.)

- cardiac impulse; apex beat and right or left ventricular heave

- auscultation of heart sounds listening for added sounds, murmurs and their radiation

- auscultation of the lungs especially for signs of pulmonary oedema

- palpation of the liver

- examination of femoral pulses

- peripheral oedema.

The history taken or aspects of the examination may point the way to other specific signs such as checking the retina for Roth's spots in suspected endocarditis or flame haemorrhages in hypertension.

Investigations will lead on from history taking and examination. An ECG (see Chapter 7) is extremely useful and as it is cheap and non-invasive is nearly always appropriate; even a baseline ECG is worth having for future reference. Chest X-ray, blood count and electrolyte assessment are all commonly performed at least once. Only the timing of the test is of significant debate since out of hours tests are generally more expensive than those performed during the normal working day. Blood cultures should always be taken if sepsis is a possibility; traditionally at least three sets of samples from different sites in the case of endocarditis and antibiotic treatment should be withheld if at all possible until this has been done so that a causative organism can be identified.

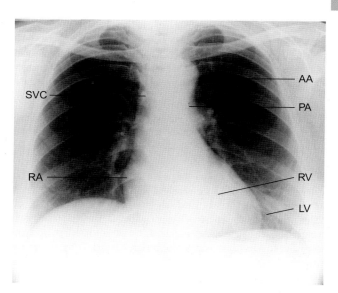

Fig. 3.9 Cardiothoracic ratio. Normal chest X-ray (posterior anterior projection). The heart is normal size with a cardiothoracic ratio (CTR) less than 50%. AA = aortic arch; PA = pulmonary artery; RV = right ventricle; LV = left ventricle; RA = right atrium; SVC = superior vena cava. (Source: Swash 2001.)

Investigations of heart disease: imaging the heart

The heart is the most dynamic organ in the body. It beats between 50 and 100 times a minute for your whole life. This movement has until relatively recently proved a barrier to accurate imaging.

Chest X-ray

A static chest X-ray does not give detailed anatomical or functional information about the heart. However it gives some information about the great vessels; the size of cardiac chambers and gross information about the function of the heart. The shape of the cardiac silhouette is determined by the contributions of the various chambers (Fig. 3.9). Where one or more chamber is grossly enlarged the silhouette will be larger than normal. The cardiothoracic ratio (CTR) is defined as the ratio of the widest total lateral dimension of the heart to the widest lateral dimension of the chest. The maximum normal CTR is 0.65 in children falling to 0.5 in adults. However cardiac enlargement may also be reflected in vertical dilatation with the heart shadow taking on a more globular outline. The secondary impact of poor cardiac function can be seen in the lungs with the signs of pulmonary oedema.

Cardiac catheterization and cine-angiography

Since the 1940s and 1950s invasive cardiac catheterization has been used to assess the physiology of the heart.

Initially used mainly in research it gradually became important in the clinical setting. A fine hollow tube or catheter is inserted via a peripheral vein or artery, usually a femoral vessel, and manipulated into the cavity of interest. This permits sampling of blood and the measurement of blood pressure from specific sites within the heart and great vessels.

Indirect measurement of left atrial pressure is achieved as a 'wedge pressure'. A catheter with a balloon at the end (Swan–Ganz catheter) is steered through the right side of the heart and into the pulmonary artery circuit. When the catheter has been advanced as far as possible the balloon is inflated. In this way the catheter tip is isolated from the right side of the heart but there is a continuous column of blood from the catheter tip, through the pulmonary capillaries to the left atrium. Wedge pressure is therefore an indirect method of assessing left atrial pressure and is a technique particularly used in intensive care settings.

As surgical and medical techniques emerged to offer treatment for cardiac pathologies the need for accurate imaging of cardiac anatomy became more important in the 1960s and 1970s. The early mainstay of cardiac imaging was ciné angiography. A radio-opaque dye is injected into a vessel or chamber via a catheter whilst the patient is exposed to X-rays from a 'camera'. The dye fills the chamber or vessel producing a radio-opaque outline of the vessel in question. Using ciné film a moving 'X-ray' can be produced so that ventricular contraction can be observed and the degree of valve regurgitation assessed.

The development of echocardiography has diminished the role of cardiac catheterization particularly in diagnostic terms. Although coronary angiography has the disadvantages of invasiveness, radiation exposure and reactions to the dye which may cause serious haemodynamic instability or renal impairment, it remains the gold standard assessment for coronary arteries in ischaemic heart disease.

Echocardiography

Ultrasound was first used in medicine after the Second World War when the development of sonar and radar allowed researchers to experiment with the effect of reflecting ultrasound generated with a piezo-electric crystal from the various boundaries within the body. In 1953 Edler and Hertz in Sweden produced the first moving images of the heart. As electronics developed it became possible to display multiple beams fired from a single transducer and a moving, two-dimensional image became possible in the late 1970s. For the first time physicians could watch the heart beat and see anatomical anomalies in real time. The technique quickly became a mainstay of cardiac assessment and remains so despite the advances in other areas of imaging. The ability to measure the structure and function of the beating heart, by the bedside if necessary, is invaluable and has extended throughout many areas of cardiac diagnosis and management including intraoperative assessment and intensive care.

The addition of Doppler—the ability to measure the speed with which blood is moving using the shift in frequency caused by the reflection from a moving target—allows blood flow velocity measurements. Blood flow velocity gives information about valve function, since at a given cardiac output the narrower the valve the faster blood must travel. Simultaneous two-dimensional imaging and blood flow may be obtained by using a colour scale to paint areas of blood flow according to the speed with which blood is moving, so-called colour flow mapping. Shades may be used to show different speeds so that dark colours are low speeds and light colours high speeds. Typically, though arbitrarily, red is used to show flow towards the imaging probe and blue for away. Turbulent flow, such as through a stenosed valve, is indicated by speckled mixtures of colour indicating the wide range of velocities present. This provides a detailed anatomical and functional assessment of the heart.

Recent advances in echocardiography have not yet become universal but show great promise. With further increases in computer processing power it is now possible to reconstruct three-dimensional images in near real time. This allows better understanding of how valves malfunction and the possibilities for repair. Tissue Doppler imaging, looking at the movement of the myocardium rather than the blood, will improve the assessment of myocardial function allowing region by region assessment. The introduction of ultrasonic contrast media will allow sensitive assessment of intracardiac shunts and myocardial perfusion.

Magnetic resonance imaging

Since its first introduction magnetic resonance (MR) imaging has become the gold standard for soft tissue imaging. Incredibly detailed anatomical reconstructions of structures are possible looking almost like sections in the dissection room. Initially the time taken to capture these images precluded the use of MR in moving organs, as the movement artefact was too great. With the advent of high-power field magnets and major increases in computer processing power, complete volumetric scans can be done in the time that an individual can hold their breath. Combining different MR modalities, 2D imaging ECG gated over multiple phases of the cardiac cycle, gadolinium-enhanced 3D angiography and direct flow measurement provides unparalleled physiological cardiac assessment. MR cine imaging provides unprecedented precision in the assessment of ejection fractions (defined as the fraction of the end-diastolic volume ejected into the aorta or pulmonary artery). By combining volumetric analysis with flow measurements precise estimates of regurgitant fractions can be made giving insight into the degree of dysfunction of ventricles and valves. MR's major limitation is that the equipment remains bulky and the scans and reconstruction time consuming. It is also significantly affected by the presence of metallic objects. In children a general anaesthetic is virtually mandatory, mainly because of the stressful environment, a noisy narrow tunnel, and the requirement to remain still and breath-hold on cue.

Case 3.1 — The heart as a pump: 2

Further development of Sammy's problem

The diagnosis was rheumatic heart disease following a streptococcal infection. Over the subsequent 15 years Sammy was seen regularly in clinic. Her exercise tolerance gradually declined and on examination she was found to have developed a mid-diastolic click and a late diastolic murmur, rumbling in character and loudest at the apex. She developed a bifid appearance of the P waves on her ECG. Echocardiography confirmed increased flow velocity across the mitral valve with reduced movement of the valve leaflets. She was commenced on diuretics and as her exercise tolerance continued to decline she was referred for mitral valve replacement following a diagnosis of mitral valve stenosis.

Interesting facts

The frequency of radio-waves in a standard 1.5 T MR scanner is 64 MHz—just a little below that of BBC Radio 4 (92–94 MHz). This frequency has a wavelength around 5 metres—so the scanner is completely unable to 'see' the subject never mind localize the heart.

High speed CT

Advances in computer-aided tomography (CT) scanning have increased the range of applications. High-speed ECG gated spiral CT scanners have provided improved imaging of cardiac structures, particularly the great vessels. The speed with which studies of the aorta can be performed make the CT scanner much safer in the case of pathologies such as acute aortic dissection where the patient may be in a precarious condition. Very fast high-resolution systems are challenging invasive coronary angiography in the assessment of coronary artery disease.

Electron beam tomography, using electrons rather than the standard X-rays, shows great promise as a technique for non-invasively imaging calcium deposits in the coronary arteries. This will allow risk stratification for atheromatous coronary artery disease.

However, despite advances in speed and image quality CT still requires a high radiation exposure, typically 20 or 30 chest X-ray equivalents, and so remains unattractive for repeat investigations.

Radio-isotope (nuclear) imaging

Radio-isotope imaging relies on the use of a radiolabelled marker which is taken up by the target tissue. Examination with a device capable of detecting radiation, a gamma camera, allows precise positioning and quantification of the labelled tissue. Technetium-99m radionuclide imaging has replaced thallium-based techniques in cardiac assessment. Injected 'dye' is taken up by perfused heart muscle. Examination at rest shows areas of myocardium which have stopped functioning. Examination during stress shows areas where perfusion is borderline and becomes inadequate during increased demand. Stress may be a simple exercise test or be pharmacologically induced by drugs such as the β-adrenoceptor agonist dobutamine. By gating the scan using an ECG it is possible to assess function throughout the cardiac cycle and to assess ejection fraction. Computer tomography allows multiplane reconstruction of the myocardium. Although technically demanding, radio-isotope scanning is extremely sensitive for myocardial perfusion problems and may even be used in the acute presentation of chest pain.

Sudden cardiac death

Sudden cardiac death is defined as an event that is non-traumatic, non-violent, unexpected and results from sudden cardiac arrest within 6 hours of previously witnessed normal health. The sudden and unexpected death of an individual is a particularly sad event coming as it does 'out of the blue'. The vast majority (>90%) of sudden cardiac deaths occur due to underlying coronary artery disease. The actual terminal event may come unexpectedly even in an individual who has known coronary artery disease and is probably the result of a severe arrhythmia such as ventricular fibrillation. Alternatively the sudden and complete occlusion of a major part of the coronary arterial tree may lead to sudden loss of function in such a large portion of the cardiac muscle that the heart is no longer capable of sustaining a sufficient output to maintain brain function. Infrequently this is the first presentation of ischaemic heart disease.

It is estimated that between 100 and 500 young people die of cardiac disease in the UK each year. Frequently the death of an affected family member is the first sign of an inherited disorder. The commonest cause of sudden cardiac death in young people is hypertrophic cardiomyopathy. This is an autosomal dominant condition in which abnormal structural proteins such as the β-myosin heavy chain cause physiological dysfunction which induces compensatory hypertrophy of the myocardium. This may be recognized at post mortem or detected using echocardiography. It is now standard practice for professional footballers to undergo routine screening to exclude this condition. Unfortunately the fact that the heart of a highly trained sportsman tends to undergo physiological hypertrophy makes screening a more difficult task. Other defects of the heart muscle such as dilated cardiomyopathy may also cause sudden cardiac death.

Post-mortem examination of the heart may be unremarkable if the underlying event leading to death is an arrhythmia as the cause is not structural. An example of this is the long QT syndrome in which defective ion channels in the myocardial cell membrane cause abnormal prolongation of the repolarization interval (beginning of QRS complex to end of T wave on the ECG). Individuals are at considerable risk of sudden cardiac death due to a particular form of ventricular fibrillation known as 'torsades de pointes'. If recorded on ECG monitoring the axis of ventricular activity is shown to rotate about the heart. The condition was first described in 1957, and some of the genes responsible for long QT variants have since been identified and include genes encoding for the proteins which form sodium and potassium channels. Typical histories include loss of consciousness with exertion, particularly swimming, possibly due to the effect of diving or exercising in cold water or cardiac arrest when startled or woken suddenly from sleep.

Medical management of these conditions involves screening families for asymptomatic but affected individuals using ECG, echocardiography and exercise testing. Significant reductions in risk may be achieved using β-blockade pointing to the adrenergically mediated initiation of the arrhythmia in these conditions. Standard advice is to refrain from vigorous exercise. For refractory or high-risk individuals, implantable cardioversion defibrillators can be used. These devices are developments of the pacemaker technology designed to detect severe arrhythmias and deliver a cardioverting DC electric shock to the myocardium. They have recently entered the National Institute for Health and Clinical Excellence Guidelines in the UK. Unfortunately though effectively lifesaving the pain and discomfort of automatic defibrillation can be extremely debilitating and may lead to morbidity of its own, particularly if the patient does not lose consciousness prior to the delivery of the life-saving shock.

Genetic testing remains a challenge in these conditions. The variability in functional molecular phenotypes means that selecting dysfunctional genotypes from the spectrum of normal variants is difficult, particularly where dysfunctional genotypes may be extremely rare. Where a number of family members are known to be affected, genetic linkage analysis may be helpful. Unfortunately the majority of cases involve a single individual within one family who has died suddenly. Screening children is particularly difficult since lack of evidence of the condition may not exclude its development in the longer term, for example with hypertrophic cardiomyopathy.

Further reading

Grubb, N.R., Newby, D.E., 2006. Cardiology, second ed. Elsevier, Edinburgh.

Haslett, C., et al., 2003. Davidson's Principles and Practice of Medicine, nineteenth ed. Churchill Livingstone, Edinburgh.

Levick, J.R., 2009. An Introduction to Cardiovascular Physiology, fifth ed. Arnold, London.

Lilly, L.S., 2006. Pathophysiology of Heart Disease, third ed. Williams and Wilkins, Baltimore.

Stevens, A., Lowe, J., 2000. Pathology, second ed. Mosby, Edinburgh.

Swash, M., 2001. Hutchison's Clinical Methods, twenty-first ed. WB Saunders, Edinburgh.

Underwood, J.C.E., 2004. General and Systematic Pathology, fourth ed. Churchill Livingstone, Edinburgh.

REGULATION OF CARDIAC FUNCTION

4

Chapter objectives

After studying this chapter you should be able to:

1. Identify heart rate and stroke volume as the two factors determining cardiac output.

2. Explain the mechanisms which aid the return of blood to the heart and the relationship of these mechanisms to cardiac output.

3. Describe the role of the sympathetic and parasympathetic nervous systems in the control of heart rate.

4. Explain the concept of preload effects on the heart and the role that preload has in determining stroke volume.

5. Outline the roles of natriuretic peptides and the renin-angiotensin-aldosterone system in regulating blood volume.

6. Discuss the role of the sympathetic nervous system in determining contractility of the ventricular muscle and the actions of drugs used as positive and negative inotropes.

7. Explain the concept of afterload effects on the heart especially in relation to arterial blood pressure.

Introduction

$$\text{Cardiac output} = \text{Heart rate} \times \text{Stroke volume}$$

When the textbook person (see Chapter 1) is at rest their cardiac output, the volume of blood pumped by each side of the heart, is about 5 L per minute. In understanding how this is achieved the 'rule of 70' might be helpful. The heart typically beats at about 70 bpm and, when the ventricle empties it goes from a volume of about 140 mL at the end of the filling phase, diastole, to about 70 mL at the end of the contraction phase, systole. The 'stroke volume' is therefore about 70 mL and about 70 mL of blood remains in the ventricle at the end of each cardiac contraction. The ejection fraction of the heart, the stroke volume expressed as a percentage of end-diastolic volume, is thus typically about 50%. When appropriate an increase in the heart's output can be achieved by a combination of an increase in heart rate and stroke volume. The maximum effective heart rate in the adult is about 180 bpm and the stroke volume can be increased both by filling the ventricle more during diastole and emptying it further during systole. In a very fit textbook person the maximum cardiac output is of the order of 25 L/min.

It must be appreciated that the circulation is a closed system with two pumps which are adjacent to each other but whose output is separated by the lungs on the one hand and the peripheral tissues on the other. Both ventricles are driven by the same pacemaker and thus the heart has to maintain 'ventricular balance', that is, over a relatively short period of time the output of the right ventricle must equal the output of the left ventricle.

Interesting facts

The heart beats about once a second for your entire life and has no opportunity to rest.

Venous return

An important feature of the closed system is that the heart can only pump out the blood it receives. Thus the cardiac output will always be limited by the venous return. If the heart rate were to increase without a concomitant increase in venous return then the result would not be an increase in cardiac output but, instead, a reduction in the volume of blood pumped at each stroke. This is seen in haemorrhagic shock when the patient has a fast heart rate but the radial pulse is not very 'full' because a smaller volume of blood is ejected from the heart at each beat.

When a person is upright, their head and shoulders are above the level of the heart but most of the rest of the body is below that level and thus gravity is largely a negative factor in determining venous return of blood to the heart. In a horizontal posture however the venous return will not be significantly opposed by gravity. For this reason if a person faints, it is usually best to leave them horizontal to aid the flow of blood back to the heart. Conversely, if a person has poor cardiac function a sitting position will decrease the venous return and hence the work load of the heart. Many people with cardiac problems sleep either in a chair or propped up in bed. The effect of gravity on venous pressure is further discussed in Chapter 10.

The main arteries, veins and nerves in the body are often in close proximity and confined within a fibrous sheath. The small to medium-sized veins, particularly in the legs, have valves which means that, as the artery pulsates, blood in the adjacent vein is displaced towards the heart. This mechanism has the advantage that if, in a period of raised cardiac output, the heart beats faster or more powerfully then the massaging action is increased and so the venous return is increased.

The skeletal muscle pump

The veins, especially in the limbs, are often to be found between major blocks of muscle. If muscle activity is increased, then the alternate compression and release of the veins will result in blood being propelled back towards the heart (Fig. 4.1). This mechanism is dependent on the presence of valves in veins in the lower limbs. This aspect of venous return is useful for guardsmen on parade. If they are standing still and upright over long periods of time there is a danger they will faint because their cardiac output, limited by the poor venous return, is not enough to supply their tissue's needs especially on hot summer days when skin blood flow may be increased. They are told to move their toes in their boots and thus use the alternate contraction and relaxation of their leg muscles to aid venous return.

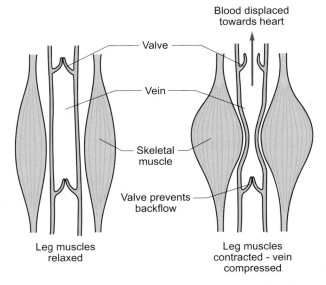

Fig. 4.1 Contraction of vessels in the legs. Contraction of vessels in the legs compresses veins and moves blood against the force of gravity back towards the heart.

The abdomino-thoracic pump

When a person breathes in, the diaphragm flattens and the rib cage moves upwards and outwards with the result that pressure in the thorax is decreased and the pressure in the abdomen rises. This increases pressure outside the abdominal vena cava and decreases it outside the thoracic vena cava encouraging blood to pass from the abdomen into the thoracic venous compartment. When the person breathes out the rise in intrathoracic pressure means blood flows from the thoracic veins into the heart and, as abdominal pressure falls, blood flows from the legs into the abdomen. This 'stirrup-pump-like' action plays a major role in aiding venous return throughout extrauterine life and again has the advantage that an increase in exercise activity and thus depth and rate of breathing is associated with an increased venous return.

Control of cardiac output

$$\text{Cardiac output} = \text{Heart rate} \times \text{Stroke volume}$$

The respiratory system has 'dead space' areas such as the nasal passages, trachea and bronchi which are ventilated but where no gas exchange takes place. This means that during exercise there is a functional advantage in keeping the respiratory rate relatively low and breathing deeply. The heart however is a through flow system and, within limits, an increase in heart rate will produce a proportionate rise in cardiac output, as long as the venous return is increased to provide the necessary blood to pump. This is true in an adult up to a heart rate of about 180 bpm. If the heart rate goes much above this value then cardiac output falls precipitously because there is an encroachment on the 'rapid filling time'—that period of time which immediately follows the end of ventricular systole and when most of the ventricular filling occurs (see Chapter 3). The result is that excessively high heart rates are associated with a reduced stroke volume. Small minute to minute changes in cardiac output, as might be associated with mild exercise such as walking, tend to be achieved largely by changes in both heart rate and stroke volume (see Chapter 13). Changes in stroke volume reach maximum levels at fairly moderate exercise intensity and the further increases during heavy exercise are achieved just with heart rate changes. The effects of exercise on cardiac function are considered in more detail in Chapter 13.

Regulation of heart rate

There is considerable variation in the resting heart rate in the adult population with a normal range of 50–100 bpm. As explained in Chapter 2 the rate of beating of the heart is normally determined by the pacemaker at the sinoatrial node (SAN). The rate of this pacemaker is modulated by both the sympathetic and parasympathetic nervous systems. At rest the parasympathetic inhibition dominates so that the typical resting heart rate of about 70 bpm is less than the natural intrinsic rate of the SAN which is about 110–120 bpm (see Chapter 2). Small increases in heart rate, such as might occur during walking, are produced by inhibition of the parasympathetic tone. If the heart rate is to go above about 110 bpm, then an increased sympathetic nerve activity is also required.

The role of the central nervous system control centres and the function of the baroreceptor reflex in the control of heart rate are further discussed in Chapter 10.

The sympathetic innervation of the heart is routed via the cervical and stellate sympathetic ganglia. It is the sympathetic fibres on the right side of the body which have the major effect on heart rate (Fig. 4.2). The fibres from the left side of the sympathetic nervous system are more concerned with the regulation of cardiac contractility. The noradrenaline (norepinephrine) released at the nerve endings acts on β_1 receptors in the SAN and increases the Ca^{++} current in phase 4 of the SAN action potential. This accelerates the rate of firing of the SAN cells (see Chapter 2).

The parasympathetic innervation of the pacemaker tissue is via the left and right branches of the vagus nerve but, like the sympathetic innervation, the fibres are distributed differentially (Fig. 4.2). The right vagus goes mainly to the SAN with a small innervation of the atrioventricular node (AVN) whereas the left vagus goes primarily to the AVN with only a small outflow to the SAN. The vagal fibres to the heart originate in the dorsal motor nucleus of the vagus or in the nucleus ambiguus (see Chapter 10).

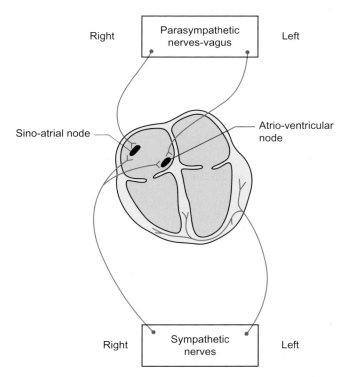

Fig. 4.2 Autonomic nerve supply (sympathetic and parasympathetic) to the heart.

The parasympathetic ganglia, the location of the nerve cell bodies, are on the cardiac surface or within the heart itself and the short postganglionic fibres release acetylcholine as their neurotransmitter. This acetylcholine acts on muscarinic (M_2) receptors in the SAN and, via an inhibitory G protein mechanism, reduces the production of cAMP within the cell. Cyclic AMP activates populations of Na^+ channels and L-type Ca^{++} channels causing depolarization of the pacemaker cells. Inhibiting cAMP formation therefore reduces the rate of depolarization and slows the heart rate. There is also a hyperpolarizing effect produced following binding of acetylcholine to M_2 receptors. This is mediated by activation of a population of K^{++} channels. As a result the membrane potential is moved closer to the potassium equilibrium potential (E_K) of $-94\,mV$ and therefore further away from the threshold at which an action potential is triggered (see Chapter 2). The right and left vagus nerves have little effect on cardiac contractility.

Interesting facts

In the animal kingdom, heart rate is inversely related to body size. Typical resting heart rates are: blue whale – 10 beats/min; elephant – 25 beats/min; adult human – 75 beats/min; mouse – 500 beats/min.

Regulation of stroke volume

The heart is an unusual form of pump in that not only is it able to change the rate at which it pumps but, if necessary, it is also able to change the volume of blood pumped at each stroke. Under resting conditions, the ventricles in the adult heart typically fill to about 140 mL (the end-diastolic volume) and empty to about 70 mL (the end-systolic volume) giving rise to a stroke volume of about 70 mL. However as the normal range of heart rate is quite wide at 50–100 bpm, individuals with a slow resting heart rate will operate with a stroke volume greater than 70 mL and people with a fast heart rate will have a correspondingly smaller resting stroke volume. Resting cardiac output will therefore be comparable between individuals with the same body size irrespective of resting heart rate. An outline of the case history of a man with increased stroke volume in his heart is described in Case 4.1:1.

It is possible to increase the stroke volume either by increasing end-diastolic volume or by decreasing end-systolic volume, or both. Both ways of changing stroke volume have a role in regulating cardiac output but the mechanisms by which they are brought about are different and they need to be considered separately. There are three key areas to be considered in relation to the regulation of stroke volume:

- preload
- contractility
- afterload.

Case 4.1 **Regulation of cardiac function: 1**

A man with aortic regurgitation

Graham is a 40-year-old man who presented to his GP with a 10-day history of malaise and intermittently raised body temperature. His GP found that he looked flushed and was febrile. His pulse was regular but rapid and of a high volume—bounding. His blood pressure was 134/42 mm Hg. Close examination revealed a number of dark lines under Graham's nails (splinter haemorrhages). On auscultation there was a soft systolic murmur with a loud decrescendo early diastolic murmur. Graham's GP suspected endocarditis and referred him for urgent cardiology assessment.

On admission the cardiology team inquired whether Graham had had any dental treatment recently. He admitted that he has not been to the dentist for some years and superficial inspection revealed extensive dental caries. Blood cultures were taken and an echocardiogram showed a bicuspid aortic valve which was mildly stenotic but which had a moderate degree of regurgitation. There appeared to be a vegetation on the aortic valve.

Initial treatment was commenced with high-dose antibiotics, penicillin and gentamicin. Blood cultures grew a streptococcus which was sensitive to penicillin. Graham's condition improved and he felt better. However the degree of aortic regurgitation remained unchanged.

This case presentation raises several questions; the answers to some of these are to be found in the text of this chapter and in Case 4.1:2.

1. What is the response of the heart to aortic regurgitation, an increase in the volume of blood contained in the left ventricle at the end of diastole?
2. What is unusual about Graham's arterial blood pressure?
3. What are splinter haemorrhages?
4. What might be the link between Graham's aortic valve problems and his dental caries?

Preload effects on the heart

The cumulative effect of the factors which determine ventricular end-diastolic volume or end-diastolic fibre length of the ventricular muscle is called a 'preload' effect on the heart. This is effectively the resting length from which the heart muscle contracts. Preload effects are often conveniently quantified as the right or left atrial pressure, the filling pressure which determines how much blood enters the ventricle during diastole. Although for most purposes this is a useful concept it is not entirely satisfactory. A ventricle stiffened by fibrotic changes for example will need a higher filling pressure than normal in order to reach a certain end-diastolic volume. Similarly, stenosis of a valve between the atria and ventricles will require a higher atrial pressure to ensure adequate ventricular filling.

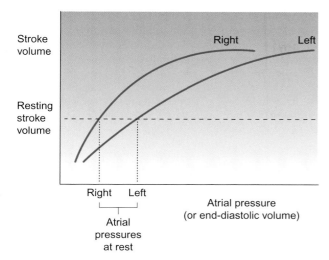

Fig. 4.3 Cardiac function curves for right and left sides of the normal heart. The left ventricle has a higher filling pressure than the right ventricle but they both reach the same maximum stroke volume.

Figure 4.3 shows the relationship between atrial pressure and stroke volume for the right and left sides of the heart. In both cases an increase in filling pressure (atrial pressure) leads to increased stretch of the ventricular muscle and results in an increase in stroke volume (stroke work). This is called Starling's law of the heart. The background to Starling's law and the mechanisms involved are explained in Box 4.1. Eventually as atrial pressure increases a maximum stroke volume is reached, imposed fundamentally by the physical size of the heart and by the presence of the pericardium as a potentially restricting bag around the outside of the heart. Under resting conditions the heart is typically operating at about halfway up the Starling curve, hence the ability to double stroke volume during exercise. Figure 4.3 also shows that the filling pressure of the left ventricle is higher than for the right ventricle. This partly reflects the thicker ventricular muscle wall on the left which requires a higher filling pressure.

During diastole the right ventricle fills as a result of the pressure gradient between the atrium and ventricle. As there is no valve between the venous system and the right atrium blood can flow from the vena cavae across the right atrium and into the ventricle. The contraction of the right atrium only 'tops up' the ventricle with a small addition of blood and in a normal heart, this is not a major component of preload effects on the heart. The relationship between cardiac output and right atrial pressure means that, to some extent, an increase in venous return can produce an increase in cardiac output (as happens when a person lies down) and a fall in venous return (such as might happen on standing up) will cause a fall in cardiac output. However the main importance of the relationship described by Starling's law is that it is the mechanism by which ventricular balance is achieved. This is of immense physiological importance—if the right ventricle output exceeded that of the left by only 0.1 mL per beat there

Box 4.1 Regulation of cardiac function

Starling's Law

If the preload to the heart increases then ventricular filling is increased during diastole and the cardiac muscle is stretched. Conversely if the preload falls then ventricular filling is reduced and the ventricular muscle fibres are less stretched. The consequences of changes in length of the ventricular muscle on cardiac performance were investigated separately by the German scientist Otto Frank (1895) working on frog heart muscle and later by the British scientist Ernest Starling (1914) working on a preparation in which a dog's heart was left connected to its pulmonary circulation but the systemic circulation was replaced by an artificial circulation made up of glass and rubber tubing.

Starling measured the volume of the ventricles whilst the isolated dog heart was beating and carried out two key types of experiment. In his first experiment he increased the venous return, the preload, by raising a reservoir of blood connected to the right atrium. He kept the 'arterial pressure' in his artificial circulation constant. When he increased the preload there was an increase in end-diastolic volume of the ventricle and Starling found that the heart continued to pump blood out to about the same end-systolic volume as before, i.e. the cardiac output increased with no change in arterial pressure. The heart was doing more work at an increased end-diastolic volume.

In his second type of experiment Starling kept the preload constant and raised the 'arterial pressure' against which the heart was pumping—the afterload. When he first increased the afterload the immediate effect was that the heart didn't empty completely but, over a few beats, he found that blood accumulated in the ventricles until eventually the end-diastolic volume had increased and by this time the heart had managed to regain its previous stroke volume and thus output. Again the heart was doing more work at an increased end-diastolic volume. Starling thus proposed his 'Law of the Heart' that the work done by the myocardium in systole is related to the resting length of the muscle fibres in diastole. This is often now given the title of the Frank–Starling mechanism.

The increased force of contraction on stretching the cardiac myocytes at rest is often explained solely as increased overlap of the actin and myosin filaments and a greater number of cross-bridges being formed within the cardiac muscle. However it appears that there is also an increase in the sensitivity of the contractile apparatus to calcium apparently achieved by an increase in the troponin C affinity for Ca^{++} (see Chapter 2).

would be 7 mL of blood trapped in the lung after a minute and 420 mL after an hour. What actually happens if right output exceeds left is that the pressure in the pulmonary circulation rises, left ventricular preload increases and, as a result, the left ventricle pumps more strongly, keeping the two sides of the heart in balance.

There are many aspects of cardiovascular function which determine right atrial pressure including pressures within the thorax and the physical characteristics of the ventricles. However, the three most important variables are blood volume, venous return and venous tone, the state of smooth muscle contraction in the walls of the veins (Fig. 4.4). Some of these key variables are discussed below. Venous return mechanisms have already been covered earlier in this chapter.

Blood volume

In the textbook person blood volume is about 5 L but it is not evenly distributed throughout the cardiovascular system. The large and small veins act as a reservoir for blood within the body and accommodate about two thirds of the total blood volume (see Chapter 14). If a person donates blood or suffers a haemorrhage then central venous pressure and preload on the heart will both be decreased. Similarly if the blood volume is expanded by infusing blood, saline or a plasma volume expander such as dextran or albumin then the central venous pressure and preload will be increased (see Chapter 14).

A family of hormones, the natriuretic peptides, of which the first to be discovered was atrial natriuretic peptide (ANP), are involved in blood volume regulation. An increase in stretch in the wall of the atria, as would occur following expansion of blood volume, leads to increased natriuretic hormone release and increased loss of salt and water via the kidneys to bring the blood volume back to normal (see Chapters 6 and 14). The major actions of ANP are firstly to increase glomerular filtration rate in the kidney. This is achieved by afferent arteriolar dilatation and efferent arteriolar constriction. In addition, ANP inhibits the actions of aldosterone. The renin-angiotensin-aldosterone system is of central importance in blood volume regulation as it is a sodium- and water-retaining system (see Chapters

6, 9 and 14). Renin secretion is promoted in response to a fall in blood pressure or a fall in blood volume. The baroreceptor reflex and activation of the sympathetic nervous system is particularly important in this context.

Regulation of blood volume is fundamental to the maintenance of a normal cardiac output. Changes in blood volume are a major factor in the compensation reactions which accompany heart failure (see Chapter 6).

Venomotor tone

The blood contained within the venous reservoir vessels is under a pressure which depends upon the blood volume but also on the extent to which the walls of the veins resist being stretched. The veins contain some smooth muscle (see Chapter 1). It is a relatively small amount compared to the smooth muscle in the walls of the arteries or arterioles but none the less if the activity in the sympathetic nerves to the veins, which act through α_1-adrenoceptors, is increased then central venous pressure will be raised and preload increased. This mechanism is activated for example when moving from a horizontal to an upright posture as this tends to redistribute about 500 mL of blood from the thoracic venous system to the lower limbs. Venomotor control opposes the tendency to venous pooling in the lower half of the body imposed by the effects of gravity. Loss of venomotor tone is frequently a clinical problem particularly in old people and results in postural hypotension, a fall in cardiac output and arterial blood pressure as a result of standing up. This results in dizziness or fainting. The effects of gravity on hydrostatic pressure in the circulation are discussed in Chapter 10.

Residual pressure

This is the pressure 'left over' from the pressure in the aorta after the blood has been forced through the peripheral tissues. However, most of the potential energy stored as arterial pressure is dissipated as the blood passes through the arterioles (see Chapter 9). The pressure in the capillaries is only about 25 mm Hg and this is reduced even further by the time the blood reaches the great veins. Thus the residual pressure, or 'vis a tergo' as it is sometimes called, contributes little to venous return.

Ventricular suction

When the right ventricle relaxes at the end of systole there is a tendency for it to 'spring open' and thus to 'suck' blood in from the atrium—the so-called 'vis a fronte'. However any attempt to drink from a glass using a floppy drinking straw will soon convince you that suction alone is not sufficient to produce a flow through thin-walled unsupported vessels such as the veins. Remember that the trachea, a body tube in which suction does occur, is held open by rings of cartilage producing a structure rather like a vacuum cleaner hose. Veins do not have this advantage and collapse if the pressure inside is less than that outside the vein. This is the normal state of the jugular

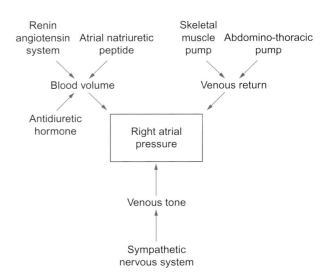

Fig. 4.4 Right atrial pressure. Major factors determining right atrial pressure, the filling pressure for the right ventricle.

vein in a person who is upright and it only becomes inflated when pressure rises in the vein, as in heart failure (see Chapter 6).

Interesting facts

Despite the fact that the normal range for resting heart rate is often reported as 50 to 100 beats per minute, the Swedish tennis player Bjorn Borg, who won Wimbledon five times, and the Spanish cyclist Miguel Indurain, who won the Tour de France five times, both have resting heart rates in the low 30 s.

Contractility effects on the heart

It is possible to increase the force of ventricular contraction without increasing the end-diastolic volume and stretching the muscle fibres. When this happens the heart empties more and there is said to be an increase in contractility (Fig. 4.5). Physiological alterations in contractility are associated with changes in the $[Ca^{++}]$ inside the cardiac myocyte (see Chapter 2). Activation of the left branch of the sympathetic nerve supply to the ventricular muscle will increase contractility through a mechanism linked to a β_1 adrenoceptor.

Many pathological mechanisms result in a decrease in contractility, often associated with an intracellular acidosis as a result of myocardial ischaemia. This is a common characteristic of heart failure (see Chapter 6). The strongest natural negative inotrope is the H^+ ion and any episode of acidosis, such as might occur with cardiac ischaemia, will have a detrimental effect on cardiac performance. The effect is seen more quickly in the case of respiratory rather than metabolic acidosis (see Chapter 1) because the entry

of CO_2 into cardiac myocytes with the subsequent generation of H^+ inside the cells is faster than the entry of the polar H^+ ions from the extracellular fluid. The mechanism by which acidic conditions inside cardiac myocytes lead to decreased force of contraction is interesting. A doubling of $[H^+]$ can halve the strength of contraction of the heart. Surprisingly there is an increase in the intracellular $[Ca^{++}]$ which would normally be expected to increase the force of cardiac muscle contraction. The complex mechanisms that actually lead to a reduced force of contraction include reduced binding of Ca^{++} to troponin and a decrease in the force developed by the cross-bridges that do form.

Pharmacological agents which increase contractility are called positive inotropes although they tend to be compounds which also have a range of other physiological actions. Many of these drugs have a sympathomimetic action resembling endogenous noradrenaline (norepinephrine) and adrenaline (epinephrine), compounds which have actions via all types of adrenoceptors (see Chapter 9). Isoproterenol (isoprenaline) is a non-selective agonist for both β_1 and β_2 receptors and it increases both contractility of the ventricles and heart rate. Dopamine has actions at several types of receptor including specific dopamine receptors and also both β_1 and β_2 receptors. It therefore has a positive inotropic action which is accompanied by an

Case 4.1   Regulation of cardiac function: 2

Comments on the clinical history

The aortic valve regurgitation means that Graham's heart is exposed to a high preload (blood returning from the lungs as normal plus blood leaking back from the aorta through the regurgitant valve). The response is an increase in the force of contraction of the ventricle which is reflected in the relatively high systolic pressure and the 'bounding' pulse. The diastolic pressure reflects the resistance to blood flowing out of the aorta (see Chapter 10), and in this case there is a low-resistance pathway for blood flowing back into the heart which incidentally generates the decrescendo diastolic murmur. The pulse pressure, the difference between systolic and diastolic pressure, is characteristically wide. The systolic murmur is generated by the forceful expulsion of blood through the partially stenosed aortic valve.

Aspects of infective endocarditis are discussed in Chapter 3. Splinter haemorrhages are small linear streaks of blood in the long axis of the finger nail caused by haemorrhages from small blood vessels. They are thought to be caused by microemboli from infective endocarditis sites (see Fig. 3.8).

There is often a link between the development of infective endocarditis and an infection which starts in the mouth. This is frequently a streptococcal infection, especially *Streptococcus viridans*. Dental procedures, including tooth extractions and even descaling, may lead to the release of organisms into the blood stream from infected areas in the mouth. A focal infection may then develop in the heart usually involving a valve.

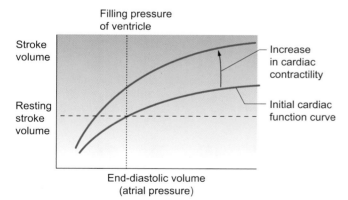

Fig. 4.5 Cardiac function curve demonstrating an increase in cardiac contractility. The whole curve is shifted upwards such that at any given filling pressure (see vertical dashed line) the increased force of contraction generates an increased stroke volume. This is distinct from preload effects on the heart which result from an increased filling pressure of the ventricle, i.e. a left to right movement along the cardiac function curve. Physiological increases in contractility are always associated with an increase in myocyte intracellular $[Ca^{++}]$.

intrarenal vasodilator action. The latter effect may be beneficial in circumstances where there is intense sympathetically driven intrarenal vasoconstriction as a result of a fall in arterial blood pressure and activation of the baroreceptor reflex. This would occur for example in many cases of heart failure and is potentially a cause of acute renal failure which may progress to chronic renal failure. Dobutamine is a dopamine analogue which has a powerful positive inotropic action but causes relatively little change in heart rate.

The inotropic actions of sympathetic nerve stimulation act through β-receptors which are coupled to cyclic AMP formation (Fig. 4.6). This second messenger activates protein kinases leading to increased transmembrane flux of Ca^{++} and increased affinity of the myofilaments for Ca^{++}. In addition there is increased reuptake of Ca^{++} into the sarcoplasmic reticulum, an effect which shortens systole and prolongs diastole with consequent beneficial effects on coronary blood flow (see Chapter 5). Cyclic AMP mediated pathways can also be manipulated using blockers of the cAMP breakdown enzyme, phosphodiesterase. Milrinone and enoximone are phosphodiesterase III inhibitor drugs which are used as positive inotropes.

The digitalis glycosides such as digoxin were discovered by William Withering in 1785 as a result of investigations of the beneficial actions of extracts of foxglove (*Digitalis purpura*) plants. They were used in the treatment of some forms of oedema, particularly in congestive cardiac failure which was known as the 'dropsy'.

Digitalis glycosides increase contractility by inhibition of the Na^+/K^+-ATPase, a mechanism which is clearly different to the sympathomimetic drugs. The mechanism by which intracellular Ca^{++} is increased is illustrated in Figure 4.7. Inhibition of the Na^+/K^+-ATPase will lead to an increase in intracellular $[Na^+]$. There is also a 3 Na^+/Ca^{++} antiporter protein in the cell membrane. A rise in $[Na^+]$ inside the cell will therefore reduce Ca^{++} expulsion from the cell and this results in retention of Ca^{++} inside the cell. This extra Ca^{++} is stored in the sarcoplasmic reticulum of the cell and is available for release when the cell is activated, hence providing a positive inotropic action.

Digitalis glycosides also produce central stimulation of the vagus nerve and enhance the sensitivity to muscarinic agonists such as acetylcholine. This inhibits the SAN and lengthens the refractory period in the AVN, both of which have an antiarrhythmic action. Although digitalis derivatives are very old drugs they are still in widespread use despite their troublesome side effects. They are not ideal drugs as they have a very narrow therapeutic index and a long half-life of 1.5 days. This means there is not much difference between a therapeutic dose and a toxic dose. Toxic doses cause an overload of intracellular Ca^{++} which can cause increased automaticity of the AVN or Purkinje fibres. This may result in ventricular ectopic beats and ventricular tachycardia. The stimulation of vagal activity will result in blockade of the AVN whilst the increased SAN automaticity causes atrial tachycardia. There may also be gastrointestinal, neurological and visual disturbances. Toxic effects include a wide range of actions around the body and regular monitoring of plasma levels of the drug is necessary.

Negative inotropes

In some clinical situations such as hypertension or angina, it may be appropriate to decrease the force of contraction of the heart muscle. This will reduce the cardiac output and

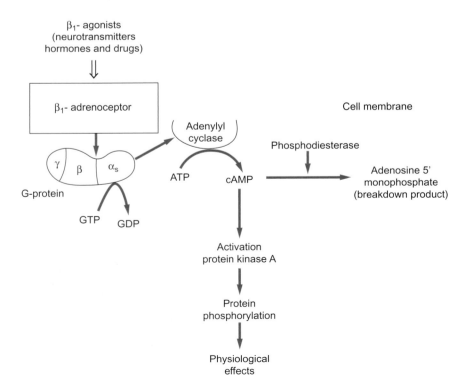

Fig. 4.6 Intracellular events following β_1-agonist binding to a receptor on a cardiac myocyte. The G-protein splits into a β_γ fragment and a α_S GTP binding fragment to produce a complex which activates adenylyl cyclase to generate the second messenger cyclic AMP. Main sites for drug manipulation are the use of β-agonist drugs (adrenaline, isoprenaline, dopamine, dobutamine) or phosphodiesterase inhibitors (milrinone, enoximone).

the work load carried out by the heart and also reduce the oxygen demand of the heart. In this case a drug with a negative inotropic action might be used. These drugs include β_1-receptor antagonists such as atenolol (see Chapter 10)

Case 4.1 Regulation of cardiac function: 3

Further investigations

Graham was reassessed echocardiographically. His left ventricular dimension was slightly above normal and the degree of aortic regurgitation was assessed as moderate. Fractional shortening was 45%. He described his exercise tolerance as less than before his illness though not severely restricted.

He was commenced on enalapril 5 mg once a day and his renal function remained unaffected as the dose was increased to 10 mg. On this dose Graham initially found his exercise tolerance improved but over the next 2 years it declined to the point where his lifestyle was restricted. Assessment in the cardiology clinic still showed a wide pulse pressure. An echocardiogram showed severe aortic regurgitation with marked dilatation of the left ventricle. Fractional shortening was measured at 35%. Graham was referred for urgent aortic valve replacement. Post valve replacement he was given the anticoagulant warfarin in addition to the enalapril. Two months after valve replacement his exercise tolerance had improved markedly and an echocardiogram showed his left ventricle to have reduced in size to slightly above normal limits. Some aspects of this case history are explained in Case 4.1:4.

---

which suppress the effects of activating the sympathetic nerves to the heart. They have the effect of slowing the heart rate as well as decreasing the force of ventricular contraction. Slowing the heart rate may also improve coronary blood flow by prolonging diastole (see Chapter 5).

Calcium-channel-blocking drugs (calcium antagonists) act on voltage-gated 'L-type' calcium channels. There are different types of calcium channel blockers, some that have predominant effects on calcium channels in the smooth muscle of blood vessels (see Chapter 10) and others that have a greater effect on cardiac muscle cells. Nifedipine and amlodipine dilate arterioles in the periphery and hence reduce blood pressure by lowering the peripheral vascular resistance. The work required of the heart to overcome the afterload (see below) is therefore reduced although there may be a reflex tachycardia. Verapamil and diltiazem tend to act more directly on the SAN and AVN to slow the heart rate and the rate of impulse conduction to the ventricle. Most calcium-channel-blocking drugs will reduce cardiac contractility and, in some cases, coronary blood flow may be improved following the relief of coronary artery spasm (see Chapter 5).

Beta-blocking drugs and calcium channel blockers have variable negative inotrope actions. This is certainly not the only pharmacological action of these classes of drugs which both have a range of effects.

Afterload effects on the heart

The aortic valve will open and allow blood to pass into the aorta when pressure in the left ventricle exceeds

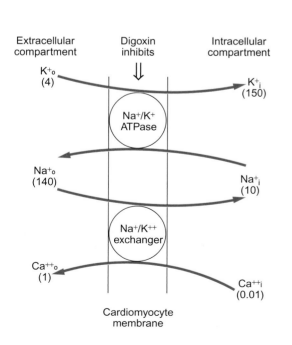

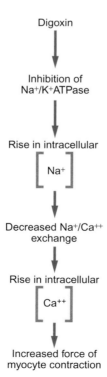

Fig. 4.7 Positive intropic action of digoxin. The cardiomyocyte membrane has two ion exchange mechanisms. The Na^+/K^+-ATPase actively expels Na^+ from the cell. Partial inhibition of the pump by digoxin leads to an increase in intracellular $[Na^+]$. The Na^+/Ca^{++} exchanger moves Ca^{++} out of the cell. This is driven by inward movement of Na^+ down its concentration gradient. A rise in intracellular $[Na^+]$ will reduce inward Na^+ flux and therefore the expulsion of Ca^{++}. The consequent rise in intracellular $[Ca^{++}]$ will increase the force of myocyte contraction. The figures in brackets indicate typical concentrations for each ion in units of mmol/L.

Case 4.1 Regulation of cardiac function: 4

Explanation of aspects

Fractional shortening of the left ventricle provides a method for quantifying the overall contractile state of the heart. This will reflect the net effect of preload, contractility and afterload effects on the heart. It is calculated from an echocardiograph recording as the difference between end-diastolic and end-systolic diameters of the left ventricle as a percentage of end-diastolic diameter.

Enalapril is an angiotensin converting enzyme inhibitor drug (see Chapter 9). By blocking the generation of angiotensin II and hence aldosterone production, it has a mild diuretic action and reduces preload on the heart. Enalapril also reduces the vasoconstrictor actions of angiotensin II thus reducing afterload on the heart. The care taken to check renal function before increasing the dose of enalapril is because angiotensin II constricts the efferent arteriole at the glomerulus and thus helps to sustain glomerular filtration rate (GFR). Excessive blockade of angiotensin II formation and therefore dilatation of the glomerular efferent arteriole may lead to acute renal failure. The reported reduction in size of the ventricle is also associated with actions of enalapril. Angiotensin II has profibrotic actions. Fibrosis is part of the process known as remodelling of the heart, an often unwanted response to many forms of cardiac disease. The fibrosis is reduced by angiotensin-converting enzyme (ACE) inhibitor drugs such as enalapril.

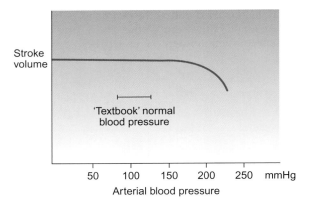

Fig. 4.8 Afterload effects on the normal heart. The stroke volume of the left ventricle remains quite constant over a wide range of arterial blood pressure. Only when blood pressure rises beyond the normal range encountered under physiological conditions does afterload on the heart start to reduce stroke volume. In a failing heart (see Chapter 6) blood pressure increases can have a much more marked adverse effect on stroke volume.

pressure in the aorta. If pressure rises in the aorta this means that the work load on the ventricle will increase. The combined effect of factors which determine ventricular wall stress (primarily chamber radius, wall thickness and the resistance to outflow of blood) are called the afterload effects on the heart. Hypertension therefore imposes an increased afterload on the left ventricle as does aortic valve stenosis. The pathological response to increased afterload is cardiac myocyte hypertrophy which may progress to cardiac failure (see Chapter 6).

In a normally functioning heart the acute changes in arterial blood pressure which occur during everyday life have little effect on the stroke volume of the heart unless blood pressure rises to very high levels (Fig. 4.8). Sustained increases in blood pressure however lead to a reduction in stroke volume and this is part of the rationale for antihypertensive therapy. In this circumstance reducing blood pressure will increase stroke volume of the heart. In cardiac failure the performance of the ventricles may be much more sensitive to afterload changes than a normal heart (see Chapter 6).

rate will rise as a result of increased sympathetic and decreased parasympathetic drive. The movement of the limbs and the increase in ventilation will increase the venous return, and hence ventricular end-diastolic volume, so that the heart will 'move up a Starling curve'. The increased sympathetic outflow will produce an increase in contractility. In very fit athletes the heart may even shrink during exercise (i.e. the end-diastolic volume decreases) as a result of the large increase in contractility and better emptying. Peripheral resistance falls during dynamic exercise and mean arterial blood pressure changes are small. Afterload effects are not therefore a major factor determining cardiac performance during dynamic exercise. This is not the case in static exercise (see Chapter 13).

Summary

During exercise, such as running, all the different ways of increasing cardiac output will come into play. The heart

Further reading

Allen, D.G., Kentish, J.C., 1985. The cellular basis of the length–tension relation in cardiac muscle. J. Mol. Cell Cardiol. 17, 821–840.

Brady, A.J., 1991. Mechanical properties of isolated cardiac myocytes. Physiol. Rev. 71, 413–427.

Fuchs, F., Smith, S.S., 2001. Calcium, cross-bridges and the Frank–Starling relationship. News Physiol. Sci. 16, 5–10.

Levick, J.R., 2009. An Introduction to Cardiovascular Physiology, fifth ed. Arnold, London.

McDonald, K.S., Herron, T.J., 2002. It takes 'heart' to win: What makes the heart powerful? News Physiol. Sci. 17, 185–190.

Molkentin, J.D., Dorn, G.W., 2001. Cytoplasmic signalling pathways that regulate cardiac hypertrophy. Annu. Rev. Physiol. 63, 391–426.

Orchard, C.H., Kentish, J.C., 1990. Effects of changes in pH on the contractile function of cardiac muscle. Am. J. Physiol. 358, C967–C981.

Waller, D.G., Renwick, A.G., Hillier, K., 2009. Medical Pharmacology and Therapeutics, third ed. Saunders, Edinburgh.

Zimmer, H.-G., 2002. Who discovered the Frank–Starling mechanism? News Physiol. Sci. 17, 181–184.

BLOOD SUPPLY TO THE HEART

5

Chapter objectives

After studying this chapter you should be able to:

1. Describe the structure of the major arterial blood supply and venous drainage vessels for the heart muscle.

2. Outline the mechanical, neural and metabolic factors which normally determine coronary blood flow.

3. Understand the concept of the autoregulation of coronary blood flow.

4. Explain the main pathological mechanisms which may impair the blood supply to the heart muscle and lead to angina pain and myocardial infarction.

5. Outline the laboratory tests used in the investigation of patients with suspected myocardial infarction.

6. Discuss the rationale for the drugs used in the management of angina and myocardial infarction.

7. Understand the use of interventions such as angioplasty and coronary artery bypass grafting in the management of patients with impaired coronary perfusion.

Anatomy of the arterial supply and venous drainage of the heart

The term 'coronary' was first conceived to describe a crown-like arrangement of the arterial blood vessels supplying the heart muscle. If the heart is considered as an upside-down cone with the flat base placed at the level of the atrioventricular groove, then the coronary arteries may be visualized as a ring at the base of the cone with branches which pass towards the tip (Fig. 5.1). This network of coronary arteries arises from two main origins in adjacent aortic sinuses. The anterosuperior sinus gives rise to the right coronary artery (RCA). This passes down the anterior atrioventricular (AV) groove. It gives rise to marginal branches which supply the anterior free wall of the right ventricle (RV). At the junction between the anterior and inferior aspects of the RV it gives off a significant branch—the acute marginal artery. It then passes inferiorly and in 70% of subjects terminates in a right posterior descending branch which supplies the inferior aspects of the RV, left ventricle (LV) and interventricular septum.

The posterior aortic sinus gives rise to the left coronary artery stem which quickly branches into the left circumflex artery. This mirrors the right coronary artery in the posterior AV groove and likewise gives off marginal branches. The other branch is the left anterior descending (LAD) artery which passes down the anterior interventricular groove to the apex and turns on to the posterior surface where it passes in the posterior interventricular groove for a variable distance. During this course the LAD gives off diagonal and septal perforating branches which supply the anteroseptal, anterolateral and apical portions of the left ventricle and the anterior papillary muscle.

The left circumflex artery gives off marginal branches, the obtuse marginal artery being a dominant feature. It passes inferiorly and usually terminates. In some individuals it turns to form a left posterior descending artery which follows the interventricular groove to a watershed with the distal portion of the LAD.

The precise arrangement of branches is variable. In about 70% of individuals the right coronary is dominant and its posterolateral and right posterior descending branches supply the inferior interventricular septum, left ventricular free wall and posterior papillary muscle. In 20% of individuals the left circumflex artery is dominant and gives rise to a left posterior descending artery and supplies the inferior portion of the heart. In 10% neither is dominant and the supply is shared.

The sinoatrial node is supplied by a branch of the RCA in 60% of cases and from the circumflex artery in 40%. The AV node is supplied by the RCA in 90% of cases. Damage to vessels supplying portions of the conducting system may lead to specific defects. In the case of damage to the sinus nodal artery it may lead to 'sick sinus syndrome' in which the frequency of generation of cardiac action potentials becomes randomly variable and inappropriate (tachy-brady syndrome). Damage to the supply to the AV node or bundle of His may lead to complete heart block (see Chapter 3) and is particularly associated with inferior myocardial infarction.

Though the arteries cross the surface of the heart, because they pass in the atrioventricular and interventricular grooves they clearly delineate the main chambers of the heart. The majority of the venous drainage is via a system of veins which run against the arterial system back to vessels which drain round the atrioventricular groove. Passing posteriorly is the great cardiac vein and passing anteriorly is the small cardiac vein, both of which drain into the coronary sinus. The coronary sinus passes under the floor of the left atrium and into the right atrium. The anterior cardiac veins drain directly to the right ventricle and atrium. The remainder of the venous drainage is in the tiny Thebesian veins which also connect mainly to the right atrium and right ventricle.

An imbalance between the oxygen demands of the heart and amount that can be supplied by the coronary blood supply leads to the development of an hypoxic pain originating in the heart which is called angina (see p. 55). An outline of a clinical case history is shown in Case 5.1:1.

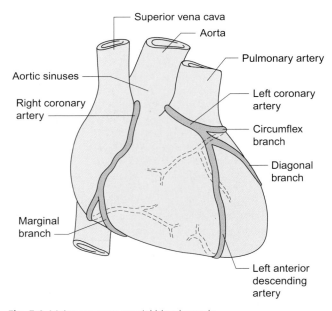

Superior vena cava
Aorta
Pulmonary artery
Aortic sinuses
Left coronary artery
Right coronary artery
Circumflex branch
Diagonal branch
Marginal branch
Left anterior descending artery

Fig. 5.1 Major coronary arterial blood vessels.

Interesting facts

Under resting conditions, the heart muscle extracts about 75% of all the oxygen which arrives in the coronary arteries. A substantial increase in oxygen delivery can only be provided by an increase in coronary blood flow not by further extraction of oxygen from haemoglobin. The corollary of this is that disease-related limitation of coronary blood flow impairs cardiac performance and leads to cardiac pain (angina).

Case
5.1
Blood supply to the heart: 1

Development of chest pain with exercise

Colin Davies is a 50-year-old smoker. Over the last 3 months he has noticed that he has became more short of breath than usual when walking to the local shops. He has a sensation of pressure and tightness in his chest. More recently he found that when he walks up the stairs in his house he gets a dull, aching pain which feels to come from the left side of his chest and extends down his left arm.

Colin saw his GP who suspected angina pectoris and arranged for him to have an exercise test at the local hospital. After 4 minutes on the treadmill Colin was feeling short of breath and had developed pain in his chest. The ECG showed ST segment depression in the lateral chest leads (V_4–V_6). The test was terminated at 4½ minutes when Colin felt he could not go on. His pain disappeared after 1 minute of rest and this was accompanied by the resolution of the ST segment changes on his ECG.

Colin's blood pressure was normal and his GP checked his fasting blood lipids and glucose which were also normal. The GP strongly recommended that he stop smoking. In view of Colin's symptoms and exercise test results his GP commenced him on oral glyceryl trinitrate (GTN) spray. He explained that this was to be used whenever Colin had chest pain symptoms.

This case history raises the following questions:

1. Why does angina pain occur and why does it get worse with exercise?
2. What is meant by ST segment depression and what does this change in the ECG suggest?
3. Why did the GP check Colin's blood pressure and fasting plasma lipids and glucose?
4. How do nitrate drugs such as GTN help to relieve angina?

Aspects of the answers to these questions are to be found in the text of this chapter. ECG changes are discussed in Chapter 7.

Regulation of coronary blood flow

At rest the myocardium receives about 5% of cardiac output. In the normal 'textbook' person there is a potential for cardiac output to increase about fivefold during exercise (see Chapter 13). This is roughly paralleled by changes in coronary blood flow and the necessity for this is largely dictated by the high oxygen extraction rate of cardiac muscle.

In skeletal muscle, under resting conditions, only of the order of 25–30% of the oxygen carried in arterial blood is extracted for use in the muscle (Fig. 5.2). The saturation of haemoglobin with oxygen in skeletal muscle

therefore decreases from about 97–98% (arterial blood) to about 70% (venous blood). Even under resting conditions the venous drainage from cardiac muscle is only 25% saturated, meaning that of the order of 75% of the oxygen in arterial blood has been extracted and used metabolically. During exercise, increased oxygen delivery to contracting skeletal muscle can be provided by a combination of increased blood flow (see Chapter 13) but also by increased (up to 80–90%) extraction of oxygen from haemoglobin. In the heart as oxygen extraction at rest is already about 75% there is limited scope for increasing oxygen delivery by this route. Studies with ^{11}C-acetate positron emission tomography (PET) scanning suggest that, in the heart, oxygen extraction from arterial blood can rise to 90% during exercise but even this is a limited way of increasing oxygen delivery. The bottom line is that if the heart needs increased oxygen supply it must be mainly provided by increased coronary blood flow. The corollary of this is that pathological mechanisms which impair coronary blood flow must limit cardiac performance.

Coronary blood flow, particularly to the left ventricle, is particularly affected by the contraction of the myocardium which crushes coronary vessels (Fig. 5.3). This mainly affects blood vessels in the subendocardial layers of the heart muscle and the blood vessels on or close to the surface of the heart are relatively unaffected. The subendocardial layers are therefore more prone to ischaemic damage. In the left ventricle, because of the high pressures developed in the contracting ventricle, coronary blood flow is much higher during diastole than during systole. In the right side of the heart intraventricular pressures are lower and so the effect of ventricular systole on coronary blood flow is less marked. When heart rate increases during exercise the duration of diastole is shortened more markedly than the duration of systole. This imposes a limitation on increases in coronary blood flow and is probably the limiting factor on maximum exercise ability in normal individuals.

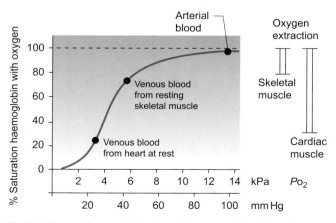

Fig. 5.2 Oxygen–haemoglobin dissociation curve. Extraction of oxygen from arterial blood in skeletal muscle is typically 25–30%. Oxygen extraction by cardiac muscle even under resting conditions is 75%.

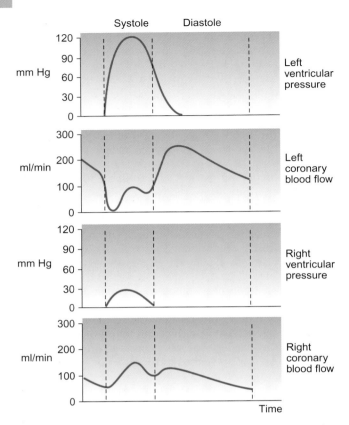

Fig. 5.3 Right and left coronary blood flow correlated with ventricular pressure.

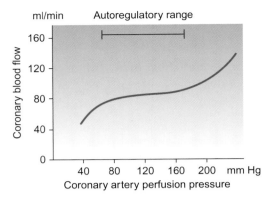

Fig. 5.4 Autoregulation of coronary blood flow.

Coronary blood flow is autoregulated (Fig. 5.4). This means that over a range of mean arterial pressures, probably in humans from about 50 to 120 mm Hg, coronary blood flow is relatively independent of arterial pressure. This is thought to result especially from responses of arterioles which are less than 150 μm diameter. Thus, as the arterial pressure increases through the autoregulatory range the smooth muscle in the wall of these arterioles contracts to maintain flow constant.

'Myogenic' effects on vascular smooth muscle mean that stretch of smooth muscle results in contraction. It is a mechanism that was first described by Bayliss in 1902 and is probably the dominant mechanism providing autoregulation of coronary flow. There are complex interactions between various blood vessel microdomains and possibly also with non-myogenic components which provide the overall autoregulatory response.

The major regulatory factor determining coronary blood flow is myocardial oxygen demand coupled to the production of vasodilator metabolites. These metabolites particularly affect blood vessels in the 150–170 μm size range. The vascular smooth muscle is thought to be particularly sensitive to changes in [adenosine], [K⁺], [H⁺] and to local changes leading to an increase in interstitial osmolarity (see Chapter 9). A major part of this vasodilator action is mediated by the opening of ATP-sensitive K⁺ channels.

This leads to hyperpolarization and consequently to relaxation of the smooth muscle.

The source of the vasodilator adenosine has been a subject of conjecture. Berne (1980) proposed that it was produced under hypoxic conditions by the complete dephosphorylation of ATP. An alternative pathway was put forward by Deussen (1989), in which adenosine was formed from ATP via the intermediate formation of *S*-adenosyl methionine and *S*-adenosyl homocysteine. Both pathways are thought to contribute to interstitial [adenosine]. The following points seem to be relevant to understanding these events. ATP, ADP and AMP are all polar molecules as a result of ionization of their phosphate groups and will not easily cross cell membranes. Adenosine is non-polar and can leave the myocardial cell once it has been formed. Adenosine in the interstitium has a very short half-life (of the order of 10 s) and so must be continuously generated. [ATP] inside cells is about 5 mmol/L but interstitial [adenosine] is about 10 nmol/L, a 500 000-fold difference in concentration. Therefore, only a very small proportion of the intracellular ATP would need to be metabolized to provide relatively big changes in interstitial [adenosine] (Fig. 5.5).

Endothelial influences on blood vessel diameter are described elsewhere (see Chapter 9). Increased shear stress on the endothelium leads to production of nitric oxide and thence to vasodilatation. This occurs particularly in large coronary arteries but it does not appear to contribute to the mechanism of autoregulation. Endothelial dysfunction leading to impaired nitric oxide release is a characteristic of a number of pathological conditions which will affect the coronary blood vessels including hypercholesterolaemia, atherosclerosis and hypertension. Assessment, prevention and treatment of endothelial dysfunction is emerging as an important area of clinical medicine, especially in relation to the coronary circulation.

Modulation of coronary blood flow via the sympathetic nervous system primarily acts through α₁-adrenoceptors on relatively large vessels. Vessels less than 100 μm diameter predominantly have α₂-adrenoceptors but α₁-receptors are also present. Activation of either of these populations of α-receptors leads to vasoconstriction and

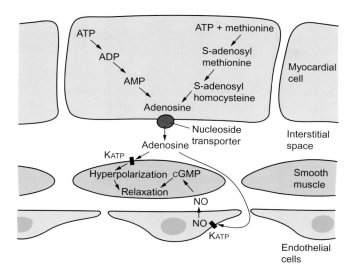

Fig. 5.5 Regulation of coronary vascular smooth muscle contraction by the metabolite adenosine and by the endothelial cell-derived mediator nitric oxide (NO).

this is the dominant sympathetically mediated response. In the past there has sometimes been confusion about the role of β-receptor-mediated vasodilatation. Although such receptors do exist in limited numbers on coronary vessels, the vasodilator response which follows β-agonist infusion is mainly a result of increased metabolite (e.g. adenosine) generation following an increased force of ventricular muscle contraction (i.e. an inotropic response). Coronary vasodilatation directly as a result of β-adrenoceptor activation is a very minor component of coronary vascular control.

The role played by cardiac sympathetic nerves in relation to coronary blood flow is still controversial. During exercise the effects of sympathetic vasoconstrictor nerves are overwhelmed by the effects of vasodilator metabolites. However, α-receptor-mediated coronary vasoconstriction may, in some circumstances, contribute to the genesis of the ischaemic pain angina.

Ischaemic heart disease

Ischaemic heart disease is the most common cause of death in the Western world. It may occur either because the coronary blood supply is reduced or because the oxygen demand of the heart has increased for instance as a result of hypertrophy. The regions of the heart most at risk are the subendocardial layers, the region most affected by vascular compression during systole.

The most frequent cause of obstruction in a main coronary artery is atherosclerosis. As this is not confined to the coronary circuit but may develop in any major vessels in the high-pressure arterial side of the circulation the details of the pathogenesis of atherosclerotic lesions are described in Chapter 8.

Occlusion of the coronary arteries may become critical in various ways:

- Progressive narrowing of vessels by atheromatous plaques.

- The plaque and the associated reduction in blood flow velocity may provide a focus for thrombus formation with consequent further reduction in blood flow. The possibility also exists of embolization of the thrombus.

- With time, a plaque becomes a rigid structure but is still surrounded by pliable blood vessel wall. There is therefore a risk of rupture (fissuring) of the plaque which provides another site for thrombus formation. The processes involved in thrombus formation are described below.

Thrombosis

Thrombosis is best considered as the inappropriate activation of the blood clotting system in a living vessel (with flowing blood) resulting in a thrombus forming inside the vessel. The thrombus may either suddenly or slowly occlude the lumen of the vessel leading to blood flow problems distal to the blockage.

A thrombus is therefore a solid mass, composed of blood constituents, which develops in a living vessel, including the heart. It is vitally important to realize that a thrombus can only form during life—this is in contrast to a clot which can occur after death or in blood taken from the circulation and put in a test tube. Thus although the key proteins and cells in thrombosis are the same as those in the clotting cascade, thrombosis is usually considered a pathological rather than a physiological process. However, this is simplistic. In reality, tiny thrombi probably form in the circulation all the time, particularly where there are small areas of trauma to the endothelium. These microthrombi are quickly removed once the endothelial defect has healed. Classically, there are three main predisposing factors, known as 'Virchow's triad', which favour the formation of a thrombus:

- changes in the intimal surface of the vessel
- changes in the pattern of blood flow
- changes in the blood constituents.

Damage to the endothelium is an important factor in thrombosis as it exposes collagen in the intima and media of the vessel wall. This will trigger platelet adhesion as a prelude to thrombus formation. Endothelial damage can be caused by atherosclerosis, trauma, inflammation, substances in cigarette smoke and hypertension, amongst others.

Change in blood flow is also an important factor. Slow flow, as occurs with incompetent venous valves and dilated veins, can lead to pooling of blood. On the arterial side of the circulation turbulent blood flow near atherosclerotic plaques or aneurysms can lead to damage to the endothelium (see Chapter 8). Both scenarios will lead to increased platelet–vessel wall interaction.

A change in blood constituents is another important factor in thrombus formation. Significant increases in total red cell or platelet numbers, as seen in polycythaemia, thrombocythaemia and leukaemia, can predispose a patient to thrombosis. Congenital deficiencies of natural anticoagulants such as protein S and protein C may also lead to thrombus formation.

Essentially, in thrombosis, the natural antithrombogenic processes in the body are overwhelmed by prothrombogenic factors. Thus, if there is damage to the endothelium, there is exposure of subendothelial collagen. By a receptor-mediated process, platelets stick to the collagen and to Von Willebrand factor found in the subintimal matrix. The platelet mass forms an aggregate, then ADP and prostaglandin A_2 are released which encourages more platelet aggregation. The platelets can bind fibrinogen causing a cellular plug to form.

The use of mechanical methods (e.g. compression stockings) and the drugs heparin, warfarin and aspirin which contribute to antithrombotic therapy are discussed later in this chapter.

As soon as the platelet plug has formed, fibrinolytic systems are activated which prevent propagation of the thrombus (Fig. 5.6). However, the presence of one or more of Virchow's triad will tip the scale towards thrombus formation.

Thrombi can form in any part of the cardiovascular system and to some extent the appearance of the thrombus depends on:

- the calibre of the vessel
- the speed of blood flow.

A thrombus forming in a small-sized vessel may cut off the blood supply. This is called an occlusive thrombus. In a large vessel such as the aorta or heart, the thrombus may be restricted to the wall only, a mural thrombus. This is much less likely to cause problems with occlusion of the vessel it has formed in, but may lead to emboli which can block subsequent smaller vessels. In a medium-sized vessel, there may be significant restriction of blood flow as a result of mural thrombus.

The speed of blood flow influences the composition of a thrombus. Thus, in very fast-flowing arterial blood, thrombi tend to be mainly composed of platelets and fibrin and therefore appear pale and laminated, whereas in slow-flowing blood in veins the thrombus is rich in red blood cells and looks more gelatinous.

Once a thrombus has formed, a number of 'events' may occur:

- lysis/dissolution
- propagation
- organization/recanalization
- embolization.

Lysis/dissolution The fibrinolytic systems (Fig. 5.6) remove the thrombus and the vessel returns to normal.

Propagation The thrombus increases in size, usually tracking along the vessel. This may lead to blockage of the entrance to several branches from the vessel.

Organization/recanalization The term organization is used to describe the process whereby granulation tissue grows into a non-living material within the body such as thrombus or dead myocardium. Ultimately, organization results in fibrosis. When a thrombus undergoes organization, granulation tissue which is made up of proliferating fibroblasts and capillary-sized vessels may form small channels in the thrombus and this network of channels may link up, restoring flow through the thrombus and therefore through the vessel. This is called recanalization.

Embolization An embolus is a solid, liquid or gaseous mass that is introduced into the circulation at one place, drifts in the blood stream and has its effect at a distant point, usually through blockage of a vessel with subsequent ischaemia.

By far the most common embolic material is thrombus-derived, hence the much used term 'thromboembolus'. Variable sized fragments of a thrombus can break off and be carried to a distant part of the circulation. The effect of the thrombus can mean sudden death caused; for example, by a massive embolus from a pelvic vein thrombus carried in the blood to the right side of the heart causing complete occlusion of the right ventricular outflow tract/pulmonary trunk. The other end of the spectrum of thromboembolic events results in no clinical effect at all; for example, a tiny embolus from a deep vein in the calf impacts in a small tributary of the pulmonary artery. Since the thromboembolus will be quickly dissolved by the lytic defences of the circulation and since the lung has a dual blood supply, it is likely there will be no anatomical or clinical effect.

It is not just thrombus that can embolize. Fragments of cholesterol debris can split off from an atheromatous

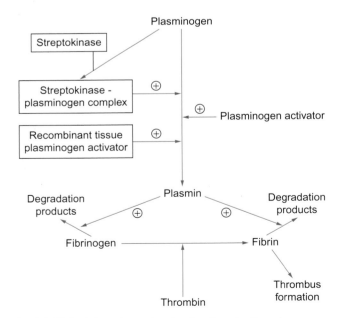

Fig. 5.6 Fibrinolytic pathway showing the sites of action of thrombolytic drugs.

plaque, as for example in carotid artery atherosclerosis leading to cholesterol emboli which pass into the circulation of the eye or brain. Air, fat (especially after trauma or a major operation such as a hip replacement), amniotic fluid, tumour cells and foreign bodies can all embolize (Table 5.1).

Anti-thrombotic therapy

In hospitalized patients the methods used to try to avoid the formation of thrombus depend on the risk involved. For moderate-risk patients mechanical methods such as elasticated stockings can be used. For higher-risk patients this may be supplemented with low-dose heparin. This is a sulphated mucopolysaccharide (glycosaminoglycan) molecule derived commercially from pig intestinal mucosa or the lungs of cattle. It forms a complex with the clotting cascade protein antithrombin which results in the activation of antithrombin. Thrombin promotes the last stage of the clotting mechanism, conversion of fibrinogen to fibrin (Fig. 5.6). Heparin also inhibits several other stages in the clotting cascade. It is inactive given orally and so must be administered by the intravenous or subcutaneous routes.

The anticoagulant warfarin is orally available. Its main activity is preventing the formation of the active form of vitamin K and thus suppressing the synthesis in the liver of factors II (prothrombin), VII, IX and X which are all part of the clotting cascade. Factor VII is the most sensitive to vitamin K deficiency. Warfarin is the most widely used oral anticoagulant but it has a narrow therapeutic index and therefore its effects must be regularly monitored.

A further step in thrombus formation, the aggregation of platelets, is inhibited by aspirin. This non-steroidal anti-inflammatory drug (NSAID) blocks cyclooxygenase (COX) pathways. Aspirin is 150 times more effective at blocking the constitutive COX-1 pathway than the inducible COX-2 pathway. The result is a decrease in prostaglandin and thromboxane production. Effects on platelet aggregation are mediated at very low aspirin dose levels by a reduction in thromboxane A_2 (TXA_2) synthesis by platelets. Prophylactic use of low-dose aspirin to decrease the risk of thrombosis has become widespread.

Thrombolytic therapy

There are a number of thrombolytic drugs available but the most commonly used are streptokinase and genetically engineered recombinant tissue plasminogen activator (rt-PA). All of the drugs activate plasminogen to form plasmin, an enzyme which promotes the breakdown of fibrin and fibrinogen into degradation products (Fig. 5.6). This leads to lysis of a thrombus and may result in some restoration of blood flow. How effective thrombolytic therapy is depends on factors such as the age of thrombus and the access of the drug to the thrombus.

The thrombolytic drugs are given intravenously or intra-arterially and have been shown in clinical trials to reduce the mortality rate after a myocardial infarction. The greatest benefits are achieved if thrombolytic therapy is commenced within 70 minutes of the onset of pain. There are a number of contraindications which must be seriously evaluated. These include a previous history of cerebrovascular events (stroke), a recent gastrointestinal bleed or a recent operation; in short, any situation where there is a risk of haemorrhage. A fall in blood pressure (hypotension) associated with release of the vasodilator bradykinin may occur with drugs such as streptokinase.

After thrombolysis with rt-PA heparin must be given intravenously for 48 hours to reduce the likelihood of re-occlusion of the vessel. This is not necessary with streptokinase as it has a longer duration of action.

Angina

Angina is pain which arises from areas of cardiac muscle which are underperfused and lack adequate supplies of oxygen. Typically it is a central, crushing chest pain, of variable severity. Classically it radiates to the left arm or into the neck. Its key feature is that it occurs on exertion

Table 5.1	Types of embolus and their characteristics
Embolic material	**Characteristics**
Thrombus (90% of major emboli)	Venous thrombosis usually from deep veins of legs (95% of cases) becomes pulmonary embolus
	Thrombus forming over an atheromatous plaque or myocardial infarct or in a fibrillating atrium can give rise to systemic embolus. This leads to infarction, e.g. brain, kidneys, gut and limbs
Atheromatous plaque debris	Frequent cause of problems in lower limbs
Infective emboli	Particularly from vegetations on heart valves produced by infective endocarditis
Fat	Generated during long bone trauma and in severe burns. Emboli travel to lungs, brain and kidney particularly
Gas	May occur during surgery (air embolus) or during rapid decompression of divers (nitrogen)
Amniotic fluid	Occurs via damaged uterine blood vessels at childbirth
Tumour tissue	Route for tumour metastasis
Foreign bodies	Small amounts of material produce a granulomatous reaction where they lodge. At-risk patients include intravenous drug users

and is relieved with rest. In some individuals the pain may be less apparent and the sensation is more of chest tightness and breathlessness (dyspnoea). Relief of the pain by the use of short-acting nitrates such as sublingual glyceryl trinitrate (GTN) (see below) is considered a useful diagnostic feature.

The hypoxia results from a discrepancy between demand for myocardial oxygen and maximum coronary blood flow capacity (Fig. 5.7). The key difference between angina and myocardial infarction is that with angina the myocardial hypoperfusion is reversible and does not cause permanent myocardial damage. A theory is that the pain is elicited by the interstitial accumulation of adenosine which activates unmyelinated nerve fibres. This is based on the observation that angina pain can be mimicked in normal individuals in a dose-related way by coronary artery infusion of adenosine. The lack of associated ECG changes shows that actual hypoxia is not occurring as a result of the adenosine infusion.

'Unstable angina' occurs at rest. It is presumably brought about by coronary vasospasm at resting levels of demand and may be difficult to distinguish from infarction, though the pain of infarction is usually more severe and prolonged. ECG changes will reflect myocardial ischaemia, i.e. ST segment depression rather than the elevation associated with infarction (see Chapter 7). Treatment should be supportive using vasodilators and anticoagulants in order to prevent progression to full infarction.

Myocardial hypoxia is also produced by an inadequacy of oxygen transport. Anaemia reduces the oxygen-carrying capacity of the blood whilst the presence of cyanosis means that the available haemoglobin is inadequately oxygenated. Both these factors may generate tissue hypoxia and angina in a borderline coronary insufficiency state.

Factors which disproportionately increase the workload of the myocardium, such as aortic stenosis or hypertension, may also precipitate angina in a patient whose coronary arteries might otherwise be adequate. The hypertensive patient may suffer a 'double whammy',

increased tendency to develop atherosclerosis and an increased afterload imposing a workload on the heart which necessitates extra oxygen delivery.

> **Interesting facts**
>
> Viagra (sildenafil) was initially developed as a potential drug for the treatment of angina. The well known uses in erectile dysfunction became apparent from side effect reports when the drug was introduced into clinical trials.

Drugs used in the management of angina

Strategies for the treatment of angina can be targeted at either increasing the coronary blood flow or decreasing the work done by the heart. In the latter case oxygen demand is decreased. This can be achieved by reducing the force of cardiac muscle contraction either by reducing preload on the heart or by reducing cardiac contractility (see Chapter 4). Other changes in workload of the heart can be achieved by reducing heart rate or arterial blood pressure (decreased afterload).

Four major classes of drugs are used:

- organic nitrates
- β-adrenoceptor blockers
- calcium channel blockers
- potassium channel openers.

The organic nitrates are exogenous sources of the natural vasodilator nitric oxide (see Chapter 9). The most widely used drug in this category is glyceryl trinitrate (GTN). There is an increasing number of other drugs including isosorbide dinitrate and isosorbide mononitrate. A major site of action of organic nitrates is on the venous capacitance vessels. Relaxing smooth muscle here leads to a reduced preload on the heart and thus reduces cardiac output (see Chapter 4). Vasodilatation on the arterial side of the circulation, particularly in this case of large arteries, leads to a reduction in blood pressure and reduced afterload on the heart. Effects of nitrates on coronary blood vessels are often minimal. Vessels may already be maximally dilated under the influence of local metabolites (Chapter 9) which have accumulated in the hypoxic cardiac tissue. Nitrates may help to improve flow through collateral vessels and also relieve coronary artery spasm when that is a cause of angina.

As many nitrate drugs undergo extensive first-pass metabolism in the liver they are not suitable for absorption in the main part of the gastrointestinal tract. Sublingual (under the tongue), buccal (between upper lip and gum) or transdermal (through the skin from an adhesive patch) routes are commonly used sites of administration.

β-adrenoceptor blockers (beta-blockers) reduce the force of cardiac contraction (reduce contractility) and lower blood pressure (reduce afterload) (see Chapter 4). These effects reduce oxygen demand by the heart and limit exercise performance. There is also a reduction in

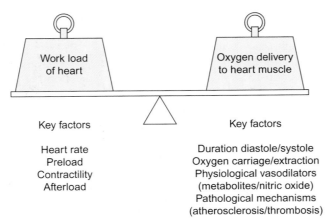

Fig. 5.7 Key factors determining the balance between the workload of the heart and oxygen delivery to cardiac muscle.

Case
5.1

Blood supply to the heart: 2

Limitations of Colin's drug therapy

Colin, whose presenting symptoms were described in Case 5.1:1, did find that the GTN relieved his symptoms. However although he gave up smoking he still found that he was using the GTN more and more frequently. He sought further advice from his GP who prescribed a long-acting oral nitrate drug. Colin's angina symptoms initially improved and he found walking to the shops and back much easier. Unfortunately, subsequently, his symptoms worsened and he sought further advice from his GP who prescribed atenolol 50 mg od. However Colin found the atenolol had too many side effects and so, after 2 weeks, he stopped taking the beta-blocker. He described the problems of the drug to his GP as a feeling of continuous fatigue and an inability to concentrate. This was made worse by a disturbed sleep pattern with vivid dreams and hallucinations.

This case history raises the following questions:

1. Why might Colin's angina be getting worse with the passage of time?
2. What was the rationale for prescribing the beta-blocker atenolol?

Aspects of the answers to these questions are to be found in the text of this chapter.

heart rate and, with the consequent lengthening of diastole, the phase of the cardiac cycle when most of the coronary perfusion occurs is prolonged. Some β-adrenoceptor blockers, such as atenolol, are referred to as 'cardioselective' as they are relatively selective for the β_1-subtype of receptors, the main type found in the heart. The first β-adrenoceptor blocker developed, propranolol, is nonselective and has approximately equivalent actions on β_1 and β_2 receptors. This drug is still widely used but is contraindicated in asthmatics as the β_2 blockade may lead to bronchospasm.

Calcium channel blockers such as nifedipine, amlodipine, verapamil and diltiazem reduce the flux of Ca^{++} ions into smooth muscle and cardiac muscle but not skeletal muscle. All of the calcium used to trigger skeletal muscle contraction is stored within the sarcoplasmic reticulum inside the muscle cells.

The main site of action of calcium channel blockers is on voltage-gated L-type (long-acting) slow Ca^{++} channels. Voltage-gated T-type (transient) channels are also blocked in pacemaker tissue of the sinoatrial and atrioventricular nodes (see Chapter 4). Beneficial effects of calcium channel blockers in the relief of angina include systemic arteriolar vasodilatation (reduced arterial blood pressure and thus reduced afterload), coronary artery dilatation (in the case of vasospasm), a reduction in heart rate and reduced cardiac contractility (reduced workload). It should be

stressed that the different drugs in this broad category have a wide spectrum of activity and they are not identical. For example, verapamil and diltiazem both reduce heart rate but the dihydropyridine drugs nifedipine and amlodipine do not. Amlodipine also does not significantly reduce cardiac contractility but, like nifedipine, it has marked effects leading to arteriolar vasodilatation.

Potassium channel opening drugs such as nicorandil open ATP-sensitive K^+ channels and hence lead to smooth muscle hyperpolarization. This inhibits the opening of L-type voltage-gated Ca^{++} channels and so produces vasodilatation in both systemic and, where possible, coronary blood vessels.

Myocardial infarction

Myocardial infarction (MI) results when there is complete interruption of blood flow to an area of myocardium. It involves necrosis of cardiac muscle followed by inflammatory cell infiltration and, because cardiac myocytes cannot regenerate, eventual fibrous repair. The subendocardial tissue in the left ventricle, which as described earlier is most prone to ischaemia, is most at risk. Figure 5.8 shows an infarcted area of tissue. The classical model for infarction is rupture of an atherosclerotic plaque (see Chapter 8) with thrombosis (see p. 53) and vasospasm completely occluding the lumen of a critical blood vessel. Frequently this is one of the major epicardial blood vessels described at the start of this chapter and shown in Figure 5.1. The infarction occurs downstream from the occluded blood vessel. As already noted, there is considerable variation in the anatomy and distribution of the main coronary arteries. However, some generalizations can be made regarding common sites of obstruction.

- Left anterior descending artery obstruction accounts for about 50% of cases. It produces infarcts in the anterior wall of the left ventricle with characteristic ECG changes in the anterior chest leads (V_1–V_3).

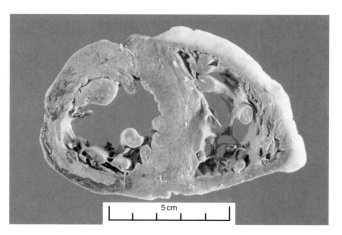

Fig. 5.8 Infarcted area of tissue. Myocardial infarct (I) in the lateral wall of the left ventricle. (Source: Stevens A, Lowe J 2000.)

Occlusion of this artery is sometimes a cause of sudden death.

- Right coronary artery obstruction occurs in about 30% of cases and leads to inferior wall infarction and sometimes posterior septum infarcts. The ECG changes are seen in leads II, III and aVF.

- Circumflex artery obstruction occurs in about 20% of cases and leads to lateral wall infarction with ECG changes in leads I, aVL and the lateral chest leads (V_4–V_6).

Depending on the vessel, the volume of muscle it supplies and the underlying structures, infarction may vary from being a mild warning sign for the individual to a terminal event. Structures which are of particular importance are the papillary muscles, the left ventricular myocardium and the conducting system. For example, rupture of a papillary muscle may result in severe mitral valve regurgitation which greatly reduces the effectiveness of an already compromised left ventricle. Infarcts can also lead to the development of arrhythmias which may be life threatening.

Interesting facts

New York Heart Association Functional Classification

This grading applies to patients with angina or heart failure:

Class I No limitations during ordinary activity
Class II Slight limitation during ordinary activity, e.g. mild or occasional angina or dyspnoea
Class III Marked limitation of normal activities without symptoms at rest
Class IV Unable to undertake physical activity without symptoms; symptoms may be present at rest.

Investigation of myocardial infarction

The clinical picture associated with MI is variable. A frequent symptom is severe crushing chest pain (angina) which may have a sudden onset or may build up more slowly. Accompanying symptoms often include nausea, vomiting and sweating. Patients may give a history of angina or non-specific chest discomfort over previous weeks but in at least 10% of patients, particularly the elderly, MI is painless.

MI is typically identified with characteristic ECG changes and increases in the serum level of proteins released from the disrupted myocardial cells. In the past plasma or serum measurements of total creatine kinase (CK), aspartate aminotransferase (also known as serum glutamic oxaloacetic transaminase, SGOT) and total lactate dehydrogenase (LDH) have been used as indicators of cardiac necrosis. However these enzymes are widely distributed in the body and lack specificity to cardiac tissue. More recently the use of other markers has increased. The MB isoenzyme of CK is found in the heart and levels

---

Case 5.1   Blood supply to the heart: 3

Colin's heart attack

Eight months later Colin was woken at 3.00 a.m. by a severe, central, crushing chest pain. It was as bad as any pain he had ever experienced. He felt cold and was sweating profusely. His wife called an ambulance and he was taken into the local hospital. A 12-lead ECG showed ST elevation in the lateral leads associated with T wave inversion. The casualty officer gave him a dose of aspirin and intravenous morphine. After review by the medical registrar Colin was moved to the coronary care unit where streptokinase was administered. Six hours from the onset of the pain blood samples were sent for measurement of cardiac enzymes. The results showed a substantial rise in creatine kinase (CK-MB) strongly supporting the clinical diagnosis of acute myocardial infarction. Following thrombolysis Colin was treated with heparin in order to maintain arterial patency. Further blood tests showed elevated levels of troponin T during the subsequent 15-hour period. The troponin T levels had returned to normal 10 days later.

After recovery from his infarction the patency of Colin's coronary vasculature was investigated by angiography. He was subsequently treated by coronary artery bypass grafting and made an uneventful recovery. Currently his exercise tolerance has improved considerably and he is free of angina pain.

This case history raises the following questions:

1. What is the basis for the use of the drugs aspirin and morphine?
2. What are the beneficial effects of streptokinase and when ideally should it be given?
3. What is the value of measurements of creatine kinase and troponin T? Why is the time course of blood sampling for these tests important?

Aspects of the answers to these questions are to be found in the text of this chapter.

---

in blood do not start to rise until 4 hours after infarction. CK-MB levels fall again within 72 hours. The CK-MB test is frequently used to provide early confirmation of a diagnosis of MI. The more specific markers troponins T and I are now the gold standard for myocardial cell necrosis as these structural proteins are found solely in myocardial cells. Their physiological function is in the coupling of a rise in intracellular $[Ca^{++}]$ to cross-bridge formation as part of the contraction of cardiac muscle (see Chapter 2). Troponin T and I levels may be modestly raised following the cardiac hypoxia associated with unstable angina. After an acute MI troponin levels are increased within 3–6 hours, reach a peak within 14–20 hours and return to normal after 5–7 days.

Since thrombosis appears to be an important component of the process of infarction the use of thrombolytic therapy, e.g. streptokinase or recombinant tissue-plasminogen activators such as alteplase or reteplase, has become a central component of care in suspected MI. These compounds, rather than being simply anticoagulant, positively promote activation of the fibrinolytic system thereby helping to break down the clot (see p. 54).

Coronary angioplasty and stenting

Percutaneous transluminal coronary angioplasty (PTCA) was first introduced as a clinical procedure in the late 1970s. A fine balloon is passed over a wire through the coronary artery until it overlies the region of narrowing. The balloon is then inflated under pressure expanding the lumen of the artery and so relieving the stenosis. Whilst much less invasive than coronary artery bypass grafting (see below) the long-term results are poor with re-stenosis occurring in a high proportion of patients in a relatively short time. To counteract this 'stenting' was introduced in which an expandable wire cage is introduced over the balloon. When the balloon is inflated it opens up the stent which then braces the arterial wall. Whilst this was an improvement over simple balloon angioplasty the re-stenosis rate initially remained high because the stent induced endothelial hypertrophy. Modern stents are coated with cytotoxic agents to prevent this and clinical results appear more promising.

Coronary artery bypass grafting

Coronary artery bypass grafting (CABG) involves replacing stenosed segments of coronary artery with vascular structures from elsewhere in the body. Two main strategies are available. Where possible the internal mammary artery may be grafted onto the blocked vessel distal to the stenosis. This gives a durable arterial supply. However the availability of such vessels is clearly limited. The other approach is to graft a vein extracted from the patient's leg, usually the long saphenous vein, between the aorta and the coronary vessel distal to the obstruction. However the vein is not structurally optimized for this function and vein grafts have a variable, but sometimes limited, lifespan. The radial artery dissected from an arm is an alternative source of graft material.

In order to achieve such delicate surgery the heart must be held still. Traditionally this has been achieved by instituting cardiac bypass in which the function of heart and lungs is taken over by a mechanical pump with an oxygenator. Blood is diverted from the right atrium or superior and inferior vena cavae through the pump and back to the aorta. The body is cooled to around 26°C to reduce oxygen demand and then the heart is stopped by instilling a cardioplegic solution of blood or crystalloid containing a high $[K^+]$ directly into the coronary arteries. This will depolarize the heart and stop contraction. The surgeon must work quickly to make the anastomoses in as short a time as possible as although cooling and cardioplegia protect the heart from the effects of ischaemia the protection is not perfect and frequently the myocardial perfusion is borderline to start with. Bypass also has an effect on cerebral function with numerous studies showing some loss in short-term memory and a reduction in IQ in patients following this form of surgery. Attempts to avoid the use of bypass techniques for coronary surgery have led to the development of devices for operating on the heart whilst it is still actively beating.

Further reading

Chilian, W.M., Gutterman, D.D., 2000. Prologue: new insights into the regulation of the coronary microcirculation. Am. J. Physiol. 48, H2585–H2586 [This paper provides an introduction to a series of specialist reviews on different aspects of coronary blood vessels.].

Cohen, M.V., Baines, C.P., Downey, J.M., 2000. Ischaemic preconditioning: from adenosine receptor to K_{ATP} channel. Annu. Rev. Physiol. 62, 79–109.

Di Carli, M.F., Tobes, M.C., Mangner, T., et al., 1997. Effects of cardiac sympathetic innervation on coronary blood flow. New Engl. J. Med. 336, 1208–1216.

Foreman, R.D., 1999. Mechanisms of cardiac pain. Annu. Rev. Physiol. 61, 143–167.

Gallagher, P.J., 2009. Cardiovascular system. In: Underwood, J.C.E., Cross, S.S. (Eds.), General and Systematic Pathology, fifth ed. Churchill Livingstone, Edinburgh.

Jones, J.H., Kuo, L., David, M.J., Chilian, W.M., 1995. Regulation of coronary blood flow: co-ordination of heterogeneous control mechanisms in vascular microdomains. Cardiovasc. Res. 29, 585–596.

Stevens, A., Lowe, J., 2000. Pathology, second ed. Mosby, Edinburgh.

Waller, D.G., Renwick, A.G., Hillier, K., 2009. Medical Pharmacology and Therapeutics, third ed. WB Saunders, Edinburgh.

Widlansky, M.E., Gokce, N., Keaney, J.F., Vita, J.A., 2003. The clinical implications of endothelial dysfunction. J. Am. Coll. Cardiol. 42, 1149–1160.

Wolfe, J.H.N., 1992. ABC of Vascular Diseases. BMJ Books, London.

HEART FAILURE

Chapter objectives

After studying this chapter you should be able to:

1. Describe the gross changes in cardiac function which may lead to the syndrome of heart failure.

2. Explain the differences between systolic and diastolic heart failure.

3. Discuss the concept of compensated cardiac failure and explain the pathophysiological changes by which compensation is achieved.

4. Describe the key metabolic changes within the myocytes of a failing heart.

5. Identify the changes in neurohormonal mechanisms which accompany heart failure often initially as a positive adaptive contribution but subsequently as a source of further decay in cardiac performance.

6. Explain the actions, advantages and limitations of the groups of drugs used therapeutically for the management of heart failure.

The typical 'textbook person' at rest has a cardiac output of about 5 L/min (see Chapter 4). The key physiological variables determining cardiac output are grouped as follows:

- preload events (filling pressure of the ventricle)
- contractility events (events inside the myocyte particularly associated with $[Ca^{++}]$ and $[H^+]$)
- afterload events (the resistance to blood leaving the heart)
- heart rate regulation.

The first three items on this list determine the stroke volume of each ventricle and the heart rate is primarily regulated by the baroreceptor reflex which keeps arterial blood pressure quite constant (see Chapter 9).

Heart failure is a complex syndrome and may be the main manifestation of practically any form of heart disorder. Many definitions of the term have been proposed and one of the most popular is as follows:

> *A pathophysiological state in which an abnormality of cardiac function is responsible for the failure of the heart to pump blood at a rate commensurate with the requirements of the metabolizing tissues*
>
> *(Braunwald 1986)*

The clinical presentation of heart failure often involves a rather vague collection of symptoms, exercise intolerance, breathlessness (particularly when supine), tiredness and ankle swelling, although not all patients necessarily have all of these symptoms. Pulmonary congestion and breathlessness will not necessarily occur unless the underlying defect is fairly substantial and/or long lasting. Ankle swelling is specifically a characteristic of right heart failure. The prevalence of heart failure in the community is age related, increasing from about 1% at age 50 to 9% at age 80. In the UK it has been reported to be responsible for about 5% of hospital medical admissions.

In Case 6.1:1 the history is outlined of a 37-year-old man who finds that his exercise capacity is becoming limited.

Interesting facts

Reduced performance of the heart muscle in systole is the most common form of heart failure but impaired diastolic function is also a common scenario.

Systolic vs diastolic failure

Impaired systolic function is the commonest cause of heart failure. However in 30–40% of all patients diastolic dysfunction is a major contributor and sometimes the primary cause of congestive cardiac failure.

In general the causes of heart failure can be attributed to one or more of the following:

- decreased myocyte contractility
- inappropriate workload due to pressure overload (e.g. hypertension causing increased afterload) or volume overload (increased preload)
- restricted filling of the ventricles (e.g. valve stenosis)
- myocyte loss.

These changes may represent either myocyte-related failure as in ischaemic heart disease or problems such as valve disease in a heart which may have normal myocyte function.

Heart failure may result from functional changes affecting either systole or diastole or both. Table 6.1 summarizes some of the key differences between systolic and diastolic heart failure. Examples of these different forms of cardiac failure are:

- Mainly systolic dysfunction:
  ischaemic heart disease
  dilated cardiomyopathy
  decreased myocyte contractility.

Case 6.1   Heart failure: 1

A builder with increasing exercise intolerance

Steven is a 37-year-old builder. Though active in his job he has noticed that over the last year he has found himself increasingly tired at the end of the day. His ability to carry heavy weights appeared to have declined substantially and occasionally he had chest pain whilst exerting himself. He sought the advice of his GP. Physical examination was largely normal apart from a high resting heart rate of 98 bpm and a loud ejection systolic murmur heard at the left sternal edge and at the apex but radiating to the neck. Steven's GP also elicited a history of unexpected death at a young age in his father's family. Two of Steven's paternal uncles had died suddenly at less than 30 years of age. The GP was concerned that there may be a familial cardiomyopathy of the obstructive type and referred him for urgent cardiology investigations. This history raises some fundamental questions:

1. Which aspects of this history might be consistent with a diagnosis of heart failure?
2. Which valves are likely to be associated with the systolic murmur and is it an indication of stenosis or regurgitation (or both)?
3. What investigations would you expect the cardiologist to carry out initially?

Answers to these questions can be found in the text of this chapter and in Chapter 3.

Table 6.1 Some characteristic differences between systolic and diastolic heart failure

	Systolic heart failure	Diastolic heart failure
Systolic BP	Low normal; hypertension	Low normal; hypertension
End-diastolic volume	↑↑	Normal or ↓
End-systolic volume	↑↑	↓
Stroke volume	Normal or ↓	Normal or ↓
Ejection fraction	↓↓	Normal
Myocardial hypertrophy	Eccentric	Concentric
LV wall thickness	↓	↑↑
Extracellular matrix	↓	↑↑

It is widely thought that cardiac myocytes cannot proliferate, only change size and shape. Some recent reports however suggest limited myocyte division is possible after myocardial infarction. In eccentric hypertrophy extra sarcomeres (see Fig. 2.1) are added in series and so myocyte length increases leading to a dilated heart. In concentric hypertrophy extra sarcomeres are added in parallel and so myocyte diameter increases.

- Mainly diastolic dysfunction:
  impaired relaxation due to fibrosis (e.g. amyloidosis)
  mitral or tricuspid valve stenosis
  constrictive pericarditis.
- Mixed systolic/diastolic dysfunction:
  hypertension
  aortic valve stenosis
  cardiac hypertrophy.

Primary left heart failure is more common than primary right heart failure and systolic failure is more common than diastolic failure. Left-sided failure is the commonest cause of right heart failure.

In order to understand the fundamental mechanisms involved we need to consider a range of topics which can be grouped under the following subheadings:

- haemodynamic events
- metabolic events
- neurohormonal aspects.

Haemodynamic events

Haemodynamic events in systolic heart failure

If the degree of functional impairment of the heart is relatively small then at rest the ventricle may be able to maintain a normal stroke volume and hence a normal cardiac output. This is achieved by an increase in filling pressure of the ventricle and hence an increase in end-diastolic volume. This increase in 'preload' causes the impaired ventricular function to move up a Starling curve (see Chapter 4) to reach a normal stroke volume (Fig. 6.1). There is however a limitation on the ability to increase stroke volume above the resting levels. This manifests itself as part of the exercise limitation experienced by heart failure patients. The increase in preload to restore resting stroke volume for a damaged heart to normal levels is referred to as 'compensation'.

The extent to which compensation can occur is limited by the shape of the cardiac function curve. If end-diastolic volume increases too much then a plateau is reached when further increases in end-diastolic volume do not produce a corresponding increase in the force of contraction of the ventricle. If the cardiac output is still inadequate when this plateau region is reached then end-diastolic volume may continue to increase and this will eventually cause the force of contraction to decrease. This is the region of 'decompensation' on the Starling curve and may rapidly lead to death (Fig. 6.2).

The commonest form of heart failure is left ventricle systolic failure. It has an annual mortality rate of 15–30% depending on disease severity. In pure left heart failure, the healthy right ventricle will continue to pump blood into the lungs until left ventricular preload is increased enough to restore ventricular balance, i.e. the same output from the two sides of the heart. This ventricular balance will be achieved at the price of raised left atrial, pulmonary capillary and pulmonary artery pressures. The raised pulmonary capillary pressure may result in pulmonary oedema (see Chapter 11) and this will cause the lungs to become 'stiff'. There will be an increased resistance to inflation of the lungs (a decreased compliance)

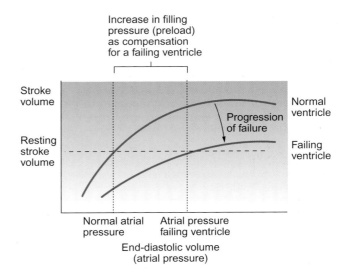

Fig. 6.1 Compensatory mechanisms in a failing ventricle. A compensatory increase in filling pressure allows a failing ventricle to achieve a normal resting stroke volume. The scope for increasing stroke volume in response to increased workload in exercise is limited. This diagram does not have numerical values on the horizontal axis and so could refer to either the right or left ventricle.

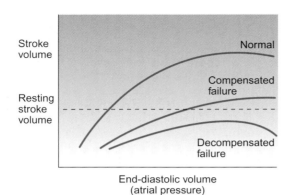

Fig. 6.2 Decompensated cardiac failure. In compensated cardiac failure the resting stroke volume and therefore resting cardiac output can reach normal levels by virtue of an increase in filling pressure (preload) for the ventricle (see Fig. 6.1). In decompensated failure increases in preload fail to achieve a satisfactory cardiac output and further increases may lead to a decline in stroke volume.

and this will produce a sensation of breathlessness (dyspnoea). The pulmonary oedema may also upset the balance between the distribution of lung ventilation and pulmonary blood flow causing a 'ventilation-perfusion mismatch' which will result in arterial hypoxaemia. This in turn will further reduce the delivery of oxygen to the heart and potentially exacerbate heart failure, producing a vicious circle of events.

The commonest cause of right heart failure is left heart failure. The right ventricle fails because of the increased afterload (increased pulmonary circuit blood pressure) produced by the left-sided failure. Right heart failure may also follow from a raised pulmonary vascular resistance (hypoxic vasoconstriction) such as may occur during decreased oxygenation of the blood in lung disease or in response to low oxygen pressures at altitude (see Chapter 9). The condition of right heart failure resulting from increased pulmonary vascular resistance or some other aspect of lung dysfunction leading to pulmonary artery hypertension is known as cor pulmonale.

In right heart failure ventricular output may be maintained by an increased preload (right atrial pressure; RAP). Clinically it is possible to assess RAP by monitoring jugular venous pressure (Box 6.1). An increase in right atrial pressure will lead to an increase in pressure back through the vena cava and peripheral veins and capillaries and will result in peripheral oedema (see Chapter 11). This is manifested by ankle oedema (if the subject is standing or seated) or sacral oedema (if they are supine). There may also be enlargement of the liver which becomes palpable below the lower ribs. However it should be remembered that the most common cause of ankle swelling in the elderly is not right heart failure but immobility or vascular disease.

The mechanisms associated with compensatory increases in filling pressure of the ventricles are largely attributable to

a combination of the sympathetic nervous system and the renin-angiotensin system. These events are discussed later in this chapter under the heading 'Neurohormonal aspects of heart failure'. The result of these compensatory changes is that, despite an intrinsic decline in some aspects of myocardial function, patients may remain asymptomatic or minimally symptomatic for years. A decline in exercise tolerance is often attributed to normal ageing rather than to developing heart failure. However at some point they are likely to develop symptoms with an associated increase in morbidity and mortality.

Haemodynamic events in diastolic heart failure

The characteristics of diastolic heart failure are delayed relaxation of the ventricle and impaired filling of the left ventricle often linked to increased stiffness of the ventricular wall. Mitral and/or tricuspid valve stenosis will also lead to diastolic dysfunction by providing an increased resistance to atrial emptying. If left-sided heart failure is purely associated with diastole then the ejection fraction (EF) of the ventricle (stroke volume expressed as a percentage of end-diastolic volume) will be normal or only slightly reduced at 40–50%. There will be an increase in left atrial pressure and pulmonary congestion secondary to raised pulmonary capillary pressure. Diastolic failure is typically seen in patients with cardiac hypertrophy (often as a result of hypertension) or restrictive problems such as the fibrotic changes which occur in amyloidosis or in pericarditis. These problems may be exacerbated by any tachycardia, as when the heart rate increases the time available for diastole is shortened more than the time available for systole (see Chapter 5).

Diastolic heart failure has a relatively high prevalence in elderly patients. Although the prognosis in terms of mortality for diastolic heart failure (annual rate about 8%) is much better than for systolic heart failure (annual rate about 19%), it is still associated with substantial morbidity.

Metabolic events in heart failure

In Chapter 5 the regulation of coronary blood flow is described. Impaired blood supply will lead to reduced ATP generation and impaired ventricular muscle performance. In Chapter 2 the roles of ATP in systole and diastole are described. Each cycle of cross-bridge formation requires the binding of a Ca^{++} ion to troponin C and the hydrolysis of an ATP molecule in order to achieve cardiac myocyte contraction during systole. ATP is also essential for myocyte relaxation during diastole as Ca^{++} must be actively pumped back into the sarcoplasmic reticulum stores. Changes in intracellular $[Ca^{++}]$ are the major factor determining the contractility of cardiac muscle (see Chapter 4).

Box 6.1 Jugular venous pressure

Right-sided heart failure is accompanied by a compensatory increase in filling pressure. This increased preload on the ventricle leads to improved stroke volume (Fig. 6.1). In a normal heart pressure in the right atrium is typically in the range −1 to +8 mmHg (mean 4). The pressure in any venous vessel above the level of the heart must be less than in the right atrium. Pressure in the jugular vein in the neck is therefore likely to be negative (less than atmospheric pressure) and so the vein is normally collapsed and in an upright posture is not visible as a bulge on the neck. However, if right atrial pressure rises then the jugular will be inflated further up the neck. This principle is used to estimate right atrial pressure.

The subject is positioned sitting but supported leaning back at an angle of 45 degrees to the horizontal plane (Fig. 6.3). The anatomical reference point for measuring how far up the neck the jugular vein is inflated is the sternal angle (angle of Louis). An approximation of actual right atrial pressure (in pressure units of cm blood/water) could be obtained by adding 5 cm to the height of jugular vein inflation above the sternal angle (note: 1.36 cm water ≡ 1 mmHg pressure because the density of mercury relative to water is 13.6).

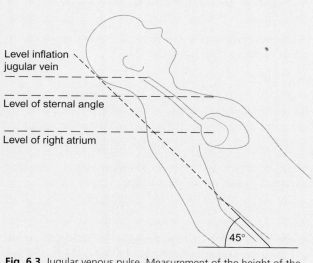

Fig. 6.3 Jugular venous pulse. Measurement of the height of the jugular venous pressure.

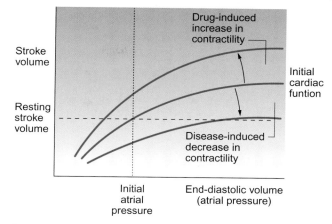

Fig. 6.4 Myocardial contractility and stroke volume. Effect of changes in myocardial contractility on stroke volume. The middle curve represents an initial starting position with a resting stroke volume achieved with an appropriate initial filling pressure (atrial pressure) or, in other words, end-diastolic volume. A disease-associated fall in contractility means that at a given filling pressure, stroke volume is reduced. Correspondingly, in response to the use of a positive inotrope drug which increases contractility, stroke volume at that initial end-diastolic volume or atrial pressure is increased.

Dysfunction of the mechanisms regulating cardiac contractility (Fig. 6.4) are important in the initiation and progression of some forms of heart failure. The defects are thought to be associated with altered sarcoplasmic reticulum uptake, storage and release of Ca^{++}. In experimental animal studies of heart failure it has been shown that maintaining contractility can prevent the development of cardiac failure. This is however a complex and still developing area. Clinical trials have shown that improving contractility by the use of positive inotrope agents (see p. 68) which increase intracellular [cAMP] have tended to increase mortality. Cardiac glycosides are drugs which increase intracellular [Ca^{++}] and hence contractility by a different mechanism compared to sympathomimetic drugs (Fig. 6.5). They are only relatively weak inotropes and neither increase nor decrease mortality among patients with congestive heart failure but do provide symptomatic relief. Further aspects of the actions of these drugs are discussed below and in Chapter 2.

Different ways of altering cardiac myocyte contractility using drugs which do not involve increased cAMP formation are being evaluated. In this context the Na^+/Ca^{++} exchange mechanism in the sarcolemma is of considerable interest (see Fig. 2.3).

In relation to drug therapy, low doses of β-adrenoceptor antagonists, which in the short term have negative inotropic actions and were therefore previously thought to be contraindicated, seem to have beneficial effects in relation to reversal of cardiac remodelling (see p. 67), increase in contractility and in improving patient survival. Some aspects of the mechanisms behind these beneficial effects of beta-blockers are still a matter for conjecture.

A further component of the metabolic changes in heart failure is the role played by H^+ ions. As described in Chapter 4, H^+ ions are the strongest naturally occurring negative inotrope and the actions involved include decreased binding of Ca^{++} to troponin C. Underventilation of the lung and the consequent increases in the P_{CO_2} of body fluids leads to respiratory acidosis (see Chapter 1). Oxidative metabolism also generates forms of acid which have to be excreted via the kidneys. Overproduction of such acids, as in diabetic ketoacidosis, or a failure of excretory mechanisms as in renal failure,

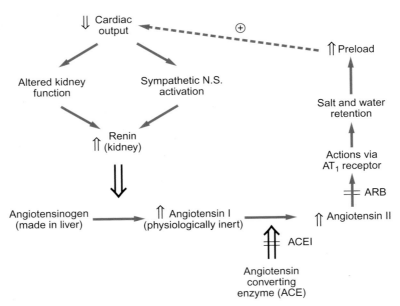

Fig. 6.5 Renin-angiotensin system. Role of the renin-angiotensin system in producing a compensatory increase in preload in response to cardiac failure. The site of action of two groups of drugs, angiotensin-converting enzyme inhibitors (ACEI) and angiotensin receptor blockers (ARB) which are used to suppress excessive actions of the renin system are also shown.

will lead to metabolic acidosis. Either form of acidosis, but particularly respiratory acidosis (as CO_2 can quickly diffuse into the myocyte), is likely to impair myocyte contraction and make heart failure worse.

Interesting facts

In earlier times heart failure was often referred to as 'the dropsy'. This word is thought to be a corruption of the term hydropsy meaning a generalized swelling of the body due to accumulation of excess water.

Neurohormonal aspects of heart failure

Activation of the sympathetic nervous system is a central component of the physiological response to heart failure and the mechanisms involved, the baroreceptor reflex, are described in Chapter 10. Sympathetic activation may be manifested as an increased heart rate, which is not necessarily helpful for a patient with a poorly functioning ventricle. Other characteristics of increased sympathetic drive include:

- Increased contraction of venous smooth muscle will contribute to increased right ventricle preload and therefore to compensation in moderate heart failure (Fig. 6.1).

- Vasoconstriction, particularly in the skin, splanchnic circulation and skeletal muscle, will help to sustain arterial blood pressure (the driving force for tissue perfusion) and divert available cardiac output to the most critical organs (heart and brain).

- Increased contractility of cardiac myocytes by a β-adrenoceptor mediated increase in intracellular $[Ca^{++}]$.

- Increased renin secretion from the juxtaglomerular cells in the kidney (see below).

It is sometimes suggested that overstimulation of pathways activated by β-adrenoceptor agonists including both the effects of neurotransmitters released by sympathetic nerves to the heart and circulating catecholamines released by the adrenal medulla may become counterproductive in heart failure. The increased mortality associated with prolonged use of β-adrenoceptor agonists as inotrope drugs is referred to above.

Figure 6.1 shows that the compensation response for cardiac failure is an increase in preload (increased end-diastolic volume or atrial pressure) on the heart. This is largely achieved by an expansion of the extracellular fluid volume, including blood volume, driven by activation of the renin-angiotensin system. Increased renin secretion occurs in response to decreased blood pressure or to any situation in which blood volume is inadequate to support the necessary preload for an appropriate cardiac output. The components of the renin-angiotensin system are summarized in Figure 6.6 and are further discussed in Chapters 9 and 14. The mechanisms regulating renin secretion from the juxtaglomerular (JG) cells in the kidney may be summarized as:

- Direct innervation of JG cells by sympathetic nerves which act through a β-adrenoceptor mechanism. Renin secretion will therefore be increased as part of the baroreceptor reflex (see Chapter 10).

Case 6.1 Heart failure: 2

Investigations on Steven's symptoms

During his cardiology appointment Steven received an ECG and an echocardiographic investigation. The ECG showed extremely large left-sided voltages. There was also evidence of abnormal repolarization with ST segment elevation and T wave inversion particularly in leads V_4–V_6.

The echocardiogram demonstrated left ventricular hypertrophy dominated by thickening of the septum which reached a maximum of 22 mm. There was outflow obstruction with a left ventricular outflow velocity of 2.8 m/s implying a high pressure gradient of 35 mmHg across the valve. The obstruction was below the aortic valve which itself appeared normal. The left ventricle was hyperdynamic with an ejection fraction of 85% but the left ventricular cavity was almost obliterated in systole and remained small even in diastole.

An exercise test was performed during which Steven managed 8 minutes 10 seconds of a standard protocol and became very breathless. He experienced some chest pain towards the latter stage of the test and the ECG at this time showed 3 mm of ST depression in leads V_5 and V_6.

The diagnosis for Steven was hypertrophic obstructive cardiomyopathy. This form of outflow obstruction imposes an afterload on the left ventricle and is therefore a form of pressure overload.

Steven was commenced on beta-blockers. He was advised to give up his job as a builder and adopt a more sedentary lifestyle particularly avoiding 'explosive' activities. His clinical history gives rise to the following questions:

1. Why, when Steven's cardiac function remains so good, does he get breathless with exercise?
2. Why was Steven's myocardium thickened?
3. What was the origin of the changes on his ECG?
4. Why were beta-blockers prescribed?
5. Why was Steven advised to adopt a more sedentary lifestyle?
6. Is this history consistent with systolic, diastolic or mixed (systolic and diastolic) heart failure?

Answers to these questions can be found in this chapter and in Chapters 3, 4 and 7.

- JG cells are intrinsically sensitive to stretch. A fall in renal afferent arteriole pressure will lead to increased renin secretion. This mechanism is independent of the sympathetic nervous system.

- A putative Na^+ and/or Cl^- load detector located at the macula densa, a group of specialized tubular cells where the ascending limb of the loop of Henle becomes the distal tubule as it passes the JG cells. It is still unclear exactly how or if this mechanism functions to control renin secretion.

- Circulating angiotensin II (Ang II) concentration exerts a negative feedback control on renin secretion via an AT_1 receptor on the JG cells.

Increased Ang II concentration increases sodium and water retention via stimulation of the synthesis of aldosterone in the zona glomerulosa of the adrenal cortex and also via direct effects of Ang II on sodium transport mechanisms in the nephron. Ang II will also increase antidiuretic hormone (ADH) secretion which further contributes to fluid retention. If the expansion of blood volume fails to generate an adequate arterial blood pressure which would eventually suppress renin secretion, this will lead to excessive expansion of the extracellular fluid compartment. This may lead to further deterioration of cardiac performance and to decompensated failure (Fig. 6.2). This scenario provides part of the rationale for the use of diuretics and blockers of the renin system (angiotensin-converting enzyme inhibitors and Ang II receptor blockers) in the management of heart failure (see p. 68). Overproduction of Ang II also contributes to the series of fibrotic changes in the heart known as remodelling. This seems to start as an adaptive response to changes in cardiac function but as failure progresses remodelling becomes counterproductive.

The potent vasoconstrictor peptide endothelin-1 (ET-1) (see Chapter 9) has also been implicated in the pathogenesis of congestive heart failure. Initially in an adaptive context ET-1 is thought to have a positive role promoting inotropic actions on the myocyte and increasing myocyte protein synthesis. Overexpression of ET-1 leads to myocardial fibrosis and myocyte necrosis in addition to local vasospasm, all of which promote the progression of failure. Endothelin production may be potentiated by the increased concentrations of Ang II which frequently occur in heart failure (see p. 66).

The two types of endothelin receptors are designated ET_A and ET_B (see Chapter 9), and drugs which block these receptors are given trivial names ending in -sentan. Drugs such as the non-selective ET_A/ET_B receptor blocker bosentan are undergoing clinical trials to evaluate their efficacy in the management of heart failure. It is not yet clear whether mixed ET_A/ET_B blockers or selective ET_A receptor blockers will be the more valuable approach.

Heart failure is also associated with the release of cytokines, particularly tumour necrosis factor alpha (TNFα) and members of the interleukin (IL) family. These cytokines appear to be particularly involved in mechanisms leading to cardiac myocyte hypertrophy.

Interesting facts

In 7th century England, blood-letting (venesection) was widely practiced because of the belief that too much blood was a cause of illness. This practice has continued in one form or other, including the use of leeches, through to the present day. Some current pharmacological therapy for heart failure is targeted at reducing blood volume.

Drug therapy for heart failure

A detailed discussion of management strategies for heart failure is outside the scope of this book, but the following generalizations can be made about the classes of drugs used.

Sympathomimetic inotropes

This group includes drugs such as isoprenaline/isoproterenol (a non-selective β_1/β_2 agonist), dobutamine (a selective β_1 agonist) and dopamine (a non-selective β-adrenoceptor agonist which is also a dopamine D_1/D_2 receptor agonist). These drugs are given intravenously to acutely ill hospitalized patients in order to provide a short-term increase in cardiac contractility. β-adrenoceptor activation leads to an increase in myocyte [cAMP] and hence an increase in intracellular [Ca^{++}] (see Chapter 2). Activation of D_1 receptors by dopamine also leads to vasodilatation within the kidney and activation of presynaptic D_2 receptors leads to peripheral vasodilatation by inhibition of noradrenaline (norepinephrine) release from sympathetic nerve endings. Dopamine-induced hypotension but with increased renal blood flow and increased cardiac contractility is often a useful combination in the management of heart failure. Dobutamine has positive inotropic actions but, compared to isoprenaline, a reduced effect increasing heart rate.

Adverse effects on patient mortality of drugs which increase intracellular [cAMP] have been referred to on page 65. In prolonged use of β-adrenoceptor agonists, downregulation of receptor number will also limit their therapeutic response.

The apparently counter-intuitive use of low dose beta-blockers in heart failure is described on page 65.

Phosphodiesterase inhibitors

Phosphodiesterase III, an enzyme in cardiac and smooth muscle which promotes the breakdown of cAMP, can be blocked with the drugs milrinone and enoximone. The increased myocyte [cAMP] increases [Ca^{++}] and hence provides useful short-term increases in myocardial contractility. Unwanted side effects include increased heart rate and arrhythmias. Unlike β-agonists, phosphodiesterase inhibitors do not cause downregulation of β-receptor number. However, as with other drugs which increase intracellular [cAMP], long-term use is associated with increased patient mortality.

Digitalis glycosides

The most widely used drug in this category is digoxin which acts as an inhibitor of the Na^+/K^+-ATPase in cardiac muscle (see Fig. 4.7). The consequent increase in intracellular [Na^+] results in reduced Na^+/Ca^{++} exchange across the plasma membrane and so Ca^{++} is retained within the cell. The increase in intracellular [Ca^{++}] provides an increase in myocardial contractility.

Although a relatively mild inotrope, digoxin can be used for an extended period provided the potential unwanted effects are kept under review. The digitalis glycosides have a narrow therapeutic window between doses which are too low to be effective and doses which are high enough to cause significant side effects. Toxicity may result from excessive increases in intracellular [Ca^{++}] which may cause various arrhythmias. There may also be increased vagal activity causing an excessive atrioventricular (AV) node block (see Chapter 2). Anorexia, nausea and vomiting are quite common side effects as are neurological disturbances including fatigue, vertigo and visual disturbances. Digitalis toxicity will be worse if it is accompanied by hypokalaemia and thus care must be taken when combining digitalis treatment with diuretics. Renal failure, hypoxaemia and hypothyroidism will also increase the risk of toxicity.

Interesting facts

In 1785, William Withering, a physician in Birmingham, described the treatment of heart failure with digoxin in his book 'An account of the foxglove'.

Blockade of the renin-angiotensin system

Angiotensin converting enzyme inhibitors (ACEI) have an established role in the management of heart failure. Increasingly angiotensin receptor blockers (ARB) which have many similar, but some importantly different, pharmacological actions compared to ACEI are being used (Fig. 6.5). The names of all of the ACEI family of drugs end in -pril (e.g. captopril, ramipril) and all the ARB family end in -sartan (e.g. losartan, valsartan).

Initially ACEI were thought to be useful in heart failure by virtue of their effects reducing preload on the heart by blocking angiotensin/aldosterone-induced salt and water retention. They also reduce afterload effects on the heart by blocking the vasoconstrictor actions of Ang II and hence lower arterial blood pressure. In a normal heart reducing afterload (arterial blood pressure in this case) has a minimal effect on cardiac performance. In a failing heart however a reduction in arterial blood pressure may significantly improve stroke volume of the heart. However, it has subsequently emerged that blockade of the renin system also results in a reversal of the cardiac hypertrophy and adverse fibrotic changes in the failing heart which together are known as remodelling. These aspects of renin system inhibition are associated with improved patient mortality. Blockade of the renin system will also reduce aldosterone and endothelin production (see Chapter 9).

Diuretics

Diuretics remain the primary group of drugs used for the management of heart failure. The selection of the diuretic used depends on the severity of the failure. For mild cases a thiazide diuretic is used, but for many patients a loop diuretic, mainly furosemide (frusemide), is necessary. A potassium sparing diuretic (amiloride or spironolactone) may be appropriate if hypokalaemia occurs. The primary aim of diuretic therapy is to return preload to the optimal level on the Starling curve (Fig. 6.6). It is important to avoid hyponatraemia, hypokalaemia, excessive volume depletion and renal impairment. On the basis of encouraging results from randomized controlled clinical trials a new group of selective aldosterone receptor antagonists which do not have the unwanted side effects of spironolactone is being developed.

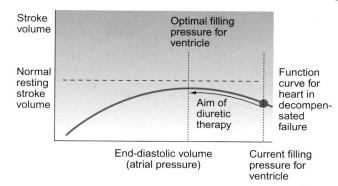

Fig. 6.6 Decompensated cardiac failure. Increases in the filling pressure (end-diastolic volume) of the ventricle have failed to reach a satisfactory output (resting stroke volume). The heart has become very dilated and further increases in the filling pressure are leading to a decline in function. The aim of diuretic therapy is to return function to the optimal point on the cardiac function curve. In the past this was sometimes achieved by venesection providing an acute reduction in blood volume. This method is still occasionally used as an emergency procedure.

Further reading

Braunwald, E., 1980. A Textbook of Cardiovascular Medicine. WB Saunders, Philadelphia.

Diwan, A., Dorn, G.W., 2007. Decompensation of cardiac hypertrophy: cellular mechanisms and novel therapeutic targets. Physiology 22, 56–64.

Gaasch, W.H., Zile, M.R., 2004. Left ventricular diastolic dysfunction and diastolic heart failure. Ann. Rev. Med. 55, 373–394.

Houser, S.R., Margulies, K.B., 2003. Is depressed myocyte contractility centrally involved in heart failure? Circ. Res. 92, 350–358.

Mandinov, L., Eberli, R.F., Seiler, C., Hess, O.M., 2000. Diastolic heart failure. Cardiovasc. Res. 45, 813–825.

Mann, D.L., Deswal, A., Bozkurt, B., Torre-Amione, G., 2002. New therapeutics for chronic heart failure. Ann. Rev. Med. 53, 59–74.

Orchard, C.H., Kentish, J.C., 1990. Effects of changes of pH on the contractile function of cardiac muscle. Am. J. Physiol. 358, C967–C981.

Schillinger, W., Fiolet, J.W., Schlotthauer, K., Hasenfuss, G., 2003. Relevance of Na^+-Ca^{++} exchange in heart failure. Cardiovasc. Res. 57, 921–933.

Timmis, A.D., Davies, S.W., 1992. Heart Failure. Gower Medical Publishing, London.

Waller, D.G., Renwick, A.G., Hillier, K., 2009. Medical Pharmacology and Therapeutics, third ed. WB Saunders, Edinburgh.

THE ELECTROCARDIOGRAM (ECG)

7

Chapter objectives

After studying this chapter you should be able to:

1. Describe how the standard 12 lead ECG is recorded.

2. Explain the origin of the various elements of the ECG trace.

3. Enumerate the basic normal values in relation to aspects of the ECG and explain the relevance of values outside these ranges.

4. Discuss how pathology impacts on the characteristic patterns of the ECG.

5. Describe the effect of certain drugs on ECG traces and their clinical significance.

Introduction

It is as important to recognize what the electrocardiogram (ECG) is not, as much as what it is. The origin of the cardiac action potential and the structure of the specialized conducting system of the heart are described in Chapter 3. The ECG is not a recording of the electrical activity of individual cells; it does not look like the action potential but reflects the activity of large numbers of cells taken en masse. It is possible to measure this activity because the heart lies in a container, the human body, which is full of a salt solution capable of carrying electrical current. Thus electrodes placed on the skin at a distance from the heart can be affected by the electrical changes within the myocardium. At rest the electrical activity of the heart dominates that of other excitable tissues such as nerve or skeletal muscle because of its relatively large mass and the coordination of its activity. A recording of the electrical activity of the heart is called an electrocardiogram. The overall net direction of the spread of excitation through the muscle mass of the left ventricle is called the cardiac axis.

It is helpful to understand the characteristics of the ECG in terms of the underlying physical process. At rest the cardiac myocytes have a resting membrane potential around −85 mV (see Chapter 2). A group of cells undergoes depolarization; the membrane potential rises to around +30 mV before repolarization. Figure 7.1 shows a schematic 'block' of myocardial tissue that has groups of cells in all phases of polarization. The wavefront of depolarization is moving from left to right in the diagram from an area of tissue that has just been depolarized towards tissue which is about to be depolarized. If we consider electrodes applied to the left and right of our block of tissue we see that there is an electrical potential difference between the electrodes. It is this potential difference between the tissue in front of the wave of depolarization and the tissue behind it that we measure as an ECG. The flow of current is from behind the wavefront of depolarization to in front of it and this is by convention taken as 'positive' and produces an upward deflection of the recorder pen.

The heart is a complex shape with depolarization spreading simultaneously in many different directions. At any one moment in time there will however be a dominant (net) direction of the spread of depolarization. By considering the heart as a battery lying in the direction of the spread of depolarization the sequential changes in deflection of the ECG pen can be more easily understood. This is equivalent to holding the battery at various orientations (Fig. 7.2). It is important to realize that it is not the heart that is changing orientation, only the direction of the wavefront of depolarization within the heart. The shape of the ECG waveform reflects the changing distribution of polarized and depolarized tissue within the heart with time.

The amplitude of the ECG deflection reflects the mass of tissue involved. Thus the atrial element of the ECG

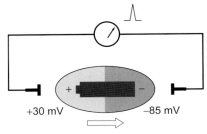

Direction of travel of depolarization wavefront

Fig. 7.1 Origin of the ECG signal.

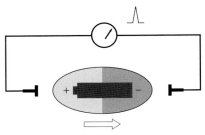

Depolarization wavefront

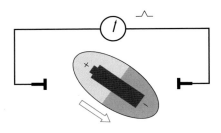

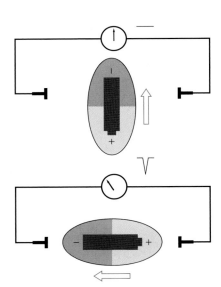

Fig. 7.2 Variation of ECG with orientation.

(P wave) is always smaller than the ventricular element (QRS complex), even though the change in membrane potential is the same in each case. Hypertrophied ventricles, for example, resulting from hypertension, will tend to give larger deflections than the average. The amplitude of the ECG deflection is also affected by other physical factors such as size, chest inflation and fat tissue.

To summarize:

- The ECG represents the spread of depolarization and repolarization through the myocardium.

- The pattern of the ECG is dependent on the net activity of the myocardium at any given instant.

- The pattern of the ECG is dependent on the relative orientation of the heart and the electrodes.

- Many pathological factors within the myocardium such as hypertrophy and ischaemic damage affect the pattern of the ECG.

- Many extracardiac factors such as posture and chest deformity may affect the ECG.

What information can be derived from an ECG recording?

- Heart rate: an ECG recording can trigger electronic ratemeters.

- Rhythm: normal and abnormal rhythms can be recorded.

- Conduction times through components of the heart can be evaluated from the duration of the components of an ECG trace.

- The direction of the mean cardiac axis of the heart in both vertical and horizontal planes can be determined.

- The extent and location of ischaemic damage.

- The effects of altered electrolyte concentration.

- The effects of drugs which affect the conducting system (antiarrhythmic drugs, digitalis glycosides, calcium channel blockers) can be monitored.

Interesting facts

British physiologist Augustus D. Waller published the first human electrocardiogram in 1887. It was recorded with a capillary electrometer from Thomas Goswell, a technician in the laboratory. Subsequently, Waller often demonstrated his technique using his dog 'Jimmy' who would patiently stand with paws in glass jars of saline.

Producing a 12-lead ECG

The electrical activity of the heart was first recorded in 1887 by A.D. Waller who concluded that such recordings would not be of clinical value. Willem Einthoven made his first recordings of the ECG in 1901. Identifying differences in the ECG made Einthoven believe that this was an investigation of value. He was awarded the Nobel Prize for his work in 1924.

Case 7.1 The electrocardiogram: 1

A patient with exercise-induced angina

In Case 5.1:1 in Chapter 5, the case history of Colin Davis, a 50-year-old smoker, was described. He suffered from chest pain on exercise. He was referred to the local hospital where he was given an exercise test on a treadmill. He developed angina during the test and an ECG showed ST segment depression in the lateral leads V_4–V_6. These ST segment changes disappeared when the exercise test was terminated.

This case history raises the following questions.

1. Why does myocardial ischaemia lead to ST segment depression?
2. What do the leads showing ST segment changes tell us about the localization of ischaemia in the heart?

Answers to these questions are to be found in the text of this chapter and they are discussed in Case 7.1:2.

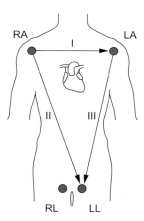

Fig. 7.3 Basic limb leads.

Recording a 12 lead ECG requires the connection of two groups of electrodes to the subject:

1. limb leads (I, II, III, aVR, aVL, aVF)
2. chest leads (generally V_1 to V_6).

The limb lead electrodes are the simplest set of electrodes and were used by Einthoven in his experiments. The basic electrode positions are on the right arm, left arm and left leg. By using the electrodes in pairs we generate sets of measurements with a specific axis or vector described as a 'lead'. Lead I utilizes the right and left arms and the axis of measurement is from right to left directly through the chest (Fig. 7.3). Lead I is taken as 0° and angles are measured clockwise from lead I. Lead II utilizes the right arm and left leg giving an axis theoretically at +60° to lead I. Lead III utilizes the left arm and left leg giving an axis which lies at +120°. These axes are

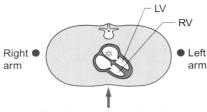

Fig. 7.4 Combining electrodes. Adapted from Hampton 2003.

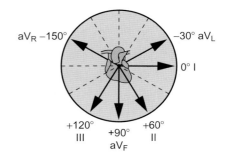

Fig. 7.5 Augmented limb leads. Adapted from Hampton 2003.

Table 7.1 A complete set of augmented limb leads produced by combining groups of three limb electrodes

Augmented limb lead	+ve electrode	−ve electrode
aVR	Right arm	Left arm + Left leg
aVL	Left arm	Right arm + Left leg
aVF	Left leg	Right arm + Left arm

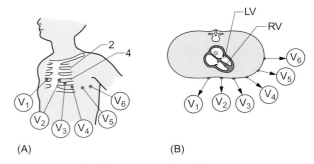

Fig. 7.6 Chest leads. (A) Position on chest. (B) Orientation in transverse plane. Adapted from Hampton 2003.

summarized in Figure 7.3. A further electrode is placed on the right leg. This is not used directly for recording but serves as a neutral reference for the other leads.

It is standard practice to use the wrists and ankles for the limb electrodes. This is convenient but not essential as the limbs effectively serve as 'wires' connected to the shoulders or hips which are the point of geometrical definition. In small children especially it is sometimes easier to use the shoulders and hips to site electrodes for leads I, II and III.

Augmented limb leads (aVR, aVL, aVF)

The augmented limb leads are produced by combining pairs of electrodes to produce 'virtual' electrodes which do not have direct physical existence. Thus, for example, by electronically combining the right arm and left arm electrodes we get a virtual electrode which appears to lie within the centre of the upper chest (Fig. 7.4). This virtual electrode can then be linked with the electrode on the left leg to give a new lead (aVF) with a new (vertical) axis. The complete set of augmented limb leads is produced by combining groups of three limb electrodes as shown in Table 7.1.

The geometry of the augmented leads is shown in Figure 7.5. The result is a new series of axes which complement the three basic limb leads. It is now possible to identify leads which come in pairs at right angles (orthogonal) to each other: lead I and aVF, lead II and aVL, lead III and aVR. This is of practical value in simplifying the analysis of the ECG (see later in this chapter).

Chest leads

The limb leads provide information about the depolarization wavefront in a coronal (vertical) plane. The chest leads give us information about the wavefront in a skewed transverse plane which approximates to the base–apex axis of the heart. The surface electrodes are applied as shown in Figure 7.6 A and as described below.

V_1: 4th intercostal space right sternal edge
V_2: 4th intercostal space left sternal edge
V_3: directly halfway between V_2 and V_4
V_4: 5th left intercostal space mid-clavicular line
V_5: anterior axillary line directly lateral to V_4
V_6: mid-axillary line directly lateral to V_4.

The limb leads are 'combined' electronically to create a virtual electrode over the spine. Thus leads V_1 to V_6 record the movement of the depolarization wavefront from the virtual electrode out in the direction of each of the chest electrodes as shown in Figure 7.6B.

12 lead ECG

We now have a total of 12 leads (I, II, III, aVR, aVL, aVF and V_{1-6}) derived from 10 electrodes. This is the standard ECG printout, an example of which is shown in Figure 7.7. Though more leads and different arrangements of presentation are possible this is the commonest form in which the ECG is presented. Note, the 'V' leads as described here may sometimes be shown as 'C' leads on a printout (see Figure 7.7).

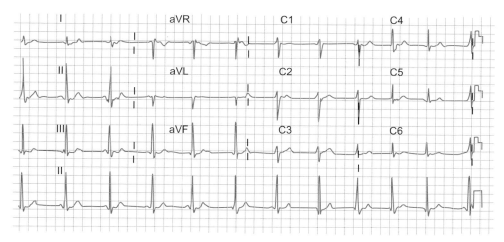

Fig. 7.7 Standard 12-lead ECG.

The components of the ECG trace

A schematic ECG waveform recorded in lead II is shown in Figure 7.8. The standard nomenclature, P, QRS, T and U waves is arcane. Originally waveforms were labelled A, B, C and D. As the equipment developed the waveforms changed shape and needed new labels. It was decided to use the second half of the alphabet starting at O for the starting point of the recording. The next features were labelled P, Q, R, S and T respectively. The flat line which precedes the P wave is equivalent to 'O' but this labelling is not used.

The P wave represents atrial depolarization. It has a relatively low amplitude because of the low muscle mass of the atrial myocardium.

There is a variable gap between the end of the P wave and the start of the QRS complex, the P–R interval. This interval represents the time taken for the atrial depolarization to reach the ventricular myocardium (see Chapter 2). It is a period of apparent inactivity but it in fact mainly represents the time needed for depolarization of the atrioventricular node (AV node) and the bundle of His. Since only a small amount of cardiac tissue is involved and this is surrounded by other, inactive, ventricular myocardium it does not produce a measurable deflection. However this region is extremely important as many clinically significant pathologies, such as heart block, have their origins in this region of the heart and cause characteristic changes in this part of the ECG.

It is crucial to remember that one of the major functions of the AV node is to control the rate of transmission of atrial impulses to the ventricles. It can only do this if there is complete insulation of the ventricles from the atria. This is achieved because the atrioventricular valve root tissue, of which the atrioventricular junction is composed, is fibrous and electrically inactive. It thus produces a natural barrier to the passage of electrical activity from the atria to the ventricles. The weakness of this control mechanism is that the heart is vulnerable to

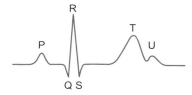

Fig. 7.8 Elements of the ECG waveform.

significant functional impairment if the AV node is compromised (see discussion of heart block below) or if there are breaks in this insulation (see discussion of Wolff–Parkinson–White syndrome below).

The QRS complex reflects the stages of mass ventricular depolarization. The initial deflection is produced by the posterior–anterior depolarization of the interventricular septum. In the normal heart the next stage is the depolarization of the bulk of the left ventricular apex and free wall. The final portion of the QRS complex is produced by the depolarization of the right ventricular free wall. The width of the QRS complex reflects the rate at which the wave of depolarization travels through the ventricles. This is largely determined by the Purkinje fibres of the specialized conducting system (see Chapter 2) which act as rapid distributors of the wave of depolarization through the myocardium.

The precise pattern of the QRS complex varies between individuals but most importantly it depends on the ECG lead being examined. For example leads V_1 and V_6 examine the heart from almost opposite directions and so usually approximate to an inverted image of each other, ventricular depolarization being dominantly negative in V_1 and positive in V_6.

During the QRS phase atrial re-polarization occurs. This is a diffuse process which lacks sufficient coherence to develop a significant waveform and is usually 'drowned out' by the QRS complex.

A further 'quiet' phase occurs: the ST segment. This phase represents the period when all of the ventricular muscle has been depolarized and myocardial contraction occurs. Myocardial contraction is not complete until the end of the T wave which represents the phase of ventricular repolarization.

Interesting facts

The Dutch physiologist Einthoven started transmitting electrocardiograms in 1905 from the hospital to his laboratory 1.5 km away via telephone cables. On March 22nd the first 'telecardiogram' was recorded from a healthy and vigorous man and the tall R waves were attributed to his cycling from laboratory to hospital for the recording.

The T wave

Why is the T wave generally an upwards deflection if it represents repolarization? Since this is the opposite process to depolarization we might expect the T wave to be a downwards deflection if repolarization spreads in the same direction as depolarization. However the wave of depolarization is distributed by specialized conducting tissues (Purkinje fibres) which have the characteristic of rapid conduction. Repolarization is not a process which can be transmitted from cell to cell but is determined by the innate electrical characteristics of the individual cells. This has the effect that the wavefront of repolarization tends to be more diffuse and travels broadly in the opposite direction to the wave of depolarization. A wavefront of the opposite polarity travelling in the opposite direction gives a deflection in the same direction on the ECG recording. The T wave is broader than the QRS complex because the process of repolarization is more diffuse and travels less rapidly.

Other elements of the ECG

U waves represent late depolarizations of the myocardium. They are often not visible on a normal trace but where they do occur they are normal features provided they are small. However they are also associated with some pathological states such as digoxin toxicity and hypokalaemia.

Practical use of the ECG

As has been discussed the ECG tracing reflects the movement of depolarization through the myocardium. By understanding the origin of its component parts we can infer a great deal of information about the structure and function of the underlying heart. The ECG is an extremely useful tool because it is quick and easy to produce at the bedside and is non-invasive.

The standard ECG is produced with a paper speed of 25 mm/s—thus each small 1 mm square corresponds to 0.04 s.

Heart rate

For the purpose of examining rate and rhythm the standard 12 lead ECG is printed with a particularly long recording of lead II (Fig. 7.7) which is referred to as the rhythm strip. Lead II is usually selected because it is one of the leads which gives particularly clear representations of the P wave. V_1 may be used for the same reason.

The heart rate may be determined by measuring the distance between R waves in successive complexes. By multiplying the distance in millimetres by 0.04 we obtain the number of seconds between complexes which may then be divided into 60 to give the number of complexes in a minute. A simpler method is to bear in mind that if there is one large square on the ECG paper between each QRS complex this is equivalent to a rate of 300 beats per minute (bpm). By dividing 300 by the number of large squares between R waves we may obtain the rate in bpm directly. A typical resting heart rate of 75 bpm would give four large squares (20 mm) between QRS complexes.

Heart rate may vary considerably from beat to beat (beat-to-beat variation). This may result from normal physiological variation or irregularity. Cardiac monitors will usually display the heart rate in bpm averaged over a number of beats. The wise, but busy, clinician will take a pulse for at least 15 s to avoid wrongly estimating the minute rate; standard textbook teaching is to count the pulse for a whole minute. The more irregular the pulse the longer it must be recorded to achieve a representative average.

Rhythm

Rhythm, as opposed to rate, is an analysis of the regularity of heart activity. The normal state of the heart is sinus rhythm, which is usually regular although the rate may vary by a factor of four even in a healthy individual. Trained athletes may have resting heart rates in the region of 40 bpm but achieve maximum heart rates of around 180 bpm depending on physiological demand and age. The criteria used to define sinus rhythm are as follows:

- single P wave precedes every QRS complex
- P–R interval is constant and within normal range for duration
- P wave axis is normal
- P–P interval is constant.

In some individuals a marked sensitivity of the sinus node to vagal tone produces a regular variation in heart rate with respiration. The heart rate increases on inspiration. This is known as sinus arrhythmia and is illustrated in Figure 7.9. It is more common in children and tends to disappear as they get older.

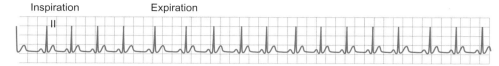

Fig. 7.9 Sinus arrhythmia. (Source:Adapted from Hampton JR, 2008.)

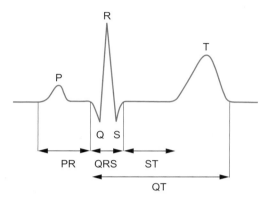

Fig. 7.10 ECG intervals.

Table 7.2	Normal ranges for ECG intervals and some pathologies	
Interval	*Normal range (msec)*	*Pathologies*
P–R	120–200	Short; Wolff–Parkinson–White
		Long; heart block (drugs, electrolytes, ischaemia)
QRS	80–120	Long; conduction abnormalities, e.g. bundle branch block, ventricular ectopics
QT$_c$	<440	Long; repolarization anomalies/ ion channelopathies, e.g., long QT syndromes

$$QTc = QT/\sqrt{RR}$$

Normal intervals on the ECG

The definition and normal ranges for various ECG intervals are shown in Figure 7.10 and Table 7.2. Most pathologies increase the length of intervals by damaging the conduction tissue. For example surgery on the right ventricle may damage the Purkinje fibres which distribute electrical activity throughout the right ventricle. This leads to delayed depolarization of the right ventricle when compared with the left ventricle. The QRS complex is slurred, with particular broadening of the latter part of the complex.

Axis

We have discussed the speed (rate) and coordination (rhythm) of electrical activity shown by the ECG. We now come to how the ECG can be used to identify the direction of travel of the wavefront of depolarization through the heart. Figure 7.2 shows how the orientation of the wavefront of depolarization with respect to the electrodes gives a different signal depending on the lead examined. Of course the heart is not a simple block of tissue but a complex tubular structure. However we can use the basic principle of Figure 7.2 to derive the following rules which allow us to define the direction of travel of depolarization;

- deflections are greatest and positive in the leads falling along the line of travel

- deflections are minimal in leads at right angles (orthogonal) to the line of travel

- the greater the amount of tissue involved the greater the deflection.

Case 7.1 — The electrocardiogram: 2

Colin's ECG changes

In Colin's case he develops chest pain and ST segment depression in the lateral leads. The ST segment depression actually represents a failure of the TP segment to return to the isoelectric state because the underlying portion of myocardium is unable to achieve full repolarization under conditions of ischaemia. ST segment depression of over 2 mm is considered significant.

As a simple rule of thumb the leads nearest the area of ischaemic change are most affected and so indicate the underlying affected myocardium. In this case the changes are likely to reflect underperfusion of the apex and posterior wall of the left ventricle. The left ventricle is the dominant oxygen consumer of the heart and stenosis in either of the coronary systems may induce ischaemia in portions of the left ventricle, particularly under circumstances of increased demand. The more proximal the stenoses the greater the volume of myocardium affected.

Thus by examining the deflection in various leads it is possible to identify the depolarization vector, a concept which tells us in what direction the wavefront is travelling, and to some extent the amount of tissue involved.

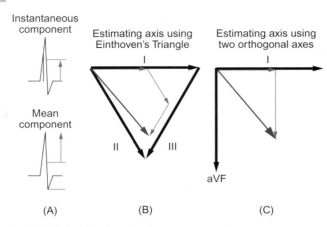

Fig. 7.11 Estimating the axis—instantaneous and mean.

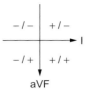

Fig. 7.12 Establishing the approximate axis—which quadrant?

There are two main forms of the depolarization vector: instantaneous and average or mean. The difference between these two is shown in Figure 7.11A. The instantaneous vector involves measurements taken at a single point in time. From the shape of the QRS complex it can be inferred that this vector varies with the cardiac cycle. The mean vector is derived from the average deflection in a lead. Thus the mean vector gives an average over the whole of the cardiac cycle.

Measuring the axis: Einthoven's triangle

In Einthoven's original work he used the geometry of the limb leads to construct an equilateral triangle (Fig. 7.11B). To estimate the axis of any part of the ECG we must measure the deflection in a given lead and by adding these components together in line with their respective leads we generate a vector which represents the direction of depolarization (Fig. 7.11B). By using the limb leads we assess the vertical (frontal) plane vector.

Einthoven's triangle has confused and intimidated many generations of students. However the concept is similar to that of vectors in mathematics. A vector in any two-dimensional plane may be described by the sum of its orthogonal components (Fig. 7.11C). The fact that the three limb leads describe a triangle makes the summation more difficult. In practice the same result can be obtained from two leads at right angles. Since the three basic limb leads are not orthogonal we must use the augmented limb leads.

To identify the depolarization vector it is only necessary to use one orthogonal pair. The simplest are I and aVF as these lie parallel to what would be natural axes for any two-dimensional plane. However it is crucial to remember that aVF points down (towards the feet) and so the frontal plane vector is positive in aVF when pointing down.

The normal range for the mean frontal QRS vector is −30° to +90° in the adult. In children the normal range is taken to be 0° to +180°. The variation in childhood is discussed in Chapter 12 but reflects the greater right ventricle workload before birth. Postnatally the left ventricle

comes to dominate the right and so the axis swings from right to left.

At a more practical level we can identify four quadrants into which the mean frontal plane vector will fall by assessing leads I and aVF (Fig. 7.12). The net deflection in each lead is estimated as positive (upward) or negative (downward).

The +/+ quadrant is within the normal range for all ages. The −/+ quadrant is normal for children but unusual for adults. The +/− quadrant is common in adults but very unusual in children and −/− is rare at any age though may be normal in children. More simply a −ve vector in lead aVF is generally pathological unless there is evidence to the contrary.

The concept of an axis can be applied separately to all parts of the ECG waveform; P wave, QRS complex and T wave. The P wave axis is frequently overlooked in the routine ECG analysis; however, it is a useful check on the function of the sinoatrial (SA) node. Since this is at the top right hand side of the heart a sinus P wave should spread to the left and down giving a P wave which is positive in leads I and II. Occasionally a second atrial focus may take over, particularly from the region of the coronary sinus (called a low atrial rhythm). Since this lies in the floor of the right atrium the P wave tends to be inverted in leads I and II. Retrograde P waves may occur in a variety of abnormal rhythms in which electrical activity is driven from 'below' the atria, e.g., 'nodal' rhythm with increased AV node automaticity or ventricular tachycardia. So long as retrograde conduction is possible the fastest initiator will drive the atrial rate. However, P waves may be difficult to discern.

The T wave axis is seldom assessed formally. However T wave inversion is a well-recognized sign of ischaemic heart disease. This is equivalent to displacement of the T wave axis from its normal alignment with the QRS axis.

The ECG and rhythm disturbances

The origin of arrhythmias

In order to understand the theoretical basis of arrhythmias it is useful to consider the prerequisites of sustaining abnormal electrical activity. Fundamental is the need to have electrically receptive tissues in which the wavefront of depolarization may propagate. Physical factors such as size and shape combine with electrical factors such as speed of propagation, refractory period and rate of spontaneous depolarization (automaticity). Structural anomalies including ischaemic damage, surgical scars, physiological state, metabolic changes, drugs and genetic variations all contribute separately and together to produce abnormal patterns of electrical activity.

A detailed discussion of arrhythmias is beyond the scope of this text. However we will cover some common examples.

Basic, clinical, analysis of arrhythmias can be commenced with decisions on the following parameters:

- rate above (tachycardia) or below (bradycardia) the expected rate for circumstances and age

- regular or irregular rhythm

- narrow or broad QRS complex (broad complex implies ventricular distribution is not via the normal conducting system)

- relation to P waves.

Atrial fibrillation

Using the criteria outlined above atrial fibrillation is associated with:

- tachycardia (usually)
- irregular rhythm
- narrow QRS complex
- no P wave.

Atrial fibrillation (AF) is the single most common rhythm disturbance. The word fibrillation is derived from the Latin for fibre or thread. The term fibrillation is descriptive of the macroscopic appearance of the atrial wall which appears to ripple like a bag of worms or threads. This common abnormal rhythm is associated with increasing age, ischaemic heart disease, mitral valve disease and hyperthyroidism. The underlying electrical activity of the atrium is completely chaotic with multiple independent foci of depolarization.

The typical 'irregularly irregular' peripheral pulse occurs because the wavefronts that activate the AV node arrive in a chaotic pattern. Further variation in the peripheral pulse occurs because premature ventricular contractions take place before ventricular filling is complete. This leads to ventricular contractions with differing ejection volumes and an associated variation in the pulse at the wrist. This is identified by auscultating at the apex and counting audible beats whilst feeling the peripheral pulse; the difference between the counted beats and the palpated pulsations is termed the apical–radial deficit.

On the ECG the characteristic pattern is a complete absence of atrial activity with no P waves identifiable in any leads combined with random ventricular activity with no beat-to-beat consistency in the R–R interval complexes.

Atrial fibrillation is not usually acutely dangerous as the refractory period of the AV node reduces the ventricular rate to below 150 bpm. Treatment with digoxin increases the AV node refractory period and thus reduces the ventricular rate but does not promote sinus rhythm. Individuals with accessory pathways (see Wolff–Parkinson–White syndrome) may die suddenly from AF as the accessory pathway has only a short refractory period and therefore may allow very high ventricular rates.

Atrial flutter

Using the criteria outlined above atrial flutter is associated with:

- tachycardia though heart rate may be normal if there is a high degree of atrioventricular block
- regular rhythm
- narrow QRS complex
- P waves usually triangular, two or three per QRS complex.

In SA node coordinated atrial depolarization the depolarization wavefront spreads out through the right and left atria and reaches the AV node leaving the atrial tissue in a refractory state. As the wavefront passes through the AV node the atrial tissue repolarizes and becomes excitable again. Usually this period of time is such that all atrial activity has ceased before the atrial myocardium is sensitized again. In atrial flutter a combination of abnormal atrial refractory period, or structural abnormality such as distension, alters the timescale in which atrial depolarization and repolarization are completed. Either a persistent wavefront travelling over an extended atrial surface returns to a point which has already become repolarized or an ectopic depolarization occurs in an atrial myocardium whose automaticity is abnormally high. The resulting wavefront may travel in a circular motion around the atrial wall, classically around the orifice of the tricuspid valve. The timescale allows the original tissue to repolarize and the wavefront becomes self-sustaining. This is called circus activity. In order to terminate the re-entrant circuit it is necessary to change the electrical characteristics of the atrial myocardium with anti-arrhythmic medication or use direct current cardioversion (electric shock) to abolish the circus activity and allow normal sinus activity to return. This may only be temporary.

Atrio-ventricular (AV) tachycardia

Using the criteria outlined above AV tachycardias, frequently called supraventricular tachycardias, are associated with:

- rate typically 140–230, lower with increasing age
- regular rhythm
- narrow QRS complex
- P waves usually not obvious—may be after the QRS complex and inverted (retrograde).

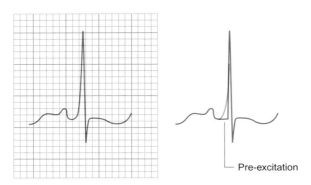

— Pre-excitation

Fig. 7.13 Origin of the Δ wave in Wolff–Parkinson–White syndrome. Myocardial bridging of the AV junction allows pre-excitation (pale line) to activate ventricular myocardium ahead of depolarization through the AV node (dark line). (Source: Adapted from Hampton JR, 2008.)

AV tachycardia is the name given to a group of arrhythmias whose origin lies above the proximal bundle of His. They are characterized by regular tachycardia, usually around 200 bpm, falling slightly with age, with a narrow QRS complex with similar characteristics to the normal ECG. These arrhythmias arise in the AV node itself or in the atrioventricular junction and are usually transmitted to the ventricles via the normal conducting tissue, hence their normal or near normal QRS complexes. The common substrate for this type of arrhythmia is a second pathway between atrium and ventricle. This may occur at the macroscopic or microscopic level.

An example of the macroscopic type of accessory pathway is the Wolff–Parkinson–White syndrome (WPW syndrome). In WPW there is myocardial bridging of the ring of fibrous tissue which acts as an insulator at the atrioventricular junction (see Chapter 2). In sinus rhythm the ECG typically shows a short P–R interval with slurring and broadening of the initial part of the QRS complex (so called Δ wave); an example is shown in Figure 7.13. In sinus rhythm the atrial depolarization is conducted to the ventricular myocardium via the normal AV nodal route but also, simultaneously, over the accessory pathway. The apparent shortening of the P–R interval occurs because the AV node slows conduction to the ventricles as normal but the accessory pathway conducts relatively rapidly initiating ventricular depolarization early with respect to the normal conducting system. Whilst the AV node is conducting it produces no obvious deflection on the ECG but the prematurely activated myocardium does. This premature activation spreads slowly through the ventricular myocardium producing the initial slurred portion of the QRS complex. However after the normal P–R interval, activation of the ventricles occurs as usual via the conducting system. Because this normal activation is distributed rapidly throughout the conducting system it overtakes the early activation of the ventricle and so 'normalizes' the QRS pattern. This is a good illustration of how the ECG may reflect simultaneous but separate events and how interpreting the ECG in the light of multiple processes aids understanding of the underlying electrical activity.

A further group of arrhythmias are the broad complex tachycardias. The broadening of the QRS complexes implies delayed conduction through the ventricular myocardium.

Ventricular fibrillation

Using the criteria outlined above ventricular fibrillation is associated with:

- tachycardia
- irregular rhythm
- broad QRS complex
- no P waves.

Similar to atrial fibrillation but applying to the ventricles, ventricular fibrillation (VF) is not consistent with an adequate cardiac output. VF is a common terminal event for many cardiac insults including ischaemic cardiac damage, electrolyte disturbances and toxins. Prompt therapy, particularly with external DC shock is essential. Even with good cardiopulmonary resuscitation prolonged VF rapidly becomes refractory due to deteriorating metabolic conditions.

> ### Interesting facts
>
> Thomas Lewis of University College Hospital, London bought a string galvanometer (invented by Einthoven) in 1909. He published a paper detailing his careful clinical and electrocardiographic observations of atrial fibrillation. Lewis identified a fibrillating horse using the string galvanometer's electrocardiogram recording. He then followed the horse to the slaughterhouse where he could visually confirm the fibrillating atrium.

Abnormalities of conduction

Abnormalities of conduction, as opposed to rhythm, apply to pathologies of the special conducting system of the heart and include heart block and bundle branch block. The term heart block refers to conditions in which the pattern of conduction through the heart is abnormal. Heart block can be divided into two major groups; pathologies affecting the AV node and proximal bundle of His (first, second and third degree heart blocks) and pathologies affecting the distributive conducting systems (intraventricular conduction disturbance, e.g. right and left bundle branch blocks). These topics are well covered in standard texts on the clinical interpretation of the ECG and have been referred to in Chapter 2. Here we shall confine ourselves to a brief overview.

Atrioventricular conduction disturbance

First degree heart block is present when the P–R interval is greater than the normal range (Table 7.2). Since conduction through the atrium is only rarely significantly prolonged an increase in the P–R interval is usually attributable to a delay in conduction through the AV node. This is occasionally found in asymptomatic individuals with normal hearts and is not of clinical significance. However some drugs such as verapamil slow AV nodal conduction and may cause first degree block.

Second degree heart block occurs in two types. Mobitz type I is also known as the Wenckebach phenomenon in which the P–R interval increases steadily over a number of beats until a P wave occurs without being followed by a QRS complex. Again the significance of this finding is determined very much by the clinical context. Mobitz type II second degree block occurs when there are more P waves than QRS complexes but the relationship between P wave and QRS complex is fixed. The degree of block is described by the ratio of the number of P waves to each QRS complex, for example 2:1 block or 3:1 block.

Third degree or complete heart block occurs when there is no relationship between the atrial and ventricular rates. Third degree block only occurs where there is loss of conduction through the AV node or proximal bundle of His and usually reflects significant damage to the conducting system which is either iatrogenic (e.g. surgical) or pathological (e.g. infarction or infection). It is possible to recover from transient third degree heart block but frequently the individual is at risk of late recurrence, particularly if there is an associated bundle branch block. In complete heart block the ventricular rate is determined by the intrinsic rate of the ventricular muscle (see Chapter 2). In most cases the ventricular rate (30–40 bpm) is insufficient to maintain an adequate cardiac output. In this case emergency pacing is required until a permanent pacing system can be implanted. Emergency pacing may be achieved either using external pads on the chest or by placing a pacing wire into the right ventricle via the subclavian, femoral or jugular vein. Permanent pacing is achieved using a battery-powered generator connected to leads which activate the right atrium and right ventricle in synchrony. Modern pacing systems are extremely sophisticated and may even involve pacing both ventricles separately.

In congenital complete heart block the damage to the AV node occurs in utero. This is associated with a wide spectrum of outcomes from fetal death due to hydrops fetalis (fetal cardiac failure) to asymptomatic individuals who may manage many years without artificial pacing.

The term AV dissociation is frequently used as if it is synonymous with complete heart block. This term describes the condition in which there is no consistent relationship between P waves and QRS complexes. However, though the term AV dissociation includes complete heart block it also applies to conditions in which AV node conduction is intact. The crucial distinction with complete heart block is that AV dissociation occurs when the ventricular rate is greater than the atrial rate, but usually only slightly faster. This may be identified by measuring the P–P and R–R intervals and comparing them. This usually happens when damage has occurred to the sinoatrial node reducing its inherent rate. The AV node or bundle of His take over as the pacemaker and generate QRS complexes which are of normal width and morphology. The atrial rate is stable but slower than the ventricular rate.

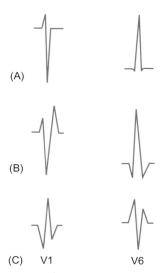

Fig. 7.14 Bundle branch block patterns. (A) Normal. (B) Right bundle branch block. (C) Left bundle branch block.

Intraventricular conduction disturbances

The width of the QRS complex is largely determined by the time taken to distribute the wavefront of depolarization through the ventricular myocardium. The structure of the conducting system is discussed in Chapter 2. The bundle of His gives rise to left and right branches which supply the left and right ventricles respectively. These fibres follow the inner surface of their respective ventricle and so normal depolarization takes place from inside (endocardium) to outside (epicardium). The earliest ventricular myocardial activation occurs in the interventricular septum and is dominantly from left ventricle to right, producing a positive deflection in V_1 on the standard adult ECG. The depolarization of the left ventricular muscle mass proceeds next leading to a negative deflection in V_1 and positive deflection in V_6. Finally the anterior free wall of the right ventricle depolarizes producing a positive deflection in V_1 and negative deflection in V_6. When conduction is normal elements may be fused to give a single deflection which is dominated by the left ventricular components producing only a large negative deflection in V_1 and positive deflection in V_6. Figure 7.14A shows schematic patterns from V_1 and V_6.

Where damage occurs to the conducting system the distribution of activity through the ventricle is slowed and the different elements may become more obvious. The QRS complex also becomes wider as distribution throughout the ventricles takes longer.

One example of damage to the conducting system is the result of surgery on the right ventricle. Frequently this may damage the right bundle branch and leads to a typical pattern in the chest leads. Since the initial postero-anterior depolarization of the septum is enhanced the initial deflection in V_1 is positive, followed by a negative deflection arising from the depolarization of the left ventricle. However the right ventricular depolarization is

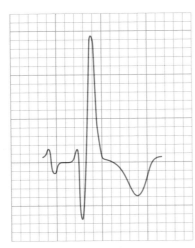

Fig. 7.15 Right bundle branch block pattern in V_1.

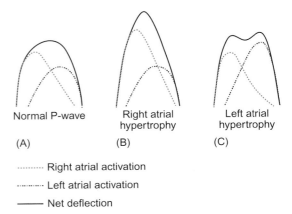

Fig. 7.16 Interaction of right and left atrial waveforms. (A) Normal P wave. (B) Right atrial hypertrophy. (C) Left atrial hypertrophy.

delayed and so the complex is typically completed with a slurred positive deflection. This typical positive, negative, positive pattern (RSr') in V_1 occurs with a complementary negative, positive, negative (QRS) in V_6 (Fig. 7.14B). This pattern is called right bundle branch block. It is important to note that the QRS complex is wider than normal, being especially broad in the latter part of the deflection. Partial right bundle branch block is a normal childhood variant in which the RSr' pattern occurs without broadening of the QRS width. A typical ECG recording from V_1 is shown in Figure 7.15.

Damage to the anterior or posterior fascicles of the left bundle branches also gives typical ECG patterns. These are commonly seen after infarction of the respective portions of the left ventricle. Theoretically the left bundle branch is a more diffuse system consisting of multiple fibres. These have been simplified to anterior and posterior fascicles. If the left bundle is interrupted early in its course then several predictable results occur. The first is that the normal postero-anterior depolarization of the septum is reversed; followed by depolarization of the right ventricle giving a QR pattern in the anterior chest leads with a mirror image in the lateral leads (Fig. 7.14C). The late depolarization of the left ventricle gives a large terminal negative deflection in the anterior leads. This results in a broad QRS pattern in V_1 with an RSr' in V_6.

Though bundle branch block may have little functional significance there are two key points to remember. Firstly, in general it is impossible to interpret the ECG in terms of acute ischaemic changes in the presence of bundle branch block. Secondly, very long prolongation of the QRS complex after surgery is associated with a significant risk of late fatal ventricular arrhythmias.

Cardiac structure and the ECG

The pattern of ECG complexes provides a variety of information about the structure of the heart. Right atrial hypertrophy is associated with tall, peaked P waves with an amplitude of more than 5 mm with standard ECG settings. Left atrial hypertrophy is characterized by a twin-peaked P wave known as P mitrale because this is most commonly associated with mitral stenosis.

Why is there this difference in the form of the P wave with hypertrophy of the different atria? This comes back to a complete understanding of the interaction between time and space which produces the ECG. Right atrial depolarization precedes left atrial depolarization because the sinus node lies in the right atrium. The right atrium is nearer the front of the chest and so, particularly in the anterior chest leads, produces a dominant deflection. Since the periods of depolarization overlap the P wave takes on a single hump, though in fact there are two separate events within it. If one or other waveform is changed the overall waveform is altered; if the right atrium is hypertrophied then the whole waveform becomes more peaked; if the left atrium is hypertrophied then the left atrial component of the P wave becomes more apparent and generates a second peak in the P wave, slightly later than that of the right atrial waveform. This is illustrated in Figure 7.16. This variation in P wave morphology emphasizes the complex interaction between cardiac morphology and function and the simplified tracing produced in the standard ECG.

As has been alluded to previously this summation of signals from different parts of the heart is important because it affects the way the ECG waveform appears and also how it changes in pathological conditions. For example, in the adult the QRS complex is dominated by the signals from the left ventricle which is much greater in mass than the right ventricle. In newborn babies this is not the case, with the right ventricle having similar mass to the left ventricle. Thus the complexes in the anterior chest leads (V_1, V_2) are very different in newborns and adults; in newborns they are dominantly positive whilst in adults they are dominantly negative (see Chapter 12). The right ventricle may be virtually ignored in interpreting the normal adult ECG.

Since the amplitude of ECG waveforms is affected by many factors, muscle mass, posture, lung volume, etc., interpreting ECG amplitudes in terms of underlying pathology is difficult. Hypertrophy of the left ventricle will tend to give increased amplitude of the S wave in V_1 and the R wave in V_6. This is essentially the same signal seen from the opposite direction. This may be increased in patients with severe hypertension or aortic stenosis where the workload of the left ventricle is significantly increased. Hypertrophic cardiomyopathy will also increase the amplitude of these voltages. The mean frontal QRS vector may also be skewed to the left by the excess signal from the left ventricle, though it is unusual for it to fall outside the normal range.

Interesting facts

In 1906, Einthoven published the first organized presentation of normal and abnormal electrocardiograms recorded with a string galvanometer. Left and right ventricular hypertrophy, left and right atrial hypertrophy, the U wave (for the first time), notching of the QRS, ventricular premature beats, ventricular bigeminy, atrial flutter and complete heart block were all described.

Ischaemia and the ECG

One of the common uses of the ECG is in acute assessment of chest pain. This may be caused by the restriction of blood flow to the myocardium, either reversible—angina pectoris—or irreversible—myocardial infarction. These two conditions produce rather different changes in the ECG which can be understood by considering the underlying processes.

Reversible ischaemia

Returning to the concept of the battery (see p. 72) the degree of deflection of the ECG signal is a function of the potential difference between the ends of the battery and the orientation of the battery with respect to the electrodes. Generally the maximum potential difference occurs when one end of the battery is fully depolarized ($+30\,mV$) and the other is fully polarized ($-85\,mV$) giving a total voltage of around $115\,mV$. If both ends of the battery are depolarized or both ends are polarized then there will be no potential difference and no net deflection. This is the condition which gives the isoelectric line on the ECG, i.e. zero displacement of the trace. Between the T and the Q wave the ventricular muscle cells are polarized. During the ST segment the ventricle is depolarized. The heart is in different states of polarization but the appearance of the ECG, a flat line, is the same.

During ischaemia, maintenance of the myocardium in its fully polarized state is compromised as it requires substantial ATP generation to maintain ionic gradients (see Chapter 1). Thus for portions of the myocardium the

Case 7.1 The electrocardiogram: 3

Unwelcome developments

Colin subsequently suffered a myocardial infarction (Chapter 5, Case 5.1:3). What are the specific ECG changes which are associated with myocardial infarction and how do they progress over time?

Initially downward curving ST segment elevation reflecting an area of myocardium that is no longer electrically active. T wave inversion occurs next. This may be seen as a deviation of the T wave axis away from tissue which no longer takes part in the repolarization process.

The appearance of Q waves is the last change which takes place in the ECG and is the change which remains longest. Q waves reflect the complete loss of myocardium in one portion of the left ventricle wall resulting in a signal being recorded which is actually from the opposite wall of the ventricle. Q waves greater than $3\,mm$ are likely to be pathological. Q waves are frequently permanent as the myocardial tissue, once killed, cannot regenerate.

resting potential is not as negative as normal. This means that in the fully polarized state there can be a current between different parts of the myocardium. However, because the depolarized state is less energy demanding, as entry of Na^+ and Ca^{++} ions are passive processes down concentration gradients, it is still possible for all myocardial cells to depolarize fully. The T–Q isoelectric line is displaced upwards by the residual flow of current between fully and partially polarized myocardium but during ventricular depolarization this is abolished. The ST segment alone therefore appears to be displaced.

Infarction

Complete loss of blood supply to the myocardium produces a typical sequence of changes. Initially there is ST segment elevation over the area which undergoes infarction. Some 24–48 hours later T wave inversion occurs along with the development of Q waves (deep negative deflections in the leads closest to the area of infarction). The specific leads involved give an indication of the location and extent of the injury.

Q waves may be understood in the context of complete loss of electrically active tissue. Since, for practical purposes, the right ventricle may be ignored in the adult because the muscle mass is swamped by that of the left ventricle the ECG can be viewed as examining the left ventricle from the outside. The conducting tissue is located on the endocardial surface of the left ventricle and thus depolarization takes place from inside to outside (Fig. 7.17). Where a portion of the ventricle is damaged and becomes fibrosed, i.e. electrically inert then it becomes electrically 'transparent' forming an electrical 'window'. Thus rather than producing a positive deflection as the

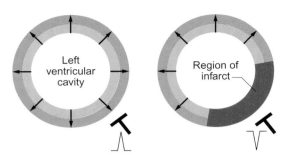

Fig. 7.17 Origin of Q waves on the ECG.

near wall of the ventricle depolarizes from inside to out-side, a negative deflection is produced as the lead records the activity in the opposite wall of the ventricle.

The change in the T wave reflects the overall change in the pattern of repolarization. This may be seen as a devi-ation of the T wave axis away from the region of infarc-tion which now has a lower muscle mass analogous to the swing of the QRS axis towards areas of greater mus-cle mass.

Interesting facts

Cremer (1906) recorded the first oesophageal electrocar-diogram which he achieved with the help of a profes-sional sword swallower. Oesophageal electrocardiography later developed in the 1970s to help differentiate atrial arrhythmias. He also recorded the first fetal electrocardio-gram from the abdominal surface of a pregnant woman.

Potassium and the ECG

Considering that potassium fluxes are so key to the mem-brane potential of myocardial cells (see Chapter 2), it is not surprising that the ECG may be altered by changes in plasma [K$^+$].

With hypokalaemia the dominant effect is flattening of the T wave and may include ST segment depression and the development of prominent U waves. ECG changes associated with hypokalaemia are not clinically significant nor do they have any particular prognostic significance. An ECG may be considered a useful adjunct but is no substitute for monitoring of plasma [K$^+$]. Hypokalaemia promotes the pro-arrhythmic effect of digoxin which acts to block the pumped inflow of K$^+$ in exchange for Na$^+$ (see Chapters 2 and 4).

As one might expect the effect of hyperkalaemia on the ECG is the opposite of hypokalaemia. The earliest feature is tall, peaked T waves. Higher levels of potassium pro-duce P wave flattening, P-R elongation and eventually slurring of the QRS complex may occur. At high concen-trations of potassium the differentiation of QRS and T wave may disappear as the ECG becomes sinusoidal in nature before sliding into ventricular fibrillation.

Case 7.1 — The electrocardiogram: 4

An overweight patient with hypertension

In Case 10.1:1 in Chapter 10 the case history of 45-year-old John Ames is described. During an insurance medical he is found to be both obese and hypertensive. How might these two factors affect his ECG?

Increasing body size tends to reduce ECG voltages, partic-ularly in the chest leads as they are most affected by dis-tance from the heart. Hyperinflation of the chest, such as occurs in emphysema, may also reduce chest lead voltages. Conversely slim people may have large voltages in the chest leads even with a normal heart.

Chronic hypertension increases the workload of the heart and leads to left ventricular hypertrophy. The increased muscle mass generates greater ECG deflections. Various cri-teria are used for diagnosing left ventricular hypertrophy. The simplest is that the sum of the S wave in V$_1$ and R wave in V$_6$ are >40 mm with standard gain settings.

ECG monitoring in hyperkalaemia is clinically useful and indeed essential. The first evidence of hyperkalaemia may be sudden and refractory ventricular fibrillation even if there is little in the way of symptoms. For this rea-son continuous ECG monitoring is mandatory during IV infusions of potassium salts.

Drugs and the ECG

All anti-arrhythmic drugs tend to promote arrhythmias as well as suppress them and should only be used where a net benefit to the patient can be identified. Some drugs such as flecainide and amiodarone may prolong the Q–T interval. Digoxin may prolong the P–R interval and causes bradycardia. Though frequently used to control ventricular rate in atrial fibrillation, digoxin tends to pro-mote atrial automaticity and may enhance or induce atrial fibrillation (see Chapter 2).

Further reading

Conover, M.B., 2003. Understanding Electrocardiography, eighth ed.. Mosby, St Louis.

Hampton, J.R., 2008. The ECG Made Easy, seventh ed. Churchill Livingstone, Edinburgh.

Houghton, A.R., Gray, D., 2008. Making Sense of the ECG, third ed. Arnold, London.

Lilly, L.S., 2006. Pathophysiology of Heart Disease, third ed. Williams and Wilkins, Baltimore.

Thaler, M.S., 2006. The only EKG Book You'll Ever Need, fifth ed. Lippincott/Williams & Wilkins, Philadelphia.

LARGE BLOOD VESSELS

8

Chapter objectives

After studying this chapter, you should be able to:

1. Describe the physical characteristics of blood flow in large blood vessels.

2. Identify the aspects of blood flow patterns which lead to turbulence, and therefore flow murmurs, in arterial vessels.

3. Explain the importance in relation to blood flow of the factors which determine the viscosity of blood.

4. Outline the fundamental aspects of atherosclerosis in arterial blood vessels including the contributing risk factors, the pathogenic mechanisms involved in the development of a plaque and the likely clinical consequences of atherosclerosis.

5. Summarize the age-related changes in blood vessel structure.

6. Outline the common pathological processes which can affect arterial and large venous blood vessels.

7. Identify the frequently used techniques for investigating peripheral vascular disease.

Case
8.1
Large blood vessels: 1

Calf pain made worse by exercise

Jamshed Patel is a 72-year-old man who has a long history of insulin-dependent diabetes mellitus (IDDM). This was mainly controlled by self-administered insulin but his doctor was aware that this treatment was not always rigorously adhered to. When he was younger he smoked a packet of cigarettes a day for about 30 years and he has been taking a beta-blocker, atenolol, and a diuretic to help control his high blood pressure for the past 20 years.

Two years ago Jamshed noticed that his right calf muscle became painful when he had walked about 800 metres. This pain subsided after a short rest and he was then able to continue walking albeit at a gentle stroll pace. The problem has gradually got worse and recently he has noticed that the pain was forcing him to rest after only about 200 metres. He countered this by adopting a more sedentary lifestyle and refusing to go shopping with his wife, much to her disgust. He is now also sometimes troubled by the calf pain when in bed and has noticed that there is some improvement in the pain if he hangs his leg out over the side of the bed.

Mrs Patel eventually persuaded her husband to visit his GP. On examining Jamshed's legs he found that there was hair loss on the right leg compared to the left. Although the femoral pulses were present for both legs the popliteal pulse was weaker on the right side than on the left. The dorsalis pedis and posterior tibial pulses were absent on the right foot but could be detected in the left. A loud bruit was heard over the femoral artery and the GP also noted that the right foot was a little swollen compared to the left and that there was a black area at the tip of two of Jamshed's toes. When questioned, Jamshed said that it was the result of him tripping over a brick whilst walking barefoot in his garden. He had not thought that this was any particular problem at the time but the toes had since become painful.

Jamshed was referred for further investigation to the vascular surgeons at the local hospital.

The following questions arise from considering this history:

1. Why is Jamshed a likely candidate for vascular disease?
2. What factors determine the blood flow characteristics in large blood vessels?
3. What does the history suggest in relation to the location of a possible vascular disorder?

Aspects of the answers to these questions are to be found in the text of this chapter.

Introduction

It is often assumed that the heart propels blood around the body but this is only true to a certain extent. When the heart goes into its refilling phase, diastole, and no more blood is entering the arterial tree, the peripheral circulation does not stop and the diastolic pressure does not fall to zero. Flow is maintained by the pressure in the large arteries which pushes blood through the small vessels. During systole, as the stroke volume of blood (about 70 mL in the resting 'textbook' person), enters the large arteries, the vessels are stretched. During diastole, the elastic recoil of the arteries helps to maintain arterial pressure and, hence, keep tissue perfusion going (see Chapter 1). The role of the heart, therefore, is to keep the arterial pressure reservoir 'topped up'.

An important functional characteristic of the cardiovascular system is that each part of the body needs to be provided with a blood flow which is appropriate to the metabolic and functional needs of that tissue. The driving force to perfuse tissues is provided by the pressure in the arteries (see Chapter 10). How much blood passes from the arterial system into the blood vessels serving a particular tissue will depend on the relative resistance to flow in the tissue. Thus, local dilatation of blood vessels will reduce resistance and increase flow, whereas constriction of vessels will increase resistance and decrease flow locally but will also serve to divert blood flow to other tissues. As this occurs throughout the microvasculature, we are provided with a precise and effective system for matching blood flow to metabolic demand. The factors regulating the microcirculation (resistance blood vessels) will be considered in Chapter 9.

In this chapter we will first consider the flow characteristics of blood as a fluid and then some of the characteristics of the large blood vessels. The common pathological changes affecting large arteries and veins will be reviewed. The case history of a man who is suffering the consequences of pathological changes in the arterial blood supply to his legs is summarized in Case 8.1:1.

Haemorheology: the physical characteristics of blood flow

It is relatively easy to describe fluid flow in simple terms by considering a homogeneous fluid flowing in a rigid tube. However, blood is not homogeneous as it consists of red and white cells suspended in plasma. Furthermore, large blood vessels are not rigid tubes—if the pressure inside them increases, they will be distended. An extensive discussion of these aspects of circulatory function is outside the scope of this book but the following fundamental points can be identified.

Blood flows down a pressure gradient

Blood, like any other fluid, will only flow from an area of relatively high pressure to somewhere where the pressure is lower. This is equivalent to pointing out that rivers only flow downhill and the water in a pond, with no outlet to a lower point, does not flow anywhere. Jamshed Patel (Case 8.1:1) has used this principle by putting his leg out of bed in order to try to increase blood flow.

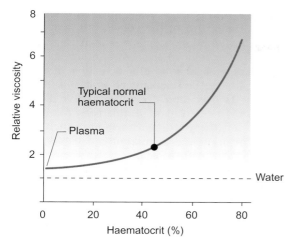

Fig. 8.1 Effect of haematocrit on the relative viscosity of blood. 'Relative' viscosity is compared to water = 1. The figure shown applies to a typical vascular bed which includes vessels of a mixture of different sizes but predominantly contains small vessels. Relative viscosity of blood is much higher when measured in a glass viscometer which has a wide bore tube (see Fig. 8.3).

Viscosity of blood

The viscosity of blood is mainly determined by the haematocrit, the percentage of blood volume which is occupied by the red blood cells. The viscosity of blood is frequently expressed as a relative viscosity, i.e. the viscosity compared to pure water taken as unity. On this basis, the relative viscosity of blood plasma, which contains protein but no red cells, is about 1.3. At a normal haematocrit, of the order of 45%, the relative viscosity of blood flowing through tissues is about 2.4 (Fig. 8.1). This assumes that the blood flow is fast enough to keep the red cells apart as, if blood flow is sluggish, the red cells tend to stick together. This is because the large plasma proteins (globulins and fibrinogen) form cross-bridges between slowly moving red cells. These bonds are disrupted in faster moving blood. Sometimes red cells pile up in a similar fashion to a pile of dinner plates and this is called rouleaux formation. Aggregation of red cells becomes an important factor increasing the resistance to blood flow in circulatory shock. It will tend to occur in the postcapillary blood vessels, the venules, when the velocity of flow is low. This may be part of the explanation for the swollen appearance (localized oedema) of Jamshed's foot (see Case 8.1:1). Blood flow may cease completely if the resistance is too high and this contributes to the localized tissue oedema which sometimes develops during circulatory shock (see Chapter 14).

Laminar and turbulent flow

Blood flow may be either laminar or turbulent. 'Laminar', otherwise known as 'streamline', fluid flow means that all the particles in the fluid are flowing parallel to the wall of the tube (Fig. 8.2). However, they are not all moving at the

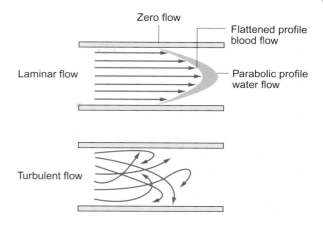

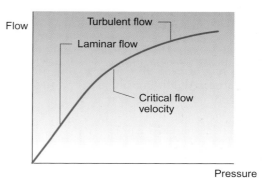

Fig. 8.2 Laminar and turbulent blood flow. When turbulent flow develops the relationship between flow and perfusion pressure changes (lower diagram).

same velocity. Those fluid particles in contact with the wall of the tube are theoretically stationary whilst those at the centre (axis) of the tube are flowing fastest (Fig. 8.2). The opposite of laminar flow is turbulent flow. In this case the fluid particles follow a much more irregular pathway and may develop vortices (whirlpools) in the blood vessel.

The conditions which result in the transition from laminar to turbulent flow were described mathematically by Osborne Reynolds in 1883. The essence of Reynolds' law is that turbulence is more likely to occur in large tubes than in small tubes. Turbulence is more likely when the velocity of flow is high and when the viscosity of the fluid is low. The blood flow velocity at which there is a transition from laminar to turbulent flow is called the 'critical velocity' (Fig. 8.2). Laminar flow is essentially silent but turbulent flow sets up vibrations in the blood vessel wall which can be heard using a stethoscope. Turbulent flow in the circulation produces the noises which are called murmurs.

As the viscosity of blood depends primarily on the haematocrit and a low viscosity makes the development of turbulence more likely, anaemic patients are more likely to have murmurs in their circulation than those with a normal haematocrit. A murmur caused in this way would disappear once the anaemia was corrected. An example of this is during pregnancy. Maternal haematocrit decreases in pregnancy because the plasma volume expands by more than the red cell volume. Flow murmurs are therefore more likely to be heard in pregnant women and may cause temporary alarm, but they normally disappear when the baby is delivered and haematocrit returns to normal. We also use the development of artificially induced flow murmurs, produced by compressing an artery with a sphygmomanometer cuff so that flow velocity increases as the basis for non-invasive measurement of arterial blood pressure (see Chapter 10).

> ### Interesting facts
>
> In 1905 the Russian army surgeon Nicolai Korotkoff described the auscultatory method for measuring blood pressure. The turbulence noises produced using an inflatable cuff to partially occlude an artery are still referred to as Korotkoff sounds. The auscultatory method allowed the measurement of diastolic pressure for the first time.

Within the normal circulation, blood flow can be thought of as approximating to a laminar flow pattern in most large vessels. The site where turbulence is most likely to occur in a normal person is in the first segment of the aorta because here the velocity of flow is high in a relatively large tube. During exercise, when the cardiac output, and therefore the velocity of flow, increases, turbulence will extend further down the aorta than at rest. Local changes in blood flow dynamics leading to turbulence are contributory factors in determining the location of endothelial cell damage which is a precursor to the development of atherosclerotic plaques in the circulation (see p. 91). Thrombus formation is more likely when blood flow is slow and there is no turbulence, i.e. in the veins.

In Jamshed's case (see Case 8.1:1) a loud bruit (flow murmur produced by turbulent blood flow) was heard over the femoral artery. The probable explanation is that a narrowing of the vessel led to locally increased blood flow velocity through the constriction and hence the development of turbulence on the downstream side.

Relationship between blood vessel radius and blood flow

Where there is laminar flow, the flow rate is proportional to the fourth power of the radius of the blood vessel. Strictly, this relationship only applies to an ideal (Newtonian) fluid. Blood is anomalous, because it is not a homogeneous fluid, it has red cells suspended in it. Despite this, the fourth power relationship, as an approximation, provides a very useful concept for both physiological and pathological considerations. The relationship 'flow is proportional to radius[4]' was first derived by the French physician Poiseuille in 1846. To illustrate the effect of the relationship we can take a simple numerical example. If a blood vessel with a radius of 4 units is

dilated to a radius of 5 units, this represents a 25% increase in the radius of the vessel. But, if we consider the effects on blood flow, if $r = 4$ then $r^4 = 256$ and if $r = 5$ then $r^4 = 625$. A 25% increase in size of the vessel would, therefore, lead to a 140% increase in blood flow.

The physiological consequence of the fourth power relationship is that small changes in the diameter of resistance blood vessels lead to relatively big changes in flow. Blood can, therefore, be diverted to match metabolic needs by constricting and dilating small blood vessels. These are known as the resistance vessels (see Chapter 9). In pathological terms, small changes in blood vessel diameter produced by, for example, atherosclerosis may result in large reductions in blood flow (see p. 90).

Narrowing of the femoral artery and hence reduction of blood flow has limited the delivery of blood to Jamshed's calf muscle (see Case 8.1:1), hence causing hypoxic pain in the muscle. This became worse during exercise because the increased oxygen demand could not be satisfied by an adequate increase in blood flow.

Red cell distribution over the cross-section of a blood vessel

'Axial accumulation' of red cells is a consequence of laminar blood flow. Red cells are dragged into the part of the blood vessel which has the fastest flow, i.e. down the middle of the blood vessel. The blood flowing slowly near the wall of the blood vessel, therefore, has a lower haematocrit than the fast flowing blood at the centre of the vessel. Small branches from a large vessel hence receive blood which has a lower haematocrit than the average for the large vessel. Because the viscosity of blood is dependent on the haematocrit, the relative viscosity of blood in small vessels will be lower than that in large vessels. Experimentally, this was shown to become significant in blood vessels with a diameter of 300 μm or less and is known as the Fåhraeus–Lindqvist effect (Fig. 8.3). It provides an explanation for the fact that the relative viscosity of blood flowing through a vascular bed (which has lots of small-diameter vessels) is

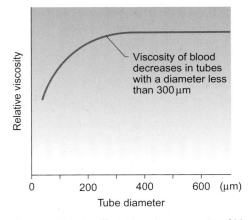

Fig. 8.3 Fåhraeus–Lindqvist effect. The relative viscosity of blood is lower in small blood vessels than in large vessels.

lower than the relative viscosity measured in a glass viscometer (which has a large tube diameter). A key point in understanding this complex phenomenon is to recognize that axial accumulation means that the red cells flow faster than the plasma in blood vessels.

Although blood does not behave as an ideal homogeneous fluid, the studies carried out by Poiseuille still provide us with a useful basis for understanding blood flow dynamics. However, Poiseuille's law does assume that the tube is rigid.

Capillary blood flow

The smallest blood vessels which have the thinnest walls behave effectively as rigid tubes. This, at first, may seem surprising. In very small blood vessels concepts such as laminar flow have little meaning as capillaries have a diameter in the range of 3–8 μm. Red blood cells have a diameter of about 8 μm which means that they are a very tight fit passing through many capillaries. Clearly, either the capillary or the red cell has to deform and it is, in fact, the red cell which changes shape (see Chapter 11). As red cells are such a tight fit in capillaries, there is a region of trapped plasma in between successive cells. This is referred to as bolus flow.

Elasticity of blood vessel walls

Large blood vessels are distensible. For a rigid (e.g. glass) tube with a laminar flow pattern, there would be a linear relationship between pressure gradient across the ends of the tube and flow down the tube (Fig. 8.4A). In a large blood vessel, Figure 8.4B shows that the relationship between flow and pressure gradient is different in two ways:

1. there is an intercept on the pressure axis (critical closing pressure)
2. there is a curvilinear relationship between driving pressure and flow.

The critical closing pressure means that there has to be a certain pressure inside the vessel in order to keep it inflated, i.e. if the pressure gradient across the wall of a blood vessel (transmural pressure) falls below a certain limiting value, then the vessel will collapse and flow will cease. Stimulation of sympathetic vasoconstrictor nerves to a blood vessel will increase the critical closing pressure and so a higher pressure will be needed inside the vessel in order to keep it open. This concept is important in understanding the shutdown of some blood vessels in circulatory shock. The fall in arterial blood pressure in shock leads, via the baroreceptor reflex, to sympathetically induced vasoconstriction in the arterioles (see Chapter 10). The pressure of blood in the vessels after this increased resistance will fall and, hence, there is a tendency for vessels to collapse (see Chapter 14).

The curvilinear relationship between blood pressure and flow (Figure 8.4B) is attributed to the fact that a blood vessel will be distended as the pressure inside it increases.

Blood flow will also therefore increase. The extent to which a blood vessel can be distended by increasing the internal pressure inside it will depend on the blood vessel size and wall structure. Figure 8.5 shows a comparison between an 'old' and a 'young' aorta and a vein. Firstly, it

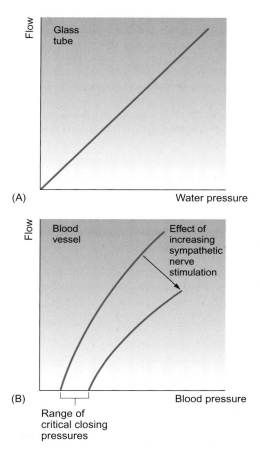

Fig. 8.4 Relationship between flow and pressure for (A) water flowing in a rigid glass tube and (B) for blood flowing in a large blood vessel.

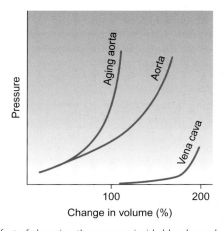

Fig. 8.5 Effect of changing the pressure inside blood vessels on the volume of the vessel. Veins are more easily distended than arteries. As arteries age they become stiffer and therefore more difficult to distend.

can be seen that the vein is more distensible than the arteries. Second, Figure 8.5 shows that an aorta from a young person is easier to distend than an aorta from an older individual. Distensibility is the increase in volume of a blood vessel per unit increase of pressure inside it. Veins have relatively thin walls which contain only small amounts of collagen compared to arteries (see Chapter 1). Veins are easily distended and are, therefore, referred to as capacitance vessels. Normally, the veins contain approximately two thirds of the body's total blood volume at any one time. Extra blood transfused into a person would primarily be accommodated in the veins and, correspondingly, blood loss would particularly result in a decrease in the volume held in the veins. Distribution of blood volume within the circulatory system is shown in Figure 1.7.

Pathology of arteries and veins

Congenital defects

Congenital abnormalities of arteries and veins are often related to an abnormal course, pattern of branching or anatomical relations of a vessel. This may be particularly important during surgery. An abnormally positioned coronary artery may predispose the patient to cardiac arrhythmias or even sudden death (see Chapter 3).

Case 8.1 Large blood vessels: 2

Investigation of the troublesome calf muscle

Palpation of the pulse sites in the leg suggested a partial blockage of the femoral artery in Jamshed's right leg (femoral pulse present, popliteal pulse reduced, dorsalis pedis and posterior tibial pulses absent). This was confirmed by an ultrasound investigation.

As the occluded section of blood vessel appeared to be relatively short a decision was taken to use percutaneous transluminal angioplasty (see Chapter 5) to try to improve the blood flow into Jamshed's leg.

After recovery from the surgery Jamshed found that he could once again walk about 1000 metres before having to stop and allow his calf muscle to recover. However, the blackened area of skin on the toes started to increase in size and a decision was later taken to amputate the gangrenous toes. Healing of the amputation site was very slow.

Issues which arise from this history are:

1. What are the probable pathological mechanisms which led to the partial occlusion of Jamshed's femoral artery?
2. What pathological processes are occurring in Jamshed's toes?

Aspects of the answers to these questions are to be found in the text of this chapter and in Chapter 1 (for Question 2).

Berry aneuryms are a consequence of a congenital abnormality of the wall of one or more cerebral arteries, usually at a junction point between two vessels in the circle of Willis. The abnormality appears to be in the media layer of the blood vessel wall. It leads to saccular aneurysm formation which may rupture. This is often related to hypertension, which may only be short term as during physical exertion. Some berry aneurysms occur in the context of other pathologies such as polycystic kidney disease, Marfan's syndrome or Ehlers–Danlos syndrome. Favoured sites for berry aneurysms include the junction of the internal carotid and posterior communicating artery and the junction of the anterior cerebral and anterior communicating arteries. Rupture of the aneurysm may lead to subarachnoid and/or intracerebral haemorrhage and possibly sudden death.

An arteriovenous fistula may also be a congenital vascular abnormality. In this case, there are well developed, abnormal communications between an artery and a vein which have the potential for thrombosis and rupture (e.g. cerebral arteriovenous fistulae).

Age-related changes in blood vessels

Many of the characteristic pathological changes seen in the vasculature of older individuals can be seen in younger populations with specific disease processes such as hypertension. The term 'arteriosclerosis' is often used to describe the 'hardened' or 'thickened' arteries of the elderly. This is due to the slow, progressive thickening of the intima, combined with medial fibrosis that occurs over many decades.

Included within the umbrella term arteriosclerosis are atherosclerosis (see below) and Monckeberg's medial calcific sclerosis. This latter disease process is characterized by areas of medial calcification in small to medium-sized arteries, especially the arteries of the upper and lower limbs. No inflammation or necrosis is involved and it usually occurs in older patients over 50 years of age. Other than being a radiological oddity, the disease usually has no clinical effects.

Atherosclerosis

Atherosclerosis is directly or indirectly the cause of death in about 50% of people in the Western world. It is a problem often associated in the public mind with modern living, but in fact the lesions were first described in 1856 by Virchow. Atherosclerotic lesions have been found in the arteries of Egyptian mummified bodies from 2000+ years ago. The intima layer of the blood vessel wall is primarily affected although development of atherosclerotic plaques appears to be secondary to altered function of the endothelial cell layer.

Atherosclerosis is the hardening and narrowing of arteries due to atheroma. This term is derived from a Greek word meaning porridge, so atherosclerosis may be thought of as hardened porridge in the artery wall. It is a problem which occurs in large blood vessels (>2 mm internal diameter) which are exposed to high blood pressures. The vessels most commonly affected are the aorta, carotid, coronary, iliac and femoral arteries. The pulmonary arteries are only affected after the development of pulmonary hypertension and veins do not develop atherosclerotic lesions unless they are transplanted to the high pressure arterial side of the circulation. This point is of particular relevance to coronary artery bypass grafting (CABG) when veins from the legs are often used to bypass diseased coronary arteries (p. 59).

> ### Interesting facts
>
> Atherosclerosis is sometimes thought of as a problem associated with modern dietary and social habits. However, lesions have been found in the arteries of Egyptian mummified bodies which are over 2000 years old.

Risk factors for atherosclerosis

A substantial number of risk factors have been identified which make the development of atherosclerotic lesions more likely. Constitutive (non-modifiable) risk factors include age, gender and some genetically determined factors such as familial hypercholesterolaemia. In the 35–55 age group fully formed atherosclerotic plaques are more common in men than in women. After the menopause there is an increased incidence and severity in women although men still remain marginally more affected than women. It is thought that oestrogens provide some protection in younger women.

Epidemiological research has identified some 'major' and some 'minor' (but still significant) modifiable risk factors. Major risk factors are diabetes, smoking, hyperlipidaemia and hypertension, all of which are treatable or avoidable. Minor modifiable risk factors include lack of exercise, obesity, personality type and stress. A number of other potential risk factors have also been proposed.

Pathogenesis of atherosclerosis

Despite the investment of large amounts of money in research budgets, the precise definition of the triggering factors for atherosclerosis remains elusive. Part of the reason for this is that atherosclerosis develops over a time course of 40+ years. This means that it is impossible to find entirely satisfactory experimental animal models of atherosclerosis. Many theories have been proposed and currently the response to injury hypothesis is particularly favoured. This theory was proposed by Ross in 1973 although it does incorporate some of the older hypotheses.

Essentially, the response to injury theory suggests that atheroma occurs because of long-term 'grumbling' injury to the endothelium. Causative factors for this endothelial injury leading to endothelial dysfunction include hyperlipidaemia (particularly low-density lipoprotein— LDL cholesterol), diabetes (damage as a result of hyperglycaemia causing glycosylation of proteins and dyslipidaemia), hypertension, toxins acquired as a result of cigarette smoking, increased plasma homocysteine and infective agents. In the latter group cytomegalovirus (CMV), *Chlamydia pneumoniae* and *Helicobacter pylori* have been particularly prominent as proposed causative organisms for atheroma formation. Many of these insults to the endothelial layer may be linked to the increased production of reactive oxygen species (ROS). This means primarily the formation of the O_2^- anion but the ROS group also includes hydrogen peroxide (H_2O_2), the hydroxyl anion (OH^-), and a range of lipid radicals formed from interaction with the peroxynitrite anion ($ONOO^-$), itself a product of the superoxide anion and nitric oxide (NO). Reduction in the availability of NO as a result of oxidative stress may be a key event in the development of atheroma at several points. Therapeutic strategies targeting a reduction in oxidative stress and an increase in NO availability are under investigation.

Altered function of the endothelial cells leads to increased permeability to LDL cholesterol and increased white blood cell adherence. Monocytes enter the intima layer and transform into macrophages. The macrophages accumulate oxidized LDL cholesterol and are then known as foam cells. Together with infiltration of T lymphocytes these events lead to the initial atherosclerotic lesion, the fatty streak. These often develop very early in life and have been found at autopsy in the arteries of stillborn babies. It is widely presumed that the fatty streak is the precursor of the later plaques but this is difficult to prove conclusively. Although high levels of LDL cholesterol present an important risk factor for atherogenesis, high levels of HDL (high-density lipoprotein) are considered to be protective.

The smooth muscle cells in the blood vessel wall are normally located in the media layer. In a normal arterial blood vessel there is a sparse population of cells with a dual contractile and fibroblast phenotype in the intimal layer. These myointimal cells start to proliferate under the influence of cytokines released from foam cells and from platelets which adhere to the damaged endothelial surface. The myointimal cells start to secrete collagen and the now stiffened atheromatous structure is referred to as a lipid plaque at this stage.

Final development of the plaque into a hard, white fibrolipid plaque (Fig. 8.6) follows further production of collagen and sometimes calcification of accumulated extracellular lipid. The damaged endothelial layer may ulcerate providing a site for thrombosis to form.

The process of atherosclerosis described above has many of the characteristics of an inflammatory response. These include invasion of monocytes which become macrophages, the involvement of T lymphocytes, the production of cytokines and growth factors and, in the later stages, focal necrosis in the blood vessel wall. Answering the question: 'An inflammatory response to what?' may prove productive in the future.

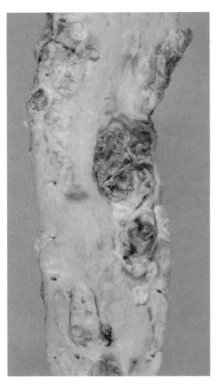

Fig. 8.6 Aortic atherosclerosis in a 73-year-old woman. (Source: Underwood JCE, 2004.)

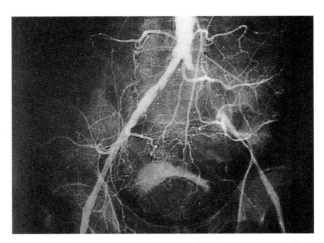

Fig. 8.7 Severe atherosclerotic narrowing of left iliac artery. Note the development of collateral circuits which bypass the region of complete occlusion. This patient presented with left sided intermittent claudication and ischaemic skin changes. (Source: Forbes CD, Jackson WF, 2002.)

Interesting facts

In 1947 the city of Framingham, near Boston, Massachusetts, was identified as representative of the American urban lifestyle. The 28 000 inhabitants were enrolled in an, initially, 20-year prospective study of vascular risk factors. This study forms the basis for a great deal of current public health approaches to cardiovascular disease.

Pathological consequences of atheroma

Major blood vessels may become narrowed by atheroma hence reducing blood flow. This may range from a fairly modest change which is insufficient to cause symptoms to almost complete interruption of flow (Fig. 8.7). This frequently results in ischaemic heart disease, or inadequacy of cerebral blood flow or peripheral vascular disease as described in the history of Jamshed in Case 8.1:1.

Exposure of collagen in the vessel wall to blood constituents when the endothelial layer is damaged initiates thrombus formation. This may suddenly totally occlude an already narrowed artery or the thrombus may embolize and block a vessel further downstream.

Weakening of the blood vessel wall as a consequence of atheroma may lead to the formation of an aneurysm, a region where the weakened wall balloons out (see p. 94). The most common site for this to occur is in the abdominal aorta (Fig. 8.8).

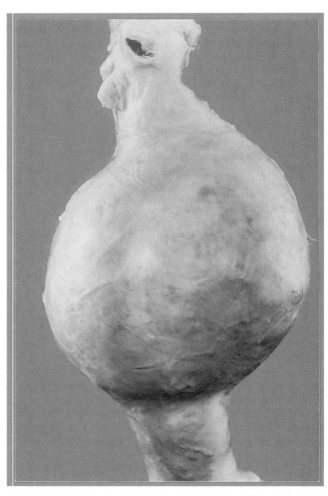

Fig. 8.8 Atherosclerotic abdominal aortic aneurysm. (Source: Underwood JCE, 2004.)

Vasculitis

Although it is relatively simple to give a definition of vasculitis as 'inflammation of the vessel wall often with accompanying mural necrosis and luminal thrombosis', the term usually excludes vessels that are inflamed or necrotic because they have been caught up in a local inflammatory process. Thus for example the vessels in the base of a gastric ulcer or the mesoappendiceal vessels in a patient with florid appendicitis would be excluded from the definition of vasculitis. It is very difficult to give an all encompassing, widely accepted classification of the diseases involved but possible ways of classifying vasculitis include: de novo (primary) vasculitic diseases (e.g. polyarteritis nodosa) and vasculitis secondary to a known systemic disease (e.g. to rheumatoid disease or systemic lupus erythematosus (SLE)).

The aetiopathogenesis of virtually all the vasculitides is poorly understood. Most theories centre on immune mediated mechanisms (immune complex or cell mediated). Perhaps the best way of classifying this group of diseases is by the size of the vessel affected:

- Large vessel vasculitis:
  Giant cell arteritis—occurs in elderly patients as a granulomatous inflammation of the aorta and its branches, often the temporal artery.
  Takayasu's arteritis—occurs in younger patients as a granulomatous inflammation of the aorta and its branches.

- Medium sized vessel vasculitis:
  Polyarteritis nodosa—often called classical polyarteritis which occurs in 40–50 year olds, mainly men. Often occurs at branch points of arteries.
  Kawasaki's disease—occurs in children. Any size vessel may be involved but there is a predilection for coronary arteries.

- Small vessel vasculitis:
  Wegener's granulomatosis—usually occurs in adults. It is a granulomatous inflammation of the respiratory tract with medium/small blood vessels also involved. Renal glomerular necrosis is common. Blood ANCA (anti-neutrophil cytoplasmic antibodies) levels are a disease marker.
  Churg–Strauss syndrome—occurs in adults and the inflammation typically includes numerous eosinophils. Respiratory tract involvement may occur and the patient may suffer from asthma.
  Microscopic polyangiitis/polyarteritis—occurs in adults and may cause glomerular necrosis. It is associated with ANCA.
  Henoch–Schönlein purpura—occurs in children and adults and is relatively common compared to other types of vasculitis. IgA is seen in vascular deposits. It may involve joints, glomeruli and the bowel.

Essential cryoglobulinaemic vasculitis—cryoglobulins are present in the blood with skin and glomerular capillaries usually involved.
Cutaneous leukocytoclastic angiitis—occurs in all age groups; skin vasculitis.

Varicose veins

Varicose veins are tortuous, dilated or stretched veins. Relatively little is known about the aetiopathogenesis of primary varicose veins. Female gender, older age, obesity and the number of pregnancies are important risk factors, particularly if more than one of these applies. There does not appear to be an abnormality in venous valves in primary cases although with the characteristic venous dilatation functional incompetence may occur. Varicose veins are nearly always in the lower limb vessels.

Secondary varicose veins may be due to a wide variety of pathologies such as congenital malformations including abnormal valves, hormone treatments, immobility and post-thrombosis. Under the microscope, the varicose vein shows intimal thickening, atrophic smooth muscle and mural fibrosis. With chronic venous congestion of the leg, oedema occurs and there are changes in the appearance and texture of the skin.

Vascular pathology of diabetes mellitus

Broadly speaking, the vascular effects of diabetes can be divided into:

- macrovasculopathy
- microvasculopathy.

Macrovasculopathy

Diabetic patients, particularly those that are poorly controlled, tend to have more severe and widespread atheroma than non-diabetics. Thus complications such as ischaemic heart disease (coronary artery atheroma), stroke (carotid and cerebral arteries), lower limb ischaemia leading to gangrene in the toes and feet and renal ischaemia tend to be more common in diabetic patients.

Microvasculopathy

Hyaline arteriolosclerosis is a frequent finding in the arteriolar (and capillary) circulation of diabetic patients. This thickening of the vessel wall, which looks very pink in a section stained with haematoxylin and eosin, may be due to increased flow of plasma proteins across the vessel wall leading to deposition of high relative molecular mass proteins such as fibrinogen and LDL cholesterol. It is important to realize that hyaline arteriolosclerosis is also seen in amyloidosis, benign hypertension and in the arterioles of the elderly. This microvasculopathic process causes ischaemic lesions in the retina associated with haemorrhage and vessel proliferation and in peripheral nerves with the resulting neuropathy leading to skin insensitivity to pain and ulceration.

Arteriolosclerosis is also responsible for renal and cerebral changes. The basement membrane of the glomerulus thickens and this is associated, paradoxically, with increased permeability of the glomerular filter leading to proteinuria. Renal failure can occur as nephrons are lost due to glomerular sclerosis. The arterioles of the kidney often show hyaline mural change.

Aneurysms

An aneurysm is an abnormal dilatation of a blood vessel, most often affecting the larger arteries or the heart. Usually the dilatation is localized, bounded by scarred and attenuated vessel wall and connects with the vessel lumen so that blood continues to flow through the dilated vessel ('true aneurysm'). However, occasionally, a 'false aneurysm' may occur and this takes the form of an extravascular blood clot which communicates with the lumen of the vessel through a defect or tear in the wall.

By far the commonest type of aneurysm is that caused by atheroma (Fig. 8.8). These aneurysms are most often located in the distal part of the abdominal aorta close to the bifurcation into the common iliac arteries. The build up of intimal atheroma weakens the arterial wall, mural fibrosis occurs and there is thrombus formation on the luminal surface. With the pulsatile arterial pressure, the artery gradually dilates and may erode on the posterior side of the aorta into the vertebral bodies giving the patient back pain. An aneurysm on the anterior side of the aorta may present as a palpable, pulsatile abdominal mass.

There are several important potential complications of an atherosclerotic abdominal aortic aneurysm, including:

- Rupture: this may lead to torrential and often fatal haemorrhage into the peritoneal cavity (haemoperitoneum).

- Embolus formation: variable sized fragments may split off from the intimal thrombus and cause occlusion of the small arteries in the legs and feet leading to gangrenous necrosis.

Other forms of aneurysm include the following:

- Infective aneurysm: also known as a mycotic aneurysm, this rare condition occurs when an infected embolus lodges in an artery and allows seeding of the vessel wall by the microbes. This classically occurs as a consequence of an embolus from an infected vegetation on a heart valve as in infective endocarditis (see Chapter 3). The vessel wall can become inflamed, soft and rupture. It is also possible for infective aneurysms to occur in septicaemia.

- Syphilitic aneurysms occur in the tertiary stage of syphilis, typically in the ascending thoracic (rather than abdominal) aorta. The disease process, which starts as an inflammatory process around the vasa vasorum of the adventitia, may lead to a thick-walled, dilated aorta which may extend back as far as the aortic root at the heart causing valvular incompetence.

- Vasculitic aneurysms. Macroscopic polyarteritis nodosa may lead to aneurysm formation by causing inflammation, necrosis, thrombosis, fibrosis and weakening of the vessel wall. With fragmentation of the elastic lamina, aneurysm formation can occur.

Dissecting aneurysm

This should be considered as a special category of aneurysm. In fact, there is not usually any significant dilatation of the vessel lumen. The pathology is due to a tear in the vessel wall. Blood enters the arterial wall through the tear in the intima and tracks into the media, shearing off the inner third from the outer two thirds. The blood may then re-enter the vessel through a second tear in the wall ('double-barrelled aorta') or may rupture to the outside of the vessel potentially causing sudden death by massive haemorrhage. Dissecting aneurysms most often occur in the thoracic aorta. The patient may present with severe chest pain (felt between the shoulder blades). Examination may reveal absent pulses in the area of dissection. The patient is often a middle-aged male with a known history of hypertension. Less commonly, dissection may occur in the context of a young patient with Marfan's syndrome. In Marfan's syndrome, there is an inherited reduction of a protein in elastic tissue. This leads to 'cystic medial degeneration' of the vessel wall, which becomes weak and can tear.

Rarely, dissection may occur in smaller calibre vessels because of invasive procedures, such as during or after coronary artery angioplasty.

Non-invasive techniques for the assessment of arteries and veins

Leading the way in the assessment of peripheral arteries and veins is ultrasound, especially Doppler ultrasound which allows the imaging of normal and abnormal flow in blood vessels. Ultrasound is 'bounced' off flowing blood and the resulting shift in sound frequency can be used to measure the speed at which the blood is moving. This corresponds to the change in tone of a siren or a train from when it is moving towards you compared to when it is moving away from you.

Magnetic resonance (MR) angiography is increasingly used for non-invasive imaging of blood flow and vessel structure. Modern systems can produce high resolution three dimensional reconstructions of vascular trees.

These are of enormous value to the surgeon or interventional radiologist.

These modalities are gradually replacing invasive angiography in which a radio-opaque medium is injected into the vessel of interest under X-ray screening. The application of all these techniques to cardiac investigations is described more fully in Chapter 3.

Further reading

Assmann, G., Nofer, J-R., 2003. Atheroprotective effects of high density lipoproteins. Annu. Rev. Med. 54, 321–341.

Bass, P., Burroughs, S., Carr, N., Way, C., 2009. Master Medicine: General and Systematic Pathology, third ed. Edinburgh, Churchill Livingstone.

Becker, A.E., de Boer, O.J., van der Wal, A.C., 2001. The role of inflammation and infection in coronary artery disease. Annu. Rev. Med. 52, 289–297.

Donnelly, R., London, N.J.M., 2000. ABC of Arterial and Venous Disease. BMJ Books, London.

Forbes, C.D., Jackson, W.F., 2002. Colour Atlas and Text of Clinical Medicine, third ed. Mosby, Edinburgh.

Gallagher, P.J., 2004. Cardiovascular system. In: Underwood, J.C.E. (Ed.), General and Systematic Pathology, fourth ed. Churchill Livingstone, Edinburgh.

Hamilton, C.A., Miller, W.H., Al-Benna, S., et al., 2004. Strategies to reduce oxidative stress in cardiovascular disease. Clin. Sci. 106, 219–234.

Hansson, G.K., Robertson, A-K.L., Soderberg-Naucler, C., 2006. Inflammation and atherosclerosis. Annu. Rev. Pathol. Mech. Dis. 1, 297–329.

Hunt, B.J., Poston, L., Schachter, M., Halliday, A.W., 2002. Introduction to Vascular Biology: From Basic Science to Clinical Practice, second ed. Cambridge University Press, Cambridge.

Jennette, J.C., Falk, R.J., 1997. Medical progress: small vessel vasculitis. N. Engl. J. Med. 337, 1512–1523.

Levick, J.R., 2009. An Introduction to Cardiovascular Physiology, fifth ed. Arnold, London.

Smith, J.J., Kampine, J.P., 1990. Circulatory Physiology—The Essentials, third ed. Williams and Wilkins, Baltimore.

Stevens, A., Lowe, J., 2000. Pathology, second ed. Mosby, Edinburgh.

Underwood, J.C.E., 2004. General and Systematic Pathology, fourth ed. Churchill Livingstone, Edinburgh.

RESISTANCE BLOOD VESSELS

9

Chapter objectives

After studying this chapter you should be able to:

1. Identify the arterioles as the main population of blood vessels posing a high resistance to blood flow and therefore the main locus for regulation of the peripheral circulation.

2. Describe the mechanism of contraction in vascular smooth muscle and explain the sources of Ca^{++} ions needed to trigger contraction.

3. Explain the beneficial and unwanted side effects of the use of calcium channel blocking drugs.

4. Discuss the role played by chemical mediators released from the endothelial cells, particularly nitric oxide and endothelins, in the control of peripheral blood vessel diameter.

5. Explain the therapeutic uses of drugs which act as exogenous sources of nitric oxide.

6. Outline the role of 'local metabolites' such as CO_2, H^+, K^+ and adenosine in matching the distribution of blood flow to the metabolic needs of a tissue.

7. Understand the role played by local hormones such as histamine, serotonin and bradykinin in the pathological responses to injury.

8. Describe the components of the renin-angiotensin system and the physiological actions of angiotensin II.

9. Discuss the therapeutic uses of drugs which oppose the actions of angiotensin II.

10. Explain the role played by catecholamine hormones adrenaline (epinephrine) and noradrenaline (norepinephrine) in cardiovascular regulation.

11. Outline the role played by the autonomic nervous system in the control of the peripheral circulation.

12. Describe the characteristics of circulatory regulation in the brain, skin, kidneys and lungs.

13. Outline the characteristics of Raynaud's disease.

Introduction

In this chapter the location of the major resistance blood vessels, the arterioles, will be identified and the properties of vascular smooth muscle, the means by which the diameter of these vessels is modified, will be described. This will provide a basis for understanding the local control mechanisms which normally allow an appropriate distribution of blood flow around the body. In many cases this means matching blood flow to the metabolic needs of tissues but in other cases a further aspect of organ function, such as glomerular filtration in the kidney, must be catered for. There are therefore variations in the ways in which blood flow to different organs of the body is regulated and a series of 'special circulations', such as the brain and muscle, will be discussed individually.

Failure to match blood flow to metabolic need will lead to loss of function of a tissue, to the development of pain and subsequently to tissue death. The case history of a lady with a problem in the regulation of the blood flow to her fingers is introduced in Case 9.1:1.

Resistance to blood flow

Where the blood flows to when it leaves the aorta depends on the relative resistance to flow in each part of

Case 9.1 Resistance blood vessels: 1

A lady with blue fingers

Sheila Duxworth is a 27-year-old lady who has always 'felt the cold' but over the last 2 years has had increasing trouble with painful fingers and hands particularly during cold weather. She sought advice from her GP who elicited a history of recurrent episodes of mild pain and numbness followed by quite severe pain lasting for up to an hour. Episodes were clearly associated with exposure of the hands to cold. Close questioning revealed that her hands became blue then white and then red and throbbing. The latter phase was particularly associated with pain.

The GP told Sheila that the problem was caused by an acute reduction in blood flow to her hands.

The GP carried out a visual examination of the capillary beds in Sheila's fingers in order to try to detect signs of a connective tissue disease such as scleroderma. She also made an appointment for Sheila to have an X-ray of her neck region to check for compression of the blood vessels supplying the arm. A blood sample was taken so that aspects of Sheila's immune system could be investigated.

Consideration of this presentation leads to the following questions:

1. How is blood flow to peripheral vessels regulated?
2. What is the explanation for the sequence of colour changes in the fingers?

the circulation. In each case, the blood flows through a series of blood vessels, arteries, arterioles, capillaries, venules and veins. The structure of the walls of all these vessels is described in Chapter 1 (see Figs 1.7, 1.8).

As noted in Chapter 8, there has to be a pressure gradient to achieve blood flow. Mean pressure in the arterial tree is typically close to 100 mm Hg and pressure in the right atrium is about 0 mm Hg (i.e. close to atmospheric pressure). Figure 9.1 shows the pressure drop going round the systemic circulation and it can be seen that the population of blood vessels through which there is the largest drop in pressure is the arterioles. These vessels, therefore, must be the segment of the circulation that have the highest resistance to blood flow. This concept is important because it means that by regulating the arterioles, we can:

- control the distribution of blood flow from the arteries
- regulate arterial blood pressure.

The product of the cardiac output and the peripheral resistance to blood flow determines the arterial blood pressure (see Chapter 10). As the arterial pressure provides the driving force to perfuse tissues, physiological control systems act to keep arterial pressure relatively constant from moment to moment and from day to day. Indeed, sustained raised arterial pressure can cause serious damage to many parts of the body (see Chapter 10). The consequence of a fall in arterial pressure is often poor brain blood flow which results in syncope (fainting).

Adjustment of the arteriolar resistance is achieved by altering the state of contraction of vascular smooth muscle. The mechanisms of smooth muscle contraction are now described.

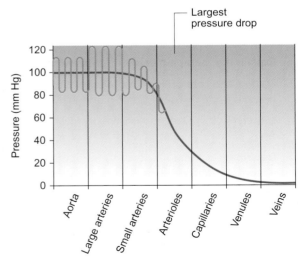

Fig. 9.1 Pressure drop during passage of blood around the circulation. The smooth line shows the fall in mean blood pressure starting from about 100 mm Hg in the aorta to close to zero in the right atrium. Blood flow in the aorta and arteries is pulsatile but this is damped out in the arterioles. The largest pressure drop occurs in the arterioles, the site of the major resistance to blood flow.

Vascular smooth muscle

Smooth muscle is located in the walls of the hollow structures of the body including blood vessels, airways, gut and bladder. The cells are spindle-shaped with a central nucleus and this is the first way in which smooth muscle cells differ from skeletal or cardiac muscle cells (see Chapter 6).

Source of Ca^{++} for smooth muscle contraction

As with the other two types of muscle, contraction of smooth muscle is triggered by a rise in intracellular [Ca^{++}]. The source of the calcium is, however, different in the three types of muscle. The calcium involved in skeletal muscle contraction is stored intracellularly. It is released from the sarcoplasmic reticulum and is pumped back into these stores during muscle relaxation. In cardiac muscle, most of the calcium used in contraction derives from intracellular stores but some enters the cardiac muscle cell down a concentration gradient from the extracellular fluid via plasma membrane calcium ion channels (see page 20).

In smooth muscle, much of the increase in [Ca^{++}] which generates contraction comes from transmembrane flux through calcium channels. A component of the rise in [Ca^{++}] is contributed by release from intracellular stores but smooth muscle does not have a structure equivalent to sarcoplasmic reticulum.

Two broad groups of stimulus-contraction coupling mechanism can be identified. In 'electromechanical coupling' depolarization of the smooth muscle cell is followed by opening of L-type voltage-gated calcium channels. The consequent rise in intracellular [Ca^{++}] leads to further release of Ca^{++} from intracellular stores (calcium-induced calcium release—CICR). This mechanism predominates in the major vascular resistance vessels which have an internal diameter less than 0.5 mm. In 'pharmacomechanical coupling' there is no change in membrane potential but the binding of a hormone or drug to a receptor leads to an increase in intracellular [Ca^{++}] either via a G-protein coupled activation of the inositol phosphate pathway and release of Ca^{++} from intracellular stores or by the opening of receptor-operated calcium channels. These mechanisms are discussed below in relation to the action of specific vasoactive mediators.

The membrane potential of vascular smooth muscle studied in vitro is close to −60 mV but in vivo it is only about −40 mV. This is because the pressure inside blood vessels stretches the smooth muscle and this stretch leads to the opening of a population of ion channels which result in partial depolarization of the cell and hence partial contraction of the smooth muscle. This is the basis for what has long been known as the 'Bayliss Effect'. Basically, if you stretch vascular smooth muscle it responds by contracting. An advantage of having partially contracted vascular smooth muscle is that physiological mediators (locally released chemicals, hormones or neurotransmitters) can either cause further contraction or relaxation of smooth muscle as appropriate. Some physiological mediators (see section 'Metabolite control of local blood flow' on p. 104) act via a population of ATP-sensitive K$^+$ channels. A decrease in [ATP] inside the smooth muscle cell increases the probability that this population of K$^+$ channels will be open. This leads to hyperpolarization and hence relaxation of smooth muscle.

Relaxation of smooth muscle requires that intracellular [Ca^{++}] is reduced. This can be achieved either by pumping the calcium back into intracellular stores or by expelling it outside the cell (see page 20 for a description of the equivalent mechanisms in cardiac muscle).

The use of different sources of calcium for contraction in the three types of muscle is illustrated by the pharmacological effects of calcium channel blocking drugs. Drugs such as nifedipine, diltiazem and verapamil will, to varying degrees, reduce heart rate and the contractility of the heart (see Chapter 5). These drugs may also be used to achieve peripheral vasodilatation as part of antihypertensive therapy (see Chapter 10). Their side effects are fairly predictable. These include facial flushing, headache and dizziness as a result of their effects on vascular smooth muscle but also constipation is a common side effect because of the effects of calcium channel blocking drugs on gut smooth muscle. Calcium channel blocking drugs have no effect on skeletal muscle function because all the calcium needed for contraction is stored within the sarcoplasmic reticulum.

The calcium channel blocking drug nifedipine was tried as therapy for the patient with Raynaud's disease described in Case 9.1:2, the aim being to cause vasodilation and improve the blood flow to the fingers.

The total calcium concentration in the extracellular fluid is normally in the range 2.1–2.6 mmol/L. Just over half of this calcium is bound to protein (particularly albumin) and so is not able to enter cells through calcium ion channels. The remaining, ionized, [Ca^{++}] is about 1.1 mmol/L. The relative amounts of ionized and bound calcium depend partly on acid–base status. Hydrogen ions displace calcium ions from anionic binding sites on albumin and therefore acidosis will increase the proportion of Ca^{++} which is in the ionized form. Routine clinical measurements of plasma calcium usually refer to 'total calcium'. This may be reported along with a 'corrected' measurement which means that allowance has been made for variations in the [albumin].

Contraction of smooth muscle

The contractile mechanism for smooth muscle is different to the two other types of muscle. In skeletal and cardiac muscle the contractile proteins, actin and myosin, are arranged in parallel layers and this is the origin of the striated (striped) appearance when these muscles are viewed under the polarized light microscope. Contraction of striated muscle (see Chapter 2) is initiated by the binding of Ca^{++} to the control protein troponin. This has the effect of moving another protein, tropomyosin, out of a

Case 9.1 Resistance blood vessels: 2

A possible diagnosis and treatment

Sheila, who has always felt the cold, returned to her GP to hear the results of the blood tests and X-ray examination all of which failed to provide any positive information.

The GP suggested that the problem was probably Raynaud's disease, which affects about 10% of women in temperate climates and is roughly ten times as common in women as in men. It is associated with an, as yet, unexplained spasm of the smooth muscle in peripheral blood vessels. Further questioning suggested that Sheila's problems were exacerbated by stress suggested that the sympathetic nerve supply to blood vessels might be involved.

The GP was unable to offer any specific treatment but advised Sheila to give up smoking and suggested that she should try a course of the calcium channel blocking drug, nifedipine.

This part of the history raises the following questions:

1. What are the mechanisms involved in vascular smooth muscle contraction and how are calcium ions involved? What would be the pharmacological actions of a calcium channel blocking drug?
2. What role is played by the nerve supply to blood vessels? How might this be linked to stress?
3. Why does the blood supply to the fingers increase above normal levels once the vascular spasm has ended? This is the basis for the redness and throbbing felt by Sheila in her fingers.

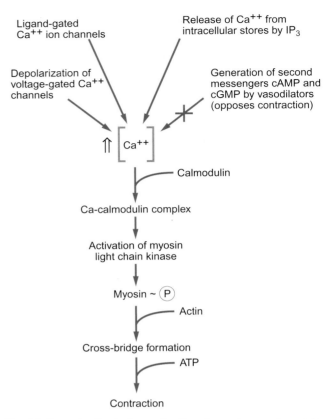

Fig. 9.2 Events leading to the contraction of vascular smooth muscle. Unlike skeletal muscles, the key event following the formation of a calcium–calmodulin complex is the phosphorylation of myosin as the trigger for cross-bridge formation.

groove on the bundle of actin filaments. Formation of a 'cross-bridge' is then achieved by the myosin head having access to a binding site on the actin filament. Muscle contraction takes place with the hydrolysis of ATP to provide the energy.

Smooth muscle does have actin and myosin as contractile proteins but does not have troponin. The Ca^{++} released into the cytosol of smooth muscle cells binds to the protein calmodulin. The calcium–calmodulin complex activates the enzyme myosin light chain kinase and this promotes phosphorylation of the myosin filament. Once this has been achieved, interaction between actin and myosin phosphate generates contraction of the smooth muscle cell. Figure 9.2 summarizes the events associated with cross-bridge formation and hence contraction of smooth muscle. When intracellular $[Ca^{++}]$ decreases, myosin is dephosphorylated by myosin light chain phosphatase. Even when dephosphorylated myosin can retain its interaction with actin. These attachments are called latch-bridges. They only detach slowly and so they maintain a level of muscle tension with little consumption of ATP.

There are several broad types of mechanism which contribute to the overall regulation of intracellular $[Ca^{++}]$. These mechanisms are illustrated in Figures 9.3 and 9.4.

Some vasoconstrictor agents such as noradrenaline (norepinephrine) act through more than one mechanism:

- Vasoconstrictor hormones such as noradrenaline, angiotensin II, endothelins, vasopressin and thromboxane A_2 bind to G-protein coupled receptors. Subsequent generation of the second messenger inositol trisphosphate (IP_3) leads to the opening of channels in intracellular calcium stores and release of Ca^{++} (Fig. 9.3).

- Vasoconstrictors also lead to membrane depolarization by several mechanisms. These include opening of ligand gated ion channels in the plasma membrane which permits influx of Na^+ and Ca^{++} accompanied by inhibition of K^+ channels (Fig. 9.3).

- Intracellular $[Ca^{++}]$ also depends on the Ca^{++} removal mechanisms. These include pumping Ca^{++} back into intracellular stores and active extrusion of Ca^{++} across the plasma membrane both of which involve Ca-ATPase enzymes. There is also a Na^+/Ca^{++} antiport exchanger. Entry of Na^+ into the cell down its concentration gradient is coupled to extrusion of Ca^{++} against its concentration gradient. The low intracellular $[Na^+]$ is of course maintained by the sodium pump (Na^+/K^+ ATPase) (Fig. 9.4).

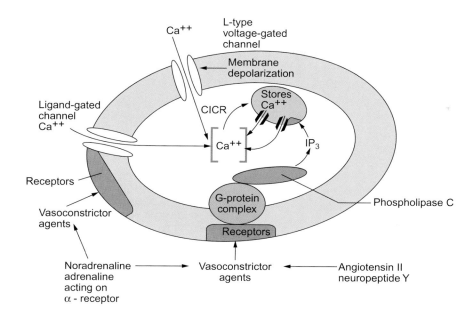

Fig. 9.3 Main pathways leading to a rise in intracellular $[Ca^{++}]$. These pathways occur in vascular smooth muscle as part of vasoconstrictor mechanisms. A rise in cytosolic $[Ca^{++}]$ results in further release of Ca^{++} from intracellular stores. This is called calcium-induced calcium release (CICR). The second messenger inositol trisphosphate (IP_3) acts via a receptor on the intracellular $[Ca^{++}]$ stores.

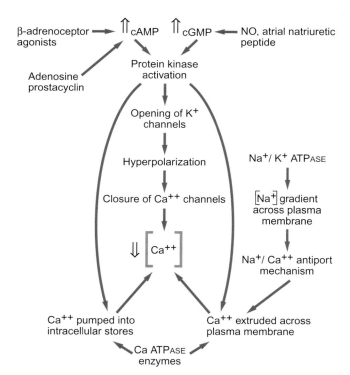

Fig. 9.4 Main pathways leading to a decrease in intracellular $[Ca^{++}]$ as part of vasodilatation mechanisms.

• Vasodilator agents act via production of either cAMP (e.g. adenosine, prostacyclin, β-adrenoceptor agonists) or cGMP (nitric oxide, atrial natriuretic peptide) as second messengers. Both cAMP and cGMP activate protein kinases and hence lead to protein phosphorylation. A reduction in plasma $[Ca^{++}]$ may then be secondary to cell hyperpolarization following

opening of K^+ channels. The hyperpolarization closes Ca^{++} channels. An alternative mechanism for vasodilatation is the activation of Ca^{++} pumps leading to either extrusion of Ca^{++} from the cell or sequestration of Ca^{++} into intracellular stores (Fig. 9.4).

Smooth muscle contracts more slowly than skeletal or cardiac muscle and has less than one third of the myosin content. However, it generates a comparable force per unit cross-sectional area to skeletal muscle. Furthermore, smooth muscle can contract to only 25% of its resting length. Smooth muscle does not fatigue and maintains tension with a low energy cost which is only 1% of the equivalent amount of ATP needed to contract skeletal muscle. It can, if necessary, contract using ATP generated anaerobically in the glycolytic pathway.

Inappropriate spasm of vascular smooth muscle is the diagnosis suggested in the case study in Case 9.1:2.

Local control of vascular smooth muscle

Endothelial factors in the control of local blood flow

The adult human circulation consists of about 60 000 miles of tubing (see Chapter 1). It is lined by a thin monolayer of endothelial cells. These cells not only provide a barrier between the blood and the other cells of the body (see Chapter 11), but they are also the source of a range of vasoactive agents which cause relaxation or contraction of underlying blood vessel smooth muscle (Figs 9.5, 9.6). One of these compounds, before it was chemically identified, was initially named endothelium-derived relaxing factor (EDRF). It is now thought that most, but not necessarily all, of the vascular effects of EDRF can be attributed

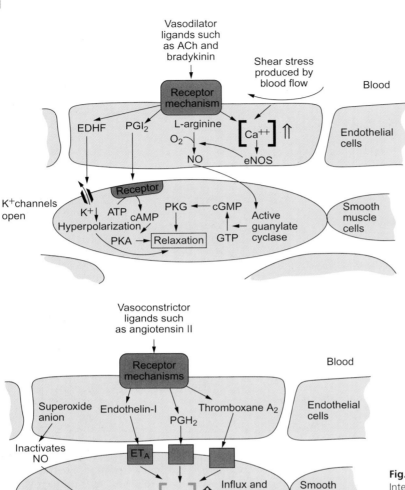

Fig. 9.5 Endothelin dependent vasodilator mechanisms. The dominant effect on NO production is probably shear stress produced by the interaction of blood flow with endothelial cells. Other agonists, in addition to bradykinin and ACh, may work through endothelial cell receptor mechanisms. Abbreviations are defined in the text.

Fig. 9.6 Endothelin dependent vasoconstrictor mechanisms. Interaction of ET-1 with the ET_A receptor on smooth muscle leads to vasoconstriction but binding of ET-1 to the ET_B receptor leads to synthesis of NO and hence vasodilatation. The vasoconstrictor response is dominant. Superoxide anion destroys NO but also generates toxic species such as peroxynitrite and hydroxyl anions.

to nitric oxide. Other factors produced by the endothelium and which also affect vascular smooth muscle contraction have been identified (see p. 103).

Nitric oxide (NO)

NO is synthesized from the amino acid l-arginine by the action of nitric oxide synthase (NOS) enzymes (Fig. 9.5). The terminology for these enzymes is a little confusing as it reflects the original site of discovery rather than current opinion of their site of importance. Endothelial NOS (eNOS) and neuronal NOS (nNOS) are both constitutively expressed in a wide range of cells, including many cell types in the cardiovascular system. These enzymes generate NO continuously. Inducible NOS (iNOS) is synthesized by cells exposed to inflammatory cytokines such as tumour necrosis factor alpha (TNFα), interleukin 1β (IL1β) and interferon alpha (IFNα). A range of other cytokines have the opposite effect and suppress iNOS expression. Overall the

balance of local cytokines determines the expression of iNOS and the rate of NO production as required. NO produced in this way in macrophages has cytotoxic actions. Excessive production of NO by iNOS also occurs in some forms of septic shock and will lead to peripheral vasodilatation and a fall in arterial blood pressure (see Chapter 14). It is assumed that iNOS generated NO does not contribute to the normal physiological control of blood vessel diameter.

Analogues of l-arginine which act as inhibitors of NOS enzymes have been developed. Much has been learnt in experimental studies about the physiological roles of NO using these inhibitors. They are also being evaluated with regard to their potential clinical uses.

NO generated constitutively by eNOS and nNOS is part of moment to moment normal vascular control mechanisms. As the physiological half-life of NO is short (a few seconds), it must be generated continuously and is available to contribute to short-term changes in blood vessel diameter. The main site of action of NO is on large diameter arterioles. The single most important trigger for NO production in relation to circulatory control is increased shear stress on the blood vessel wall (Fig. 9.5). If blood flow velocity in an artery increases, this leads to increased NOS activity in the endothelial cells and hence vessel dilatation. The existence of flow dependent vasodilatation was first reported by Schretzenmayr in 1923 but the mechanisms involved only became apparent when NO was recognized as an important vasoactive compound in 1986. NO synthesis can also be triggered by blood borne agonists such as bradykinin, acetylcholine and thrombin acting via receptors on the endothelial cell (Fig. 9.5). This has applied importance, for example, when considering the action of the angiotensin converting enzyme inhibitor (ACEI) group of drugs (see Chapter 10). The ACE enzyme is responsible for the inactivation of bradykinin as well as for the activation of angiotensin II. ACEI drugs, therefore, lead to increased bradykinin concentration and so increased NO synthesis. Part of the antihypertensive action of ACEI drugs is, therefore, related to NO induced vasodilatation.

NO produced in endothelial cells diffuses out of these cells and through the plasma membrane of underlying smooth muscle cells. Within smooth muscle NO binds to the haem part of guanylate cyclase and thereby increases the rate of production of cyclic GMP. In smooth muscle cells this mediator, via activation of protein kinase G, leads to a reduction in intracellular $[Ca^{++}]$ and hence smooth muscle relaxation (Fig. 9.5).

Endothelial dysfunction is important in many disease mechanisms including diabetes, hypertension (see Chapter 10) and atherosclerosis. This dysfunction is not, however, simply explained by alterations in the rate of NO production by endothelial cells. The superoxide anion O_2^- inactivates NO and forms the peroxynitrite anion ($ONOO^-$). This highly reactive anion has many different adverse effects on cell function. Countering the effects of superoxide anion is the strategic basis for many new approaches to therapy for chronic vascular disease. In the absence of NO, superoxide anion leads to the production of hydroxyl anion (OH^-) which can also have damaging effects.

Drugs which are sources of NO The group of drugs known as organic nitrates or nitrovasodilators have been in clinical use since the nineteenth century. They either spontaneously release NO (e.g. sodium nitroprusside) or are enzymically degraded and release NO (e.g. glyceryl trinitrate (GTN), amyl nitrate, isosorbide mononitrate and isosorbide dinitrate). These drugs therefore mimic the effects of endogenous NO. Nitric oxide and the nitrosothiols which are produced by the interaction of NO with sulphydryl compounds such as glutathione activate guanylate cyclase (see above) and lead to vasodilatation. The rationale for the use of these drugs in the management of angina is further discussed in Chapter 5 but the fundamentals are as follows. The drugs have their actions on three particular populations of blood vessels.

1. Capacitance vessels (mainly small veins): dilatation of these vessels leads to venous pooling of blood and a reduction in preload on the heart (see Chapter 4).

2. Arterial resistance vessels (mainly arterioles): vasodilatation in this case leads to a reduction in arterial blood pressure and consequently a drop in afterload effects on the heart (see Chapter 4).

The combined effect of nitrovasodilators working on capacitance vessels and arterial resistance vessels is a reduction in work done by the heart and, hence, a drop in cardiac oxygen demand.

3. Coronary arteries are often, mistakenly, thought to be the major site of action of nitrovasodilator drugs. In an ischaemic heart these vessels may well be nearly maximally dilated as a result of the accumulation of local metabolites (see p. 104). There is therefore little remaining vasoconstriction which could be reversed by nitric oxide donor drugs. However, nitrovasodilators may improve blood supply within the heart by actions on collateral blood vessels and can also be useful in the relief of coronary artery spasm (see Chapter 5).

As mentioned above, NO has a very short half-life and nitrovasodilator drugs are also subject to extensive first pass metabolism in the liver. These factors severely limit the duration of action of the drugs. The first pass metabolism effects can be reduced by using appropriate drug administration routes. These are sublingual (under the tongue), buccal (tablets held between the inside of the cheek and the gum) and transdermal (steady absorption from a skin patch for up to about 24 hours). Intravenous administration of GTN may be used to obtain acute effects of the drug.

The side effects of nitrovasodilator drugs are fairly predictable. Effects on the venous capacitance vessels will lead to pooling of blood in the veins and hence to postural hypotension, dizziness, fainting (syncope) and a reflex increase in heart rate (see Chapter 10). Arterial dilatation leads to headache as a result of dilatation of cerebral blood vessels and raised intracranial pressure (see p. 108) and to increased skin blood flow, which appears particularly as facial flushing.

Tolerance, a reduction in effect with sustained high plasma levels of the drugs, is also a problem with nitrovasodilator drugs. Possible mechanisms for tolerance include an increase in superoxide anion production within smooth muscle cells and a reduction in the availability of thiol groups to produce nitrosothiols. There are also other probable effects which contribute to the development of tolerance. The problems posed by tolerance can be reduced by adopting appropriate dosing strategies.

Other endothelium derived relaxing factors

The chemical structure and precise physiological role of endothelium derived hyperpolarizing factor (EDHF) is as yet unknown. It is thought to cause smooth muscle relaxation by promoting the opening of K^+ channels (Fig. 9.4).

Prostacyclin (prostaglandin I_2, PGI_2) is released from endothelial cells and is a potent inhibitor of platelet aggregation. PGI$_2$ is also a vasodilator and acts by increasing the production of cyclic AMP and hence activating protein kinase A (PKA) in smooth muscle cells (Fig. 9.5).

> ### Interesting facts
>
> Legend has it that Queen Cleopatra was killed in 30 BC when bitten by an asp. The venom of this snake contains a peptide, sarafotoxin 6c. Only when the endothelins were discovered in 1988 was the structural homology between sarafotoxin and endothelins recognized, thus providing an explanation for how Cleopatra died, by intense coronary vasoconstriction.

Endothelins

The endothelins are a group of peptides which were first discovered in 1988. There are three endothelins designated ET-1, ET-2 and ET-3. Of these three compounds, ET-1 is considered the most important in humans and it has its action predominantly on the ET$_A$ type receptor but it also has actions on the ET$_B$ receptor. Interaction of ET-1 with ET$_B$ receptor on the endothelial cell leads to increased NO production (a vasodilator), but the dominant action of ET-1 is vasoconstriction following binding to an ET$_A$ receptor on vascular smooth muscle (Fig. 9.6).

The initial product of gene expression is a preproendothelin molecule with 212 amino acids. This is enzymatically cleaved to form a 38 amino acid peptide—'Big endothelin 1'. Final processing of this peptide to the main biologically active compound ET-1 involves endothelin-converting enzyme (ECE).

ET-1 is the most potent naturally occurring pressor agent known and, as the name implies, endothelin gene expression does occur in the vascular endothelium. However, this is not the only site of synthesis. Vascular effects of ET-1 are widespread and are thought to contribute to normal cardiovascular regulation with the coronary, kidney and brain blood vessels being particularly sensitive. An interesting historical footnote is that structural analogues of ET-1, the sarafotoxin peptides, occur in the venom of a snake, the Israeli burrowing asp. In 30 BC, Queen Cleopatra of Egypt died after being bitten by this snake. We now know that the cause of her death was likely to be intense coronary vasoconstriction following interaction of the snake venom sarafotoxin with ET$_A$ type receptors.

In addition to a role in normal vascular control, there is much interest in the involvement of endothelins in disease mechanisms. Sustained endothelin induced vasoconstriction has been implicated in the mechanisms of essential hypertension, congestive heart failure and chronic renal failure amongst others. Intermittent vasoconstriction produced by endothelins is thought to occur in a range of conditions including unstable angina, acute renal failure, subarachnoid haemorrhage, Raynaud's disease and migraine. In addition to the intrinsic vasoconstrictor effects, endothelins augment the effects of other vasoconstrictors such as angiotensin II, noradrenaline (norepinephrine) and serotonin (Fig. 9.6).

The roles of endothelins in these disease mechanisms are not confined to vasoconstrictor effects. ET-1 has effects on gene expression and protein synthesis, and the outcomes of this include smooth muscle and cardiac myocyte hypertrophy. Effects on fibroblasts lead to increased deposition of fibrotic proteins such as collagen. ET-1 is also a co-mitogen leading to an increased rate of cell division in some tissues.

At the time of writing, there are no specific drugs targeting the endothelin system in routine clinical use. However, there are many compounds in various stages of development by the drug companies. These include selective ET$_A$ and ET$_B$ receptor antagonists, non-selective (mixed) ET$_A$ / ET$_B$ blockers and endothelin converting enzyme (ECE) blocking drugs. These drugs are potentially useful as antihypertensive agents and also in the management of heart failure, pulmonary hypertension and renal failure.

Other endothelium derived constricting factors

Endothelial cells can synthesize the vasoconstrictor prostanoids thromboxane A$_2$ and prostaglandin H$_2$ (Fig. 9.6). Other contributions of endothelial cells to blood pressure elevation include the production of superoxide anions which inhibit the dilator actions of nitric oxide (see p. 102) and the activation of the physiologically inert peptide angiotensin I to the potent pressor agent angiotensin II. The enzyme involved, angiotensin-converting enzyme (ACE), is present on the surface of the endothelial cells (see p. 106).

The bottom line on the role played by the endothelial cells in circulatory control is that they produce a mixture of compounds with a number of actions including both dilator or constrictor effects. The endothelium plays an important role in both physiological and pathological mechanisms involved in circulatory control.

Metabolite control of local blood flow

A major rationale for endothelial involvement in vascular control mechanisms (described above) appears to be to adjust arterial and arteriolar diameter to match changes in blood flow velocity. Increased flow velocity leads to increased shear stress between blood and the endothelial wall. This is an important factor regulating production of both NO and ET-1. The equivalent rationale for metabolite control of blood vessel size is that it enables matching of blood flow to the metabolic needs of a tissue. A local increase in metabolic rate will lead to an accumulation of metabolites which will in turn cause vasodilatation. The principle of metabolite induced vasodilatation is outlined in Figure 9.7. Metabolite effects, therefore, provide the major mechanism for regulating the distribution of blood flow. Metabolite-based regulation appears to be particularly important both in tissues, such as the brain, which

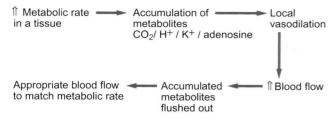

Fig. 9.7 Pathway for metabolite regulation of peripheral blood flow.

require a fairly constant blood flow and in tissues in which metabolic needs may fluctuate widely, such as the heart or skeletal muscle. The kidney, which has excretion and fluid volume regulation as its main functions, has a high blood flow compared to the tissue's metabolic needs. Metabolites therefore play little role in blood flow regulation in the kidney. The major target vessels for metabolite based control are arterioles and precapillary sphincters. The main site of metabolite effects is on small, rather than large, arterioles.

What are metabolites? Common examples are CO_2, H^+, adenosine and K^+. Local changes in the osmolarity of the interstitial fluid also contribute to blood flow regulation. It is perhaps surprising that oxygen concentration does not directly figure in this context but distribution of blood flow is normally regulated by the accumulation of waste products rather than by changes in oxygen availability. Under hypoxic conditions the low O_2 levels can have some effect by opening ATP-sensitive K^+ channels and hence causing vasodilatation but this is not relevant to normal physiological circumstances. Release of vasodilator prostaglandins is also linked to Po_2-dependent processes. Increased production of CO_2 in a tissue leads to increased H^+ production from the dissociation of carbonic acid.

It is thought that H^+, rather than CO_2 directly, is the effective agent as, in isolated tissues, dilute HCl infusion produces similar vasodilator responses. Increased $[H^+]$ ions work through opening ATP-sensitive K^+ channels on smooth muscle and, following hyperpolarization of the smooth muscle cell, relaxation of smooth muscle leads to increased blood flow.

Adenosine is a potent vasodilator in skeletal and cardiac muscle cells. It is formed in the muscle cells either by the complete dephosphorylation of ATP to adenosine or in a parallel pathway which involves the intermediate formation of *S*-adenosyl methionine from ATP (see Fig 5.5). It should be remembered that the normal [ATP] inside a muscle cell is of the order of 5×10^{-3} mol/L whereas [adenosine] outside the myocyte is about 1×10^{-8} mol/L, a 500 000-fold difference. Significant accumulation of adenosine, therefore, only requires the use of a minute proportion of the available ATP. Adenosine, a non-polar molecule, can cross myocyte membranes. The action of adenosine as a dilator is partly mediated by ATP-sensitive K^+ channels on the endothelial cells which increase NO production and partly by similar actions on K^+ channels leading to hyperpolarization of the underlying smooth muscle.

K^+ ions leave skeletal and cardiac muscle cells and also neurons during the repolarization phase of action potentials. Changes in extracellular $[K^+]$ contribute to the initiation of the cardiovascular responses to exercise (see Chapter 13).

In summary, accumulation of 'metabolites' in a tissue leads to vasodilatation. In terms of tissue selectivity, in the brain CO_2/H^+ levels are particularly important, whereas in skeletal and cardiac muscle adenosine and K^+ are of greater significance. Metabolite control is discussed in more detail in relation to specific tissues later in this chapter. There is still much to be discovered in this area.

Hormonal control of blood vessel diameter

Mechanisms concerned with hormonal control of vascular smooth muscle can be grouped under two headings.

- Local hormones (autocoids) are mainly involved in local responses as part of pathological events. Specific examples (see this page) include histamine, bradykinin and serotonin but the definition could arguably also include the endothelium-derived mediators NO, PGI_2 and the endothelins described above.

- Systemic hormones circulate in the blood and have an effect all round the circulation. The most important examples here are the renin-angiotensin system and the catecholamines adrenaline (epinephrine) and noradrenaline (norepinephrine) released from the adrenal medulla.

Local hormones

Histamine

Histamine has widespread physiological actions which are mediated via three types of receptor. It is involved as a neurotransmitter in the central nervous system (action on H_3 receptors) and in the control of gastric acid secretion (action on H_2 receptors). The vascular actions of histamine, which form part of the inflammatory responses to trauma and allergic responses, are mediated by the H_1 receptor type. Histamine is synthesized and stored in mast cells, particularly in those tissues which come into contact with the outside world (skin, lungs and gut). It is also found in basophils where it again forms part of tissue defence mechanisms.

The major vascular responses to H_1 receptor stimulation include a transient increase in capillary permeability which can lead to oedema (see Chapter 11). If this occurs to a substantial extent, it can lead to a reduction in circulating blood volume and, consequently, hypotension. This may be accompanied by histamine induced arteriole and capillary dilatation which will also contribute to blood pressure lowering. In severe allergic reactions, such as an anaphylactic reaction to a bee sting, these responses may be life threatening. Treatment includes the rapid use of antihistamine drugs, together with glucocorticoids as anti-inflammatory agents and adrenaline (epinephrine) as a vasoconstrictor (see p. 107). Actions of neurally released

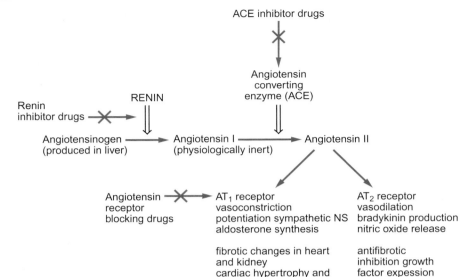

Fig. 9.8 Renin-angiotensin system and drugs. Main components of the renin-angiotensin system and the site of action of drugs which inhibit it. Some of the physiological actions of the renin system may be mediated by peptides other than angiotensin II (angiotensin III, angiotensin IV and angiotensin 1–7).

histamine in the skin contribute to the weal and flare response which is part of local allergic responses.

Antihistamine drugs (H_1 receptor antagonists) suppress most of the vascular effects of histamine. Some of the older drugs in this class, such as chlorphenamine (chlorpheniramine) and promethazine, have sedative side effects. Newer antihistamines, such as terfenadine, do not cause marked sedation.

Bradykinin

The nine amino acid peptide bradykinin causes dilatation of arterioles and an increase in venule permeability. It is generated by the enzyme kallikrein from kininogen during inflammatory responses. Bradykinin also binds to receptors on the endothelial cells and increases the production of nitric oxide (see p. 102). Interest in this area has been stimulated by the development of angiotensin converting enzyme (ACE) inhibitor drugs (see p. 107). ACE inactivates bradykinin and so ACE inhibitor drugs increase the physiological half-life of bradykinin. Bradykinin is also the most potent autocoid in pain responses, an action shared by histamine (acting on H_3 receptors) and by serotonin.

Serotonin (5-hydroxytryptamine, 5-HT)

Serotonin causes constriction of large arteries and veins and increases the permeability of venules. It contributes to inflammatory responses. Platelet released serotonin causes local vasoconstriction at the site of blood vessel injury, thus helping to limit blood loss. Serotonin released from argentaffin cells in the intestine contributes to the local regulation of blood flow. In the cerebral circulation, serotonin induced vasoconstriction contributes to the arterial vasospasm associated with the onset of migraine and with the response to subarachnoid haemorrhage.

Systemic hormones

Renin-angiotensin system

Renin is a systemic hormone secreted by the kidney. It is an enzyme which generates angiotensin I as shown in Figure 9.8.

Angiotensin I (Ang I), is physiologically inert but it is the precursor of angiotensin II (Ang II) which is produced as a result of the actions of angiotensin converting enzyme (ACE). This enzyme is mainly bound to vascular endothelial cells. There is also evidence of locally generated Ang II, which has actions as a paracrine hormone within a number of tissues in the body including blood vessel walls. The main physiological actions of Ang II on AT_1 receptors can be summarized as follows:

- Direct pressor action via receptors on vascular smooth muscle. In addition Ang II promotes the formation in endothelial cells of vasoconstrictors such as ET-1 and thromboxane A_2.

- Potentiation of sympathetic nervous system activity by several mechanisms. This contributes to the pressor effect of Ang II.

- Stimulation of aldosterone synthesis by actions on the zona glomerulosa of the adrenal cortex. This role of Ang II contributes to blood volume regulation (see Chapter 14).

- Increase in antidiuretic hormone (ADH) secretion.

- Potentiation of thirst responses (dipsogenic actions) by effects within the brain.

The full range of responses to a second receptor type, the AT_2 receptor, is not yet clear but it appears to oppose the pressor actions of Ang II mediated by the AT_1 receptor.

Although Ang II is still regarded as the dominant peptide mediating the actions of the renin-angiotensin system, there is now considerable interest in related peptides. These are designated Ang III, Ang IV and Ang (1–7).

> ### Interesting facts
>
> The pressor compound produced by renin was discovered at the same time by two separate research groups. It was referred to as hypertensin by a group in Argentina and as angiotonin by an American team. They subsequently compromised on the name angiotensin.

Ang II has an important role in pathological events as well. It can promote cell hypertrophy and hyperplasia and also promotes fibrotic changes in many tissues. An example is in the series of changes referred to as 'remodelling of the heart' during progressive cardiac failure (see Chapter 6).

Pharmacological blockade of the renin-angiotensin system Blocking drugs for the renin-angiotensin system were initially conceived as antihypertensive agents, which act by reducing peripheral resistance, and as drugs for the management of congestive heart failure. In the latter case, the beneficial effects include reduction in fluid retention by reducing aldosterone synthesis (reduced preload on the heart) and reduction in arterial blood pressure (reduced afterload on the heart). However, more recently, the value of 'organ protective' effects of renin blockade have become recognized. Renin system blockade reduces the rate of progression of the fibrotic changes associated with the development of chronic renal failure, for example in diabetic patients, as well as the fibrotic changes in heart failure.

What drugs are available to block the renin angiotensin system? β-adrenoceptor blocking drugs (see p. 106) provided the earliest, but rather non-specific, form of renin blockade. Renin secretion from the juxtaglomerular cells in the kidney is partly regulated by circulating catecholamines and by sympathetic nerves acting through β-adrenoceptors. However, beta-blockers have many other components to their pharmacological spectrum of activity.

Angiotensin converting enzyme inhibitors (ACEI) were developed during the 1980s. There are now over 30 drugs in this class available internationally. The first drug clinically available was captopril and the second was enalapril. All of the drug names in this class end in -pril. They not only block the formation of the active hormone Ang II but also block the breakdown of bradykinin to inactive peptides (see p. 106).

The antihypertensive actions of ACEI therefore include blockade of the direct vasoconstrictor effects of Ang II and a modest diuretic action mediated by reduced aldosterone production. The drugs are also described as being sympatholytic as Ang II potentiation of the sympathetic nervous system is blocked. A further component of the antihypertensive action may be linked to increased levels of the vasodilator bradykinin. Certainly, increased [bradykinin] is the basis for the major side effect of these drugs, a dry

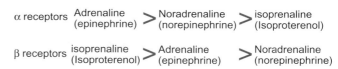

Fig. 9.9 Catecholamine receptors. Original division of catecholamine receptors (adrenoceptors) into α and β subtypes by Ahlquist (1948). Subsequently a more sophisticated classification (α_1, α_2, β_1, β_2 and β_3) has evolved. Beyond this further subdivisions are sometimes used.

cough in 10–30% of patients. Bradykinin is also an agonist on endothelial cells for the production of nitric oxide (Fig. 9.5). This is also thought to contribute to the hypotensive action of these drugs.

In the 1990s non-peptide angiotensin receptor blocking (ARB) drugs became available. These act on the AT_1 receptor and have a similar profile of action to ACEI except that bradykinin metabolism is not affected and the actions of Ang II on the AT_2 receptor are not blocked. The first clinically available drug in this class was losartan and this was followed by valsartan and a number of other drugs, all with names ending in -sartan.

Renin inhibitor drugs which block the enzymatic actions of renin have been developed and are now entering clinical use.

Adrenal medullary hormones

The human adrenal medulla produces a mixture of catecholamine hormones which is approximately 80% adrenaline (also known as epinephrine) and 20% noradrenaline (also known as norepinephrine). These two hormones are also released from sympathetic nerve endings although in this case the relative proportions are reversed and noradrenaline is the major component. The effects of the neuronally released hormones are much more significant in the control of circulatory function under normal physiological conditions than the effects of the hormones from the adrenal medulla. Chromaffin cell tumours, phaeochromocytomas, which are often, but not necessarily, in the adrenal medulla, secrete excessive amounts of adrenaline and noradrenaline which have marked effects on the cardiovascular system.

Receptors for catecholamines were originally divided into two types, α and β, classified on the basis of agonist potency as indicated in Figure 9.9. Subsequently, following the development of selective antagonist drugs, the receptor types were subdivided into α_1 and α_2, β_1, β_2 and β_3. Sometimes further subdivisions of this basic classification based on pharmacological and gene cloning studies are used.

The main receptor type on the heart is the β_1 receptor. Stimulation leads to an increase in the force and rate of cardiac contraction (see p. 45). The dominant catecholamine receptor on blood vessels is the α_1 receptor and this mediates vasoconstriction. In some parts of the peripheral circulation postsynaptic α_2 receptors also exist on vascular smooth muscle and stimulation leads to vasoconstriction.

Presynaptic α_2 receptors modulate the release of neuro-transmitters into the synaptic cleft. Thus, a rise in transmitter concentration in the synapse stimulates presynaptic α_2 receptors and shuts off further transmitter release. Blood vessels also have a limited distribution of β_1 and β_2 receptors which, when activated, lead to vasodilatation.

The dominant effects of excessive adrenal medulla activity or of exogenous adrenaline (epinephrine) are inotropic and chronotropic actions on the heart (β_1 receptor effects) and vasoconstriction on peripheral blood vessels (α_1 receptor effect). This is the basis for the use of drugs such as adrenaline in emergency situations involving circulatory collapse.

Interesting facts

The classification of catecholamine receptors into α and β subtypes was proposed by the Swedish pharmacologist Ahlquist in 1948. Further refinement of the classification followed later with the synthesis of selective blocking drugs and advances in gene cloning techniques.

Autonomic nervous system and peripheral circulation control

The autonomic nervous system has two branches, the sympathetic (SNS) and parasympathetic (PNS) nervous systems. Various attempts have been made to define the difference between SNS and PNS on either a functional or a chemical (neurotransmitter) basis. The only satisfactory definition, however, has an anatomical basis determined by where the nerves enter or leave the central nervous system.

Sympathetic nerves pass through the roots of spinal cord thoracic (T) and lumbar (L) segments. Specifically, this involves segments T_1 to L_2 and the SNS can be described as thoracolumbar in origin. The nerves emerging from the spinal cord (preganglionic nerves) are relatively short and form a synapse in a ganglion (a collection of nerve cell bodies outside the central nervous system). The postganglionic nerves are relatively long and run to the tissue being supplied.

Parasympathetic nerves originate in or enter the cranial (brain) segments III, VII, IX and X and the sacral segments (S2–S4) of the spinal cord. The PNS can, therefore, be described as being craniosacral in origin. Each of the branches of the autonomic nervous system has both sensory (afferent) and motor (efferent) functions.

The dominant vascular response to SNS activation is vasoconstriction mediated by α_1 receptors. Skeletal muscle and coronary blood vessels have a limited distribution of β_1 and β_2 receptors which exert a vasodilator effect but this is a minor response compared to α_1-mediated vasoconstriction even in these tissues. The existence of a sympathetic cholinergic nerve supply to blood vessels in skeletal muscle has been demonstrated in some experimental animals but is still a matter for conjecture in humans.

There is no parasympathetic nerve supply to most of the peripheral circulation as it is confined to erectile and secretory tissues. Activation of a PNS supply to blood vessels leads to vasodilatation as part of the erectile response in the genitalia. PNS induced vasodilatation also occurs in the pancreas and salivary glands as part of their secretory functions. In the pancreas vasoactive intestinal polypeptide (VIP) is a major neurotransmitter for the parasympathetic nerve supply.

In summary, the major characteristics of the nerve supply to blood vessels are that they are sympathetic in origin releasing noradrenaline (norepinephrine) onto α_1 receptors and resulting in vasoconstriction. Regulation of these nerves is further discussed in relation to blood pressure regulation in Chapter 10. A possible role for sympathetically induced vasoconstriction in patients with Raynaud's disease is discussed in the case history in Case 9.1:3.

Special circulations

The gross distribution of blood flow to the various parts of the body is discussed in Chapter 13. The regulation of some specific vascular beds is discussed here. Coronary blood flow regulation is described in Chapter 5.

Brain (cerebral) circulation

The brain receives about 15% of resting cardiac output, for the textbook 70 kg person a flow rate of about 750 mL/min. This is a relatively high flow rate as the brain, which typically weighs 1.4 kg in a textbook adult, only represents

Case 9.1 — Resistance blood vessels: 3

Problems with the calcium channel blocking drug

Sheila, discussed in Case 9.1:1 and 9.1:2, returned to her GP after two weeks of taking the prescribed nifedipine and told her that there was some good news but mainly bad news. The good news was that Sheila had not had problems with her blue, white and red fingers but the bad news was a series of other problems. Her face was always flushed and she seemed to have a continuous headache. On several occasions, she had felt dizzy and had to sit down. This had forced her to give up taking the nifedipine 3 days previously and the side effects had now disappeared.

This part of the history raises the following questions:

1. How is the blood flow to 'special circulations' such as the brain and skin regulated?
2. What is the explanation for the drug side effects experienced by Sheila?
3. What are the possible pathological consequences of sustained poor perfusion of tissues?

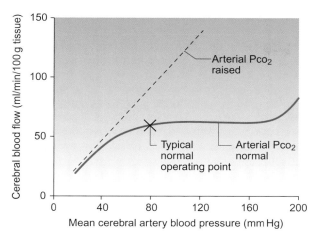

Fig. 9.10 Autoregulation of cerebral blood flow. Over an arterial pressure range between 60 and 175 mm Hg flow remains quite constant, provided arterial P_{CO_2} is within the normal range. Autoregulation breaks down when there is chronic CO_2 retention.

about 2% of body weight. Flow rate is substantially higher to the grey matter (mainly cell bodies) than to the white matter (mainly nerve axons) of the brain. The brain has a high oxygen consumption rate and a high heat generation rate. Interruption of the blood supply to the brain results in loss of consciousness within a few seconds and permanent damage within a few minutes.

A detailed discussion of the vascular anatomy of the brain is outside the scope of this book but is fundamental to the diagnosis and management of cerebrovascular problems. Two pairs of blood vessels, the basilar and internal carotid arteries, enter the cranium and anastomose beneath the optic chiasma to form the circle of Willis. The brain is supplied by branches from the circle of Willis, the anterior, middle and posterior cerebral arteries. Arterioles within the brain are quite short and so much of the vascular control occurs at the level of the small arteries.

Brain blood flow is autoregulated (Fig. 9.10) such that flow is kept fairly constant at about 55 mL/min/100 g tissue and this is independent of fluctuations in mean arterial pressure across the range 60–175 mm Hg. Although the brain has a rich sympathetic nerve supply, stimulation of these nerves makes little difference to autoregulation. However, the autoregulation mechanism is very sensitive to the P_{CO_2} of arterial blood. If a subject hyperventilates and therefore reduces arterial P_{CO_2}, then brain blood flow will decrease substantially. This is the reason behind the feeling of 'light headedness' following a period of voluntary hyperventilation. The autoregulation response is abolished by hypercapnia (high P_{CO_2}) and brain blood flow then increases in proportion to arterial pressure (Fig. 9.10). As the brain is encased in the cranium and cannot expand, retention of CO_2, as in chronic obstructive pulmonary disease, results in cerebral vasodilatation and raised intracranial pressure. The patient may therefore complain of headache. Increased metabolic activity in specific parts of the brain will lead to local increases in blood flow (functional hyperaemia).

As humans have an erect posture, the brain is above the level of the heart. Mean cerebral artery pressure is therefore typically of the order of 77 mm Hg. Figure 9.10 shows that if arterial pressure falls below about 50 mm Hg the autoregulation mechanism fails. If the perfusion pressure of the brain falls below about 40 mm Hg then syncope (fainting) occurs. Such a fall in blood pressure may occur as a result of a sudden drop in cardiac output (e.g. because of venous pooling of blood in the limbs) or because of excessive peripheral vasodilatation (e.g. because of the effects of a high ambient temperature). However, when fainting occurs in response to psychological stress associated with fear, pain or shock, the mechanisms are less well understood. In the period immediately before a faint the subject becomes pale and sweats profusely. They tend to hyperventilate, leading to hypocapnia, and then often yawn. Loss of consciousness follows a sudden increase in vagal outflow leading to a slowing of heart rate (bradycardia). This is accompanied by dilatation of peripheral vascular vessels, particularly in skeletal muscle. This is attributed to an inhibition of sympathetic vasoconstriction outflow which originates in the hypothalamus. This series of events is sometimes referred to as a 'vasovagal attack'.

Skeletal muscle blood flow

Under resting conditions, skeletal muscle receives about 20% of the cardiac output even though muscle accounts for 50% of body weight. Only a relatively small proportion, about one third, of capillaries are being fully perfused at any one time in resting muscle. Access of blood to the remaining capillaries is limited by the closure of precapillary sphincters. These sphincters have no nerve supply but are sensitive to changes in local metabolite concentration and so will open during exercise. Terminal arterioles are also dilated by metabolite accumulation. During vigorous exercise, muscle blood flow can increase more than 20-fold and may account for 80–90% of the increased cardiac output. This can mean an increase in muscle blood flow from about 1 L/min at rest to 20–22 L/min in intense exercise for the textbook person (see Chapter 13).

There is a rich sympathetic vasoconstrictor nerve supply to blood vessels in skeletal muscles. Under resting conditions, this maintains muscle blood flow at a relatively low level. Cutting the sympathetic nerves to a resting muscle leads to a doubling of blood flow. During exercise, the sympathetic vasoconstrictor nerves continue to be active but their effects on vascular tone are opposed by local accumulation of metabolites. Interstitial $[K^+]$ is particularly important as a metabolite in skeletal muscle. During muscle action potentials, K^+ ions leave the muscle and local interstitial fluid $[K^+]$ may rise from a resting value of about 4 mmol/L to as high as 9 mmol/L at the start of exercise before blood flow has fully increased. A concurrent rise in local osmolarity of up to 10% and a rise in inorganic [phosphate] also contribute to vascular regulation. The magnitude of any adenosine-mediated effects is related to the extent of local tissue hypoxia.

Skin (cutaneous) blood flow

Unlike tissues such as skeletal and cardiac muscle, the metabolic requirements of the skin for oxygen are fairly constant. Under resting conditions the skin, which weighs about 2 kg in the textbook person, has a blood flow of 200 mL/min or about 4% of cardiac output. Skin blood flow is regulated particularly by sympathetic vasoconstrictor nerves which are more profuse in some areas of the skin than in others. The skin of the hands and feet is more richly supplied than the trunk and limbs.

A major feature of the cutaneous circulation is its role in body temperature regulation. Heat loss is promoted by increasing the blood flow through capillary loops which run close to the surface of the skin. Shunting of blood towards or away from these capillary loops is achieved by opening and closing arteriovenous anastomoses, thick wall coiled vessels which link arterioles and veins in the skin. These anastomoses, together with cutaneous arterioles and veins, are controlled by the sympathetic nerve supply acting through α_1 receptors. Central control of these nerves originates in the hypothalamus, the location of the body's thermostat. Aspects of the regulation of skin blood flow in a person with Raynaud's disease are described in Box 9.1 in this chapter.

Kidney (renal) blood flow

Under resting conditions renal blood flow, at about 20–25% of cardiac output, is high compared to the size of the kidneys which only account for about 0.5% of body weight. Flow is autoregulated and is controlled particularly in relation to the need to maintain glomerular filtration rate (GFR).

The renal vasculature has an intense sympathetic vasoconstrictor nerve supply. At times of activation of the sympathetic nervous system, as in exercise (see Chapter 13) and during circulatory shock (see Chapter 14), renal blood flow is reduced substantially below resting levels. If this period of reduced blood flow is prolonged during circulatory shock situations and GFR is reduced, this may lead to pathological changes within the nephron (acute tubular necrosis—ATN) which can compromise patient survival.

Renal blood flow is not determined by metabolite effects. Indeed, with such a high resting blood flow rate, it is difficult to see how such a mechanism could function effectively.

Splanchnic blood supply

Under resting conditions the splanchnic blood supply (gastrointestinal tract and liver) receives about 24% of the

Box 9.1 Raynaud's syndrome

Skin blood flow is partially regulated by temperature; exposure to cold leads initially to vasoconstriction. In 1862 Raynaud described abnormalities of this mechanism, an exaggerated reaction which he attributed to overactivity of the sympathetic nervous system. This explanation still exists as a possibility today and some patients have been successfully treated by cutting the sympathetic nerve supply to the arms. However, the problem does not necessarily permanently resolve following sympathectomy and this treatment is now seldom used. Roles for other vasoconstrictor mechanisms, such as the endothelins, have also been proposed. It is suggested that at least part of the problem is not the result of an exaggerated initial response to cold but a failure to recover normally from cold exposure. Usually, skin blood returns to appropriate levels quite rapidly after cessation of cold exposure, but in patients with Raynaud's syndrome there is a delay.

Raynaud's syndrome is about ten times as common in women as in men. As in the case of Sheila in the previous case history boxes, the phenomenon may be exaggerated by stress, which also leads to activation of the sympathetic nervous system.

In some patients Raynaud's phenomena are an early feature of the autoimmune disease scleroderma. This is a problem for which the aetiology is unclear but it is associated with the excessive deposition of collagen and mucopolysaccharide in various parts of the body including the face. Later this may spread to the arms, legs and trunk. Within the cardiovascular system there is intimal fibrosis in small and medium-sized

arteries hence leading to diminished skin blood supply. Of the order of 10% of patients with Raynaud's phenomena will develop overt scleroderma but about 90% of patients with scleroderma have Raynaud's syndrome.

The colour changes which occurred in Sheila's hands following exposure to cold (blue, white and then red) can be explained as follows. The initial blue phase represents peripheral cyanosis associated with inappropriate vasoconstriction and sluggish blood flow. There is excessive deoxygenation of the available haemoglobin leaving higher than normal concentrations of deoxyhaemoglobin and hence cyanosis (see Chapter 1). Normally this is followed by metabolite-induced vasodilatation (red phase). In people displaying Raynaud's syndrome however there is a phase of intense vasoconstriction (white phase) in which there is insufficient blood flow to even give discernable cyanosis. Ultimately when the vasospasm is released, metabolite induced vasodilatation does occur (red phase) but there may also have been sufficient accumulation of metabolites to cause a pain response, perhaps mediated by the excessive release of pain mediating neurotransmitters.

With regard to therapy for mild cases of Raynaud's syndrome, treatment can be targeted at minimizing the problem by avoiding the cold, stopping smoking and dressing appropriately. This may include using gloves with a built-in heating mechanism. Use of a mixed α_1/α_2-adrenoceptor antagonist may be helpful. It is vitally important to avoid tissue necrosis leading to ulceration and gangrene.

cardiac output. The venous drainage from most of the gastrointestinal (GI) tract enters the hepatic portal vein and this supplies 70% of the hepatic blood flow. The remaining 30% is provided by the hepatic artery. During exercise and other situations when the baroreceptor reflex is activated, sympathetically mediated constriction of the veins and venules displaces blood from the splanchnic beds so that more blood volume is available for use in other parts of the circulation. This constriction which raises the local resistance to flow also contributes to the maintenance of arterial blood pressure.

The liver has a major role in drug metabolism and orally administered drugs which are absorbed in the gastrointestinal tract will be taken in the hepatic portal vein to the liver and subjected to 'first pass metabolism'. An anatomical point of pharmacological significance is that the venous drainage from the extreme ends of the GI tract, the buccal cavity and the anal canal, does not enter the hepatic portal vein. Drugs absorbed in these two regions of the GI tract are not therefore subject to first pass metabolism.

Lung blood flow

The lungs normally receive a blood flow which is the same as the cardiac output. During exercise, when there is an increase in cardiac output, lung vascular resistance must fall otherwise there would be a marked rise in pulmonary artery pressure. The fall in resistance is largely achieved by passive dilatation in response to any tendency to an increase in pressure. There is a sympathetic vasoconstrictor nerve supply to the lungs but the effects of increased sympathetic activity during exercise appear to be swamped by the passive dilatation effects.

An interesting aspect of the control of the lung circulation is hypoxic vasoconstriction. In regions of the lung which are poorly ventilated and fall below a threshold level of Po_2, vasoconstriction occurs. The oxygen sensor mechanism is located within the pulmonary smooth muscle, possibly in the mitochondria. A signal produced in this way activates a population of K^+ channels and, via a change in membrane potential, increases Ca^{++} entry and causes constriction of local pulmonary vascular smooth muscle.

Further reading

Born, G.V.R., Schwartz, C.J., 1997. Vascular Endothelium. Physiology, Pathology and Therapeutic Opportunities. Schattauer, Stuggart.

Braddock, M., Schwachtgen, J.-L., Houston, P., et al., 1998. Fluid shear stress modulation of gene expression in endothelial cells. News Physiol. Sci. 13, 241–246.

Hobbs, A.J., Higgs, A., Moncada, S., 1999. Inhibition of nitric oxide synthase as a potential therapeutic target. Annu. Rev. Pharmacol. Ther. 39, 191–220.

Kelm, M., 2002. Flow-mediated dilatation in human circulation: diagnostic and therapeutic aspects. Am. J. Physiol. 282, H1–H5.

Ledoux, J., Werner, M.E., Brayden, J.E., Nelson, M.T., 2006. Calcium activated potassium channels and the regulation of vascular tone. Physiology 21, 69–79.

Levick, J.R., 2009. An Introduction to Cardiovascular Physiology, fifth ed. Arnold, New York.

Pohl, U., de Wit, C., 1999. A unique role of NO in the control of blood flow. NIPS: News Physiol. Sci. 14, 74–80.

Tomita, T., Bolton, T.B., Bolton, T.B. (Eds.), 1996. Smooth Muscle Excitation. Academic Press, London.

Waller, D.G., Renwick, A.G., Hillier, K., 2009. Medical Pharmacology and Therapeutics, third ed. WB Saunders, Edinburgh.

Wolfe, J.H.N., 1992. ABC of Vascular Diseases. BMJ Books, London.

ARTERIAL BLOOD PRESSURE

10

Chapter objectives

After studying this chapter you should be able to:

1. Identify cardiac output and the peripheral resistance to blood flow as the major variables determining the dynamically generated arterial blood pressure.

2. Describe the central mechanisms regulating arterial blood pressure including the sensory inputs and the motor outputs via the autonomic nervous system which together make up the baroreceptor reflex.

3. Explain the background to the methods used for routine measurements of arterial blood pressure.

4. Understand the problems inherent in trying to establish what is a normal blood pressure and at what stage a diagnosis of hypertension is established.

5. Explain the major pathological effects of untreated hypertension.

6. Describe the actions of the major classes of drugs available for treating hypertension.

7. Discuss what is meant by hydrostatic pressure in the circulation and explain how it will vary with posture.

Introduction

Pressure developed in the arterial tree depends on the amount of blood being pumped into it, the cardiac output, and the resistance to blood flowing out of the arteries, the peripheral resistance. The resistance of the entire systemic circuit between the aortic valve in the left side of the heart and the right atrium where the blood returns to the heart is called the total peripheral resistance (TPR).

The relationship between the mean arterial blood pressure, cardiac output and resistance can be summarized as follows:

Mean arterial blood pressure (MABP) = Cardiac output (CO) × Total peripheral resistance (TPR)

This equation is directly analogous to Ohm's Law which is concerned with electrical current flow along a wire, i.e. $V = I \times R$. Blood pressure and voltage (V) represent the driving force (potential energy) to move blood or drive current flow. Cardiac output and current flow (I) are equivalent as are the two types of resistance.

A simple model of the arterial circulation is shown in Figure 10.1. Blood pressure can be regulated by changes in either cardiac output or the peripheral resistance.

Arterial blood pressure provides the driving force to perfuse the tissues of the body with blood. This driving force is dissipated as blood moves round the circulation and there is a continuous fall in pressure between the arteries and the right atrium (see Fig. 9.1). Mean aortic

pressure is typically about 95 mm Hg whereas right atrial pressure is about 0–5 mm Hg. Although the output of the heart is phasic, i.e. blood enters the circulatory system during cardiac systole and this ceases when the heart refills during diastole, circulation of blood around all the tissues of the body is continuous. This is driven by the head of pressure maintained in the arterial tree (see p. 86). Blood pressure in the arteries is pulsatile but by the time blood reaches the capillaries, where the important functions of the circulatory system take place, the pressure fluctuations have been damped out (see Fig. 9.1).

It is important that arterial pressure is maintained quite constant, as a fall in pressure below a critical level leads to underperfusion of the brain and the subject faints (see Chapter 9). A sustained rise in arterial blood pressure—hypertension—leads to the pathological changes in blood vessels described later in this chapter. Moment to moment fluctuations in arterial blood pressure are minimized by the baroreceptor reflex. This reflex is summarized in Figure 10.2.

An outline of a case history of a patient with hypertension is shown in Case 10.1:1.

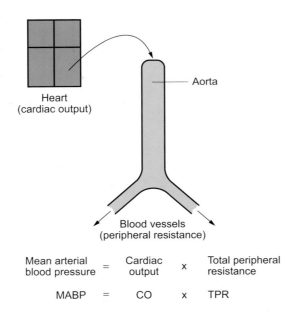

Mean arterial blood pressure = Cardiac output × Total peripheral resistance

MABP = CO × TPR

Fig. 10.1 Simple model of the circulation. Blood pressure in the arterial vessels (the driving force to push blood around the body) depends on the input of blood from the heart (cardiac output) and the resistance to outflow (total peripheral resistance).

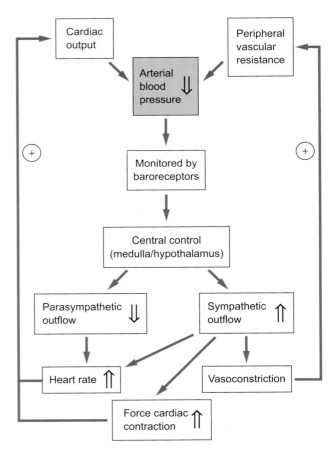

Fig. 10.2 The baroreceptor reflex. The response to a fall in arterial blood pressure is an increase in both cardiac output and peripheral resistance that will restore blood pressure.

The factors determining cardiac output have been discussed in Chapter 4. The essential features are that the heart has an intrinsic contractile rate which can be modified by the parasympathetic (vagus) nerve to slow the heart or by the sympathetic nerves to increase heart rate. The force of contraction of the heart and, therefore, the stroke volume is determined by a combination of preload effects (blood volume, venous return, venous tone), contractility effects (changes in myocyte [Ca^{++}] produced physiologically by sympathetic nerve stimulation) and afterload effects (mainly opposition to opening the aortic valve produced by the arterial blood pressure).

The factors determining peripheral blood vessel resistance to flow have been discussed in Chapter 9. Some of the mechanisms (metabolite, endothelial and local hormone effects) ensure an appropriate distribution of flow within tissues to match the local metabolic activity.

Case 10.1 Arterial blood pressure: 1

An insurance medical

Mr John Ames is a 45-year-old smoker who is overweight (body mass index 28) but he has been feeling well and has no symptoms of cardiovascular disease. He applied for life insurance cover and was referred for a medical examination. His blood pressure was found to be 188/106 mm Hg. Examination of the cardiovascular system showed no evidence of cardiac disease with no murmurs and with normal pulses all round. His GP arranged a blood test for serum fasting lipids (LDL and HDL cholesterol and triglycerides) and also to check renal function (urea, creatinine and electrolyte concentrations). A urine sample was checked using a dipstick test for glucose and protein. A renal ultrasound test to assess kidney size was arranged at the local hospital.

While waiting for the results of these tests to return the GP insisted that John should come to the surgery to have his blood pressure measured twice more by the practice nurse in the coming 10 days. The blood, urine and ultrasound tests all provided normal results but John's blood pressure was still high on the subsequent checks and the GP told him he had essential hypertension. A thiazide diuretic was prescribed. This history raises the following questions.

1. John was told he had essential hypertension. What does this mean? At what level of blood pressure elevation should therapy be considered?
2. Why was it important to check John's blood lipid levels?
3. What was the reason behind the repeated blood pressure measurements?
4. Why was John's renal function checked?
5. What does body mass index mean?

Aspects of the answers to these questions are to be found in the text of this chapter and in Box 10.1.

Adjustment of the overall resistance to maintain arterial blood pressure at a relatively constant level is achieved by the autonomic nerve supply to peripheral blood vessels. This has the fundamental characteristics that it is sympathetic in origin, using noradrenaline (norepinephrine) as the main neurotransmitter which, acting primarily through α_1-receptors, leads to vasoconstriction (see Chapter 9). Although there are parts of the circulation where one or other of these characteristics does not apply, these are very limited and specialized aspects of vascular control and are not major factors determining the total peripheral resistance.

In order to link all these components together we need a baroreceptor mechanism to continuously provide central control mechanisms in the brain with information about the current arterial blood pressure.

Interesting facts

In 1733 the Englishman, the Reverend Stephen Hales, made the first successful measurement of blood pressure by inserting a long glass tube into the carotid artery and jugular vein of a horse. Blood in the arterial cannula rose 2.92 metres up the tube, but in the venous cannula it was only 0.5 metres.

Arterial baroreceptors

Baroreceptors are actually modified nerve endings buried in the blood vessel wall. An increase in pressure within the vessel stretches the blood vessel wall and therefore distorts the nerve endings. This leads to the opening of ion channels and the generation of action potentials in the baroreceptor nerves. If the blood vessel is experimentally prevented from expanding in response to a change in internal pressure, then there is no change in action potential number. This demonstrates that the baroreceptor does not directly monitor pressure as such but rather pressure is sensed indirectly as stretch produced in blood vessel walls.

Anatomical location of baroreceptors

The location of the main arterial baroreceptors is shown in Figure 10.3.

The carotid sinus is a thin-walled dilatation of the internal carotid artery which occurs just after the bifurcation of the common carotid artery into the internal and external carotid arteries. The carotid sinus baroreceptor is a bundle of nerve fibres which is a part of the glossopharygeal (IX) cranial nerve.

The aortic arch baroreceptor is a part of the vagus (X) cranial nerve and the nerve endings are distributed in the wall of the aortic arch.

Information from these two groups of baroreceptors enters the brain at the level of the medulla.

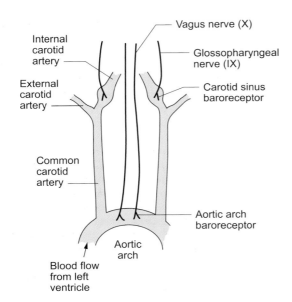

Fig. 10.3 Location of major arterial baroreceptors.

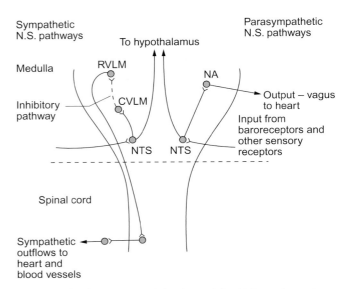

Fig. 10.4 Blood pressure regulation by medulla. Major pathways in medulla which are concerned with blood pressure regulation. CVLM = caudal ventrolateral medulla; NA = nucleus ambiguus; NTS = nucleus tractus solitarius; RVLM = rostral ventrolateral medulla.

Central control of the cardiovascular system

The view that the cardiovascular system is regulated from a 'vasomotor centre' located in the medulla is now obsolete. This concept implies an anatomically distinct part of the brain which could be demonstrated in a dissection room. In practice cardiovascular control involves interaction between diffuse parts of the medulla, hypothalamus, cerebral cortex and cerebellum.

The initial processing of information from the baroreceptors occurs in the nucleus tractus solitarius (NTS) in the medulla. The NTS has connections to the regions of the medulla which organize the outflow to the two divisions of the autonomic nervous system. The cell bodies of the preganglionic parasympathetic nerves, which slow heart rate, are located in the nucleus ambiguus and the dorsal motor nucleus. There are also neural connections from the NTS to the rostral ventrolateral medulla, a region of the brainstem controlling the sympathetic outflow to the heart (increases rate) and to the peripheral blood vessels (mainly leading to vasoconstriction). Figure 10.4 summarizes the main pathways in the medulla involved in the control of arterial blood pressure.

The hypothalamus functions effectively as the site within the brain which contains information about the 'set point' for arterial blood pressure i.e. what the pressure should normally be held at. The hypothalamus has a number of regions involved in cardiovascular control. The hypothalamic depressor area receives an input from the NTS. It is therefore informed about the arterial blood pressure and plays a very significant role in the baroreceptor reflex. The defence area of the hypothalamus plays a part in the cardiovascular responses to acute stress. The response to stress is an increase in heart rate and sympathetically mediated vasoconstriction particularly in the skin, the splanchnic (gut and liver) and the kidney

circulations. An acute rise in blood pressure occurs in response to stress which means that the normal baroreceptor reflex, which keeps blood pressure constant, has been overridden. The brain regions involved in this include the amygdala, part of the limbic system. The series of responses to acute stress, which include changes in blood pressure, has been given various names including the term 'alerting response'. The cardiovascular responses are reversed quite quickly when the perceived threat is removed.

A further function of the hypothalamus in vascular control relates to the fact that the temperature regulating area in the anterior hypothalamus controls the changes in skin blood flow which are part of the response to changes in body temperature.

The cerebellum is involved in the coordination of muscle movement in exercise and is also involved in the circulatory responses to exercise. Aspects of this are discussed in Chapter 13.

The baroreceptor reflex

A flow chart summarizing the baroreceptor reflex for the regulation of arterial blood pressure is shown in Figure 10.2. The responses to a fall in blood pressure are illustrated. The reflex response is an increase in heart rate, an increase in the force of cardiac contraction and an increase in peripheral vasoconstriction, all of which will help to restore blood pressure to normal levels. It has been said that regulation of heart rate is the primary role of the baroreceptor reflex and that responses leading to vasoconstriction and venoconstriction are of secondary importance.

The functional characteristics of the carotid sinus and aortic arch baroreceptors are essentially similar. Both consist of a mixture of large myelinated nerve fibres (A fibres) and a greater number of small, unmyelinated C fibres. The A fibres have a lower threshold response (30–90 mm Hg) than the C fibres (70–140 mm Hg). Thus, at normal pressures, A fibres are all stimulated to generate action potentials but only about a quarter of the C fibres are active. The A fibres reach a maximum firing rate before the C fibres. A generalization would therefore be that the myelinated A fibres are most important at normal pressure ranges but the C fibres become increasingly activated as pressure rises above the normal level. The arterial baroreceptors provide an input to the brain relaying pulse pressure, i.e. rate of change of pressure, as well as mean arterial pressure.

Baroreceptor reflex resetting occurs during the long-term rises in blood pressure known as hypertension and also during the changes in blood pressure which occur with increasing age. The site of these adaptive changes is in the central control mechanisms. The changes in baroreceptor function are a consequence of raised blood pressure rather than a primary cause of hypertension. Sensitivity of the baroreceptor mechanism may decrease when there are changes in the arterial wall compliance which sometimes occur as a consequence of atherosclerotic changes (see Chapter 8).

In humans, circulatory control mechanisms are dominated by the baroreceptor reflex but there are also other reflex responses which contribute to overall control.

Cardiopulmonary reflexes

Sensory inputs from receptors in the heart and lungs contribute to overall circulatory regulation. The receptors are located mainly, but not exclusively, on the low pressure side of the circulation. The effect of these reflexes under normal circumstances is thought to be to elicit a tonic (continuous) reduction in heart rate and to reduce peripheral vasoconstriction. Several different reflex mechanisms have been identified, some of which have opposing effects. They have been studied mainly in animals and their role in humans is poorly understood.

Groups of receptors located at the junction of the atria and the great veins effectively monitor blood volume. Approximately two thirds of blood volume is contained in the veins and changes in this volume will alter the stretch in the wall of the veins. This stretch is detected by myelinated vagal afferent nerves. In the control of blood volume this information is supplemented by an input from the arterial baroreceptors and by hormonally mediated changes in kidney function. An increase in blood volume leads to decreased secretion of antidiuretic hormone (ADH) and therefore a diuresis. Concurrently a decrease in renin secretion from the kidney leads to a decrease in aldosterone mediated sodium retention (see Chapter 9). An increase in the secretion of atrial natriuretic peptide

(ANP), released in response to increased atrial stretch, also contributes to a diuretic and natriuretic response. All of these endocrine responses to increased blood volume help to return blood volume to normal. There is also a neurally mediated component to the response. Increase in blood volume leads to reflex inhibition of sympathetic vasoconstriction within the kidney. The resulting vasodilatation leads to an increase in glomerular filtration rate (GFR) and contributes to the diuretic response. These hormonal mechanisms which regulate kidney function effectively control blood volume and therefore play a major role in the long-term control of arterial blood pressure (BP). The mechanisms for acute control of BP (primarily the baroreceptor reflex) are superimposed on this background.

Stretch receptors at the vena cava–right atrium junction provide the sensory component of the Bainbridge reflex. A rapid infusion of saline, and consequent stretch of the great veins, leads to a reflex increase in heart rate. This reflex would help to shift blood from a congested venous system through to the arterial side of the circulation. The reflex may be important in the early stages of exercise when the skeletal muscle pump first produces an increase in venous return (see Chapter 13).

Chemoreceptor reflexes

The aortic bodies and carotid bodies are chemoreceptors which are primarily involved in the control of lung ventilation but they also have a role in cardiovascular regulation. These peripheral chemoreceptors respond to changes in Po_2, Pco_2 and pH and their afferent nerves run with the nearby baroreceptor afferents to enter the brain at the medulla. Although the contribution of chemoreceptor reflexes to circulatory control under normal circumstances is small, under conditions of low arterial Po_2 (hypoxaemia) or high arterial Pco_2 (hypercapnia) they elicit a sympathetically driven vasoconstriction and an increase in heart rate. The physiological role of the chemoreceptor reflex is thought to be to protect brain blood flow when arterial blood pressure falls.

Measurement of arterial blood pressure

The first recorded measurement of arterial blood pressure was made in 1773 by the Reverend Stephen Hales. The measurement was made by direct cannulation of an artery in a horse. Although derivatives of this approach are still used in, for example, intensive care units or for experimental studies, direct artery cannulation is certainly not the basis for routine blood pressure measurements. Historically much effort was devoted to finding non-invasive methods. In 1896 the Italian physician Riva-Rocci produced a sphygmomanometer with an inflatable cuff. This heralded the modern method for blood pressure measurement, the auscultatory method developed by the Russian surgeon Korotkoff in 1905.

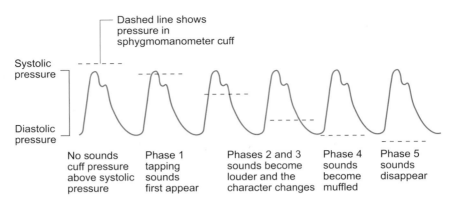

Fig. 10.5 Korotkoff sounds. Generation of Korotkoff sounds during measurement of arterial blood pressure using a sphygmomanometer cuff.

The fundamental physical principle used is the transition from laminar flow to turbulent blood flow in an artery. Laminar flow (see Chapter 8) is essentially silent but turbulent flow sets up vibrations in the blood vessel wall which can be heard using a stethoscope placed over the artery. These flow murmurs are known as Korotkoff sounds. The conditions for the development of turbulence are that it is more likely to develop when the flow velocity is high and when the tube has a large diameter.

During blood pressure measurement, the sphygmomanometer cuff is placed over an artery, usually the brachial artery in an upper arm, and inflated. When the pressure within the cuff exceeds the pressure in the artery, the blood vessel is compressed and no blood flow occurs (Fig. 10.5). The peak of the arterial pressure wave is called the systolic pressure. If the pressure in the cuff is allowed to fall slowly, eventually the point is reached at which the cuff pressure is slightly below the systolic pressure. At this peak of the pressure wave, the blood will flow, at increased velocity, through the still greatly narrowed section of blood vessel and emerge into the uncompressed section of downstream blood vessel. This is a situation in which turbulence will develop and Korotkoff sounds will be generated. Systolic pressure is recorded as the cuff pressure at which Korotkoff sounds are first heard (phase 1).

Interesting facts

The French physician Laennec invented the stethoscope in the early 19th century. His prototype was a tube of rolled up paper.

As the pressure in the cuff is allowed to fall further the vessel will only be completely occluded for progressively shorter periods of time (Fig. 10.5). Although Korotkoff sounds are still produced, the character of the sounds changes (phases 2 and 3). The problem now becomes to record the diastolic pressure, the trough pressure reached in the arterial tree. This pressure is reached just before the aortic valve reopens and a further volume of blood enters the arteries. The best correlation with direct (arterial cannulation) methods for blood pressure measurement is when the Korotkoff sounds become muffled (phase 4). This is often very difficult to discern, especially in an environment such as a hospital ward where there may be considerable background noise. Disappearance of the Korotkoff sounds (phase 5) is routinely used even though it occurs slightly below the true diastolic pressure. In some situations, for example sometimes in pregnancy when blood viscosity is reduced, the Korotkoff sounds do not disappear and so phase 4 (muffling) must be used to record diastolic pressure.

The upper part of the arm is normally used for blood pressure measurements. This is not just a convenient appendage to wrap the cuff around with a convenient artery, the brachial artery, in which to listen for Kortkoff sounds. Using the upper arm means that the pressure is recorded at the level of the heart, a useful reference point.

Mercury in glass manometers have traditionally been used to record blood pressures. This is of course the reason for the convention of recording blood pressure in units of millimetres of mercury (mm Hg). Pressure is determined as the height of the column of mercury in the manometer tube. Concerns regarding possible safety hazards associated with mercury have led to the progressive adoption of alternative pressure recording devices. However, the fundamental principle of generating Korotkoff sounds in order to record systolic and diastolic pressures remains unchanged.

Mean arterial blood pressure is often calculated. Because of the shape of the arterial pressure wave (Fig. 10.6) mean pressure is not the same as the average of the systolic and diastolic pressures. The mean pressure through the duration of the arterial pressure wave is weighted more towards the diastolic pressure. A convenient way to calculate mean arterial blood pressure (MABP) is therefore:

$$\text{MABP} = \frac{(\text{systolic pressure}) + (2 \times \text{diastolic pressure})}{3}$$

This is the same as the alternative formula:

$$\text{MABP} = 1/3 \text{ systolic pressure} + 2/3 \text{ diastolic pressure.}$$

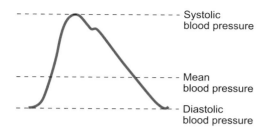

Fig. 10.6 Mean arterial blood pressure. Because of the shape of the arterial pressure wave, mean pressure is closer to the diastolic pressure than to systolic pressure.

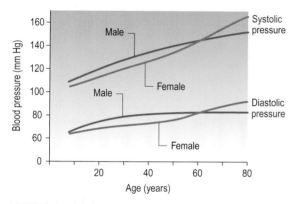

Fig. 10.7 Relationship between age and arterial blood pressure in males and females.

Normal arterial pressure

A typical 'normal' blood pressure measurement is often quoted as 120/80 mm Hg (systolic/diastolic). While this value is appropriate for the textbook subject (male, 20–25 years old weighing 70 kg), it is not appropriate for the entire population. There is firstly a gender-related difference. Considering large population groups, blood pressures in premenopausal females are a little (5–10 mm Hg) lower than in males. There are also changes in blood pressure with age with lower than 'textbook' values in children (see Chapter 12) and higher pressures in older people (Fig. 10.7).

Acute rises in arterial pressure occur frequently in normal people. These may happen in response to stress or even events such as having a full bladder. During sexual intercourse systolic blood pressure may sometimes rise towards 300 mm Hg. After short term acute fluctuations blood pressure will return to basal levels, normally without any pathological damage occurring.

The fact that blood pressure is labile and that there are age and gender related differences in blood pressure clouds the issue over defining what normal blood pressure is and therefore what constitutes an abnormally high pressure, i.e. hypertension.

Hypertension

There is a continuous spectrum of arterial blood pressures within the population. It is not a bimodal distribution with one group in whom blood pressure is 'normal' and a clear dividing line to the 'abnormal' pressure group. There is disagreement as to whether systolic pressure or diastolic pressure is the most important indicator for a decision to initiate treatment for hypertension. There is also no clear internationally agreed definition as to what constitutes hypertension. Effectively it is a question of making a judgement about whether blood pressure is sufficiently high to be likely to result in significant end-organ damage. Initiating treatment with drugs carries with it its own set of risks and side effects. The pragmatic definition of hypertension advanced in 1971 by Professor Geoffrey Rose is still appropriate, i.e. 'that level of blood pressure above which investigation and treatment do more good than harm'.

There are various sets of guidelines which suggest when treatment for raised blood pressure should be initiated. One such set of guidelines was published by the British Hypertension Society in 2004. It suggests that antihypertensive drug therapy should certainly be initiated in anyone with a systolic blood pressure >160 mm Hg or a diastolic pressure >100 mm Hg. In people with systolic pressures between 140 and 159 mm Hg or diastolic pressures between 90 and 99 mm Hg other factors must be part of the decision to treat. These other factors include evidence of damage to tissues such as the cerebral circulation, the heart or kidneys and also whether the patient is diabetic. The pathological consequences which result from hypertension are discussed later in this chapter. Where evidence of end organ damage exists, treatment should be started at the lower ranges of blood pressure outlined above. Note that this is only a brief illustrative summary of some much more complex recommendations. Other sets of guidelines have been published by the World Health Organization (WHO) together with the International Society of Hypertension (ISH) and also by the European Society of Hypertension (ESH).

The prevalence of 'mild hypertension' within the population changes with age. In Europe and the USA it is approximately 2% in the under 25 year old group and rises to 25% in the 50–59 year old group and to 50% in the 70+ year old group. 'Malignant or accelerated hypertension' is fortunately rare. In this case patients may present with uncontrolled hypertension and blood pressures perhaps in excess of 220/120 mm Hg. It is vitally important to initiate treatment immediately in this group.

Interesting facts

Despite the widespread recognition that high blood pressure is 'bad for you', it is still impossible to provide a universally acceptable quantitative definition of hypertension.

Box 10.1 Plasma lipids and body mass index

Lipoproteins are the form in which lipids circulate in the blood. Triglycerides and cholesterol are absorbed from the gut into the lymphatic system of the intestinal villi in the form of chylomicrons and reach the circulation via the thoracic duct (see Chapter 11). In muscle and adipose tissue the triglycerides are hydrolysed by lipoprotein lipase and absorbed into the tissues. The residue of the chylomicrons which includes cholesterol is taken up by the liver. Further cholesterol is synthesized by the liver itself, a process for which the activity of the enzyme hydroxymethylglutaryl coenzyme A reductase (HMG CoA reductase) is the rate limiting step. The use of 'statin' drugs which block this enzyme and therefore reduce circulating cholesterol lipid levels is widely advocated to reduce the risk of atherosclerosis related cardiovascular disease.

The 'endogenous pathway' shuttles lipids between the liver and peripheral tissues, thus creating a family of lipid–protein complexes. Low density lipoprotein (LDL) contains mainly cholesterol esters and uptake into tissues is mediated by LDL receptors. High levels of LDL increase the risk of cardiovascular disease. Conversely high density lipoprotein (HDL) functions to remove cholesterol from tissues and so cardiovascular risk is inversely related to the HDL levels. The beneficial effects of statin drugs include reduction of circulating LDL cholesterol and a modest rise in HDL.

Body mass index (BMI) is calculated as the weight (in kilograms) divided by the height (in metres) squared. It is frequently used as an index to define obesity. The normal range for BMI is 19–24.9 and 25–29.9 is considered to be overweight.

A figure greater than 30 is considered to be obese. John would therefore be considered overweight but not quite obese. Obesity is a risk factor for cardiovascular disease.

One of the problems of managing hypertension is in deciding whether the patient truly has raised blood pressure, especially as hypertension is often asymptomatic until end-organ damage becomes apparent. A proportion of patients have a higher blood pressure when it is measured in a clinic or surgery than when going about their daily life. It is clearly the blood pressure which the subject has for most of their daily life, rather than the short time spent in a doctor's surgery, which is the relevant figure to consider. To gain more information, blood pressure may be monitored throughout the day by using ambulatory blood pressure monitoring (ABPM) devices. A significant difference between clinic and ABPM recorded pressures is called 'white-coat hypertension' or 'isolated office hypertension'. Interestingly, patients with white coat hypertension, although their blood pressure is normal during most of their daily lives, are at higher risk of adverse cardiovascular events than patients whose blood pressure is normal in the surgery.

Mechanisms of hypertension

$$\text{Mean arterial blood pressure} = \text{Cardiac output} \times \text{Total peripheral resistance}$$

All forms of established hypertension are primarily associated with an increase in the resistance to blood flow. There may be changes in cardiac output in the early stages of the development of some forms of hypertension but, fundamentally, raised resistance in the arterioles is the basic mechanism for established hypertension. Nevertheless, drugs which act by reducing cardiac output may be used therapeutically to reduce blood pressure.

There are some forms of raised arterial pressure, mainly involving renal or endocrine disorders, for which it is possible to attribute a mechanism based on disturbances of known physiological mechanisms. These include several forms of renal disease (linked to increased activity of the renin-angiotensin system), phaeochromocytoma (linked to raised adrenal medulla catecholamine secretion) and Conn's syndrome (linked to raised adrenal cortex aldosterone secretion). When all of these mechanisms of hypertension with a physiologically definable cause are put together they only account for about 5% of the total hypertensive population. The remaining 95% of hypertensive people are said to have essential (or idiopathic) hypertension. In this group there is no single definable mechanism but there have been a large number of theories put forward.

Interesting facts

Although hypertension affects about a quarter of adults in the Western world, we can still only provide a suggestion of the altered physiological mechanism involved in about 5% of cases. This group of patients have 'secondary hypertension'. The remaining 95% are described as essential hypertensives.

There is evidence that essential hypertension may be associated with a reduction in the number of nephrons within the kidneys. How precisely this links to peripheral vasoconstriction is not entirely clear. A possibility is that reduced renal function leads to a failure to adequately excrete a sodium load. This could trigger the release of a hypothalamic natriuretic peptide which has a cardiac glycoside structure. This is variously described as a digoxin-like or ouabain-like glycoside. As with the action of digoxin on the heart (see Chapter 4), the hormone inhibits Na^+/K^+-ATPase. In the smooth muscle cell membrane there is also a Na^+/Ca^{++} passive exchange co-transporter (see Chapter 9). This is driven by the $[Na^+]$ gradient across the membrane, with Na^+ moving into the cell and Ca^{++} moving out. Inhibition of the Na^+/K^+-ATPase would lead to increased intracellular $[Na^+]$ and hence reduced Ca^{++} extrusion from the cell. Such an action on vascular smooth muscle would raise intracellular $[Ca^{++}]$, promote contraction and hence raise the peripheral resistance. Other popular mechanisms for the pathogenesis of hypertension

Case
10.1 Arterial blood pressure: 2

Initially John was advised to lose weight, give up smoking and take more regular exercise. Over the next 6 months he joined a gym, managed to lose a significant amount of weight and gave up smoking. However over this period of time his BP fluctuated between 155 and 180 systolic and 85 and 95 diastolic.

Although John was feeling more healthy, the GP was concerned that his blood pressure was still not adequately controlled. A beta-blocker was therefore added to the prescribed diuretic. However this made John feel lethargic and tired. He was changed to slow release nifedipine (a calcium channel antagonist). Whilst this move effectively controlled John's BP he found that he did get more frequent headaches whilst taking the drug. A further change in medication was made and he was switched to the ACEI drug enalapril supplemented with the thiazide diuretic bendroflumethazide. A check was made of his renal function profile after 5 days' medication.

John found that he tolerated the enalapril well and had no problems with it. His BP was well controlled with systolic pressure generally in the range 140–155 mm Hg and diastolic pressure below 95 mm Hg. The drugs prescribed for John raise the following questions:

1. Why was John unable to tolerate the side effects of beta-blocker therapy?
2. Why should nifedipine give John a problem with headache?
3. How do angiotensin converting enzyme inhibitors lower blood pressure and why was it important to check renal function after a period of 5 days on the drug?

Answers to these questions are to be found in the text of this chapter and in Chapter 9 (p. 106).

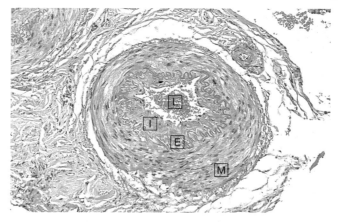

Fig. 10.8 Structure of a small artery from a patient with benign hypertension. The smooth muscle in the media (M) has undergone hypertrophy. The intima (I) and the elastic lamina (E) have become thickened. The lumen (L) is reduced in size. (Source: Stevens A, Lowe J. 2000.)

include some aspect of overactivity of the renin-angiotensin system or the sympathetic nervous system. No one mechanism can currently explain all of the experimental data. Essential hypertension in any one individual may eventually prove to be the cumulative effect of a number of genetic, lifestyle and environmental factors.

Pathological consequences of raised arterial pressure

Worldwide, hypertension is estimated to cause 7.1 million premature deaths per year. Longstanding essential hypertension results in left ventricular hypertrophy. In this 'pressure-overload' effect on the heart additional sarcomeres are added in parallel to the original sarcomeres (see Chapter 2). However hypertrophy may progress to congestive failure with dilatation of the heart. This 'volume overload' means additional sarcomeres are added in series. Changes in the architecture of the heart which involve both the myocytes and the extracellular matrix are referred to as remodelling (see Chapter 6).

Hypertension is a risk factor for the development of atherosclerosis (see Chapter 9) and will accelerate its development in large arterial blood vessels. However, the structure of the lesions produced is the same as in normotensive subjects. In addition there are changes in the vascular wall which are selective responses to hypertension. These include thickening of the media layer of muscular arteries as a result of smooth muscle hyperplasia and collagen deposition. The latter changes occur in small arteries and arterioles rather than the large vessels affected by atherosclerosis (Fig. 10.8).

Small arterial and arteriolar blood vessels within the kidney show intimal proliferation and deposition of large proteins such as fibrinogen, a process known as hyalinization, in the media layer. These pathological changes lead to nephron loss and the ultimate development of chronic renal failure. The nephron loss leads to exacerbation of the hypertension, a vicious circle.

Other vascular disorders associated with hypertension include intracerebral haemorrhage, dissecting aneurysm of the aorta and subarachnoid haemorrhage due to the rupture of berry aneurysms (see Chapter 8). Globally, data suggest that about 62% of cerebrovascular disease and 49% of ischaemic heart disease can be attributed to inadequate management of hypertension. However, in patients with hypertension 80% of strokes are caused by intra-arterial thrombosis or embolism from the heart or large arteries. Intuitively one might expect hypertension to be linked to haemorrhagic events as a cause of stroke, but in fact this represents only 20% of the total.

Endothelial dysfunction is characteristic of hypertension and also many other disease mechanisms associated with altered vascular function. The changes in the endothelium appear to be a response to hypertension rather than a cause of hypertension linked to reduced production of vasodilator mediators (nitric oxide or prostacyclin) or increased production of a vasoconstrictor (endothelins).

Treatment of hypertension

Treatment strategies for essential hypertension cannot be directly targeted at the disordered physiological mechanism because it is unknown. Good management includes the use of non-drug based methods. Weight reduction, reduced salt intake, limiting alcohol intake, increasing physical exercise, increasing fruit and vegetable consumption and reducing total fat and saturated fat intake are all thought to help to lower arterial blood pressure. Furthermore, failure to adopt these lifestyle changes may limit the response to antihypertensive drugs. Attention must also be given to other cardiovascular risk factors, smoking, control of diabetes and blood lipid levels. The use of statin drugs to reduce hepatic cholesterol synthesis should be considered. However, the extent to which blood pressure can be reduced purely by lifestyle changes is limited.

A considerable range of drugs is available to reduce blood pressure and a detailed discussion of these is outside the scope of this book. Individually each drug will only produce fairly modest (5–15 mm Hg) reductions in blood pressure and so combinations of different classes of drugs may be necessary to achieve adequate blood pressure control. Common strategies include the use of beta-blockers and/or thiazide diuretics as first line treatments. More recently, calcium channel blocking drugs (also called calcium antagonists) have been added to this list and angiotensin converting enzyme inhibitors (ACEI) (see Chapter 9) also have their advocates as first line drugs. Brief further details of all these groups of drugs is shown below.

Thiazide diuretics, e.g. bendroflumethiazide (bendrofluazide)

The initial diuretic response is produced by inhibition of a Na/Cl co-transporter on the lumenal membrane of the distal tubule of the nephron. Compensatory activation of the renin-angiotensin-aldosterone axis however limits salt and water depletion as a basis for blood pressure lowering. Longer term hypotensive actions of these 'diuretic' drugs come from direct effects on Ca^{++} entry into vascular smooth muscle.

Other diuretics such as the loop diuretic furosemide (frusemide) and the potassium sparing diuretics spironolactone, amiloride and triamterene, which block the sodium retaining actions of aldosterone, can also be used to help lower blood pressure but are not normally used as first line drugs.

Beta-blockers, e.g. atenolol (β_1 selective) propranolol (β_1/β_2 non-selective)

Beta-blockers have a number of pharmacological actions. Reductions in heart rate and myocardial contractility through actions on β_1 receptors lead to a decrease in cardiac output (see Chapter 4). Blockade of juxtaglomerular cell β receptors in the afferent arteriole of the kidney suppresses the secretion of renin. In addition to their role as antihypertensive agents, beta-blockers have other beneficial effects in relation to heart disease (see Chapter 6). β-adrenoceptor blocking drugs have a wide range of side effects. These include tiredness, exercise limitation, dizziness, nausea, anorexia and bradycardia. In patients with asthma the use of a β_1 selective drug is preferable as a non-selective β_1/β_2 blocker may contribute to bronchoconstriction.

Calcium channel blocking drugs, e.g. nifedipine, verapamil and diltiazem

These drugs block the entry of Ca^{++} ions into voltage gated (L-type) calcium channels in vascular smooth muscle (see Chapter 9) and hence reduce the peripheral resistance. Nifedipine and structurally related drugs are mainly used in hypertension management. As these calcium channels exist in a number of tissues there are predictable side effects. They may include headache (cerebral vasodilatation), and constipation due to effects on gut wall smooth muscle. Some calcium channel blocking drugs also have a negative inotropic action on the heart (see Chapter 4).

Angiotensin converting enzyme inhibitors (ACEI)

These compounds, together with the more recently developed angiotensin receptor blockers (ARB), have been discussed in Chapter 9. In addition to their blood pressure lowering vasodilator effects and their mild diuretic actions, they have beneficial effects in relation to the prevention of fibrotic changes in the heart and slowing the progression of renal disease (renoprotective actions).

Other antihypertensive drugs

Alpha-blockers (e.g. prazosin, doxazosin) reduce sympathetic tone and therefore dilate both arteriolar and venous blood vessels. This reduces the peripheral resistance directly but also reduces cardiac output by an effect on the preload of the heart. A potential side effect of α_1 receptor blockade is postural hypotension as a result of venodilation.

Imidazoline I_1 receptors are concentrated in the medulla of the brain in areas concerned with the central regulation of arterial blood pressure (see p. 116). Moxonidine is a drug which blocks imidazoline I_1 receptors and hence decreases sympathetic outflow and increases vagal tone.

The centrally acting α_2-adrenoceptor agonists such as methyldopa and clonidine now have only limited use as blood pressure lowering drugs. They reduce sympathetic outflow by actions in the medulla, particularly on the nucleus tractus solitarius (NTS) (see p. 116).

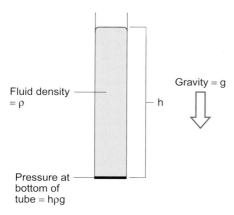

Fig. 10.9 Hydrostatic pressure in a glass tube. Pressure at the bottom of the tube depends on the height of the fluid column, the density of the fluid and gravity.

Hydrostatic pressure in the circulation

So far we have been considering pressure in the arterial system as being 'dynamically' generated through an interaction between the pumping action of the heart and the resistance to blood flowing out of the arterial tree.

Mean arterial blood pressure
= Cardiac output × Total peripheral resistance

Or:

$$MABP = CO \times TPR$$

We also need to consider a second type of pressure, often referred to as a 'hydrostatic' pressure, generated simply by the height of a column of blood. This is illustrated in Figure 10.9. Pressure at the bottom of a tube containing a fluid depends on the height of the column of fluid (h), the density of the fluid (ρ) and gravity (g). Pressure = $h\rho g$.

The circulatory system also has tubes containing a fluid and the hydrostatic fluid pressure generated is illustrated in Figure 10.10. Thus, in an upright person, the actual pressure in an artery in the ankle will be the sum of the 'dynamic' pressure (mean approximately 95 mm Hg) generated by the pumping action of the heart and the 'hydrostatic' pressure (about 90 mm Hg) produced by the height of the column of blood from the level of the tricuspid valve in the heart (the notional zero point) to the feet. This gives a total ankle artery pressure of about 185 mm Hg in an upright person. Note: the density of mercury is 13.6 times the density of water. Thus, as the convention is to express blood pressures in units of mm Hg, a column of 13.6 mm of blood will exert a pressure of 1 mm Hg. (This assumes that the density of blood is the same as the density of water.)

On the venous side of the circulation, consideration of the impact of the hydrostatic pressure gradient is a little more complicated. If we imagine a person suspended by a

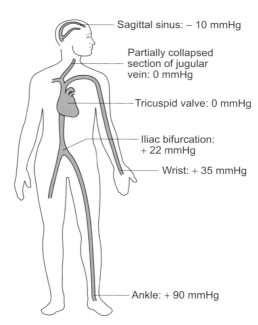

Fig. 10.10 Hydrostatic pressures within the human circulation.

harness under the armpits, so that their feet are off the floor and there is no need for skeletal muscle contraction in the legs, hydrostatic pressure in the veins of the feet would be similar to the arterial side of the circulation. However, skeletal muscle contraction in the legs compresses the veins, an important aspect of maintaining venous return to the heart (see Chapter 4). The column of blood in the venous system is therefore separated into shorter lengths and so, during walking, the effective hydrostatic pressure in the veins of the ankle might only be about 25 mm Hg.

In an upright person, if the hydrostatic pressure at the right atrium (tricuspid valve) is zero (i.e. the same as atmospheric pressure), pressure in the jugular vein, which is above the heart, is negative. The jugular vein is therefore partially collapsed and has an oval cross-section in the normal upright person. It is only when pressure rises in the jugular, as in heart failure (see Chapter 6), that the jugular vein becomes visible. This is the basis for using the height of the column of blood inflating the jugular vein as an index of right atrial pressure. Pressure in the sagittal sinus (just under the top of the cranium) in an upright normal person is about −10 mm Hg.

Hydrostatic pressures in the circulation change markedly with changes in posture. In a supine person the maximum hydrostatic pressure in the circulation would change from about 90 mm Hg (upright) to only a few mm Hg (horizontal). Moving from a supine to an erect posture requires the activation of reflexes which oppose venous pooling of blood in the lower half of the body. This involves sympathetically mediated venoconstriction, particularly in the small veins.

As the hydrostatic pressure in the veins depends on the effect of gravity (hydrostatic pressure = $h\rho g$), there has been considerable interest in the effects of higher gravitational forces on the circulatory system. This is particularly important in the context of space flight and for the pilots of fighter aircraft making fast changes in direction. In a normal 'inside' turn there will be an increased gravitational force towards the feet. Venous pooling can be prevented in this case by using a G-suit, a tightly fitting garment which opposes expansion of the lower half of the body. Although these considerations of space travel and fighter planes may not affect the majority of the population, a considerable number of people do try bungee jumping. In this case, during the initial dive head-first, the hydrostatic pressure in the lower half of the body will increase with a corresponding decrease in the upper part of the body. Blood volume will be pooled in the lower half of the body and venous return to the heart will fall. As the major baroreceptors are located in the upper part of the body in the carotid sinus and aortic arch (see section on arterial baroreceptors in this chapter), this will contribute to the already excitement induced fast heart rate. However, once the fall is increasingly restrained by the elastic properties of the 'ropes', the person will rapidly decelerate but the hydrostatic pressure in the top half of the body will increase as the blood moves up the circulatory system. This will tend to bring about a rapid fall in heart rate.

Further reading

Beevers, G., Lip, G.Y.H., O'Brien, E., 2007. ABC of Hypertension, fifth ed. BMJ Books, London.

Donnelly, R., London, N.J.M., 2009. ABC of Arterial and Venous Disease, second ed. BMJ Books, London.

ESH/ESC Hypertension Guidelines Committee, 2003. Practice guidelines for primary care physicians. J. Hypertens. 21, 1779–1786.

Field, M., Pollock, C., Harris, D., 2010. The Renal System, second ed. Churchill Livingstone, Edinburgh.

Gallagher, P.J., 2009. Cardiovascular system. In: Underwood, J.C.E., Cross, S.S. (Eds.) General and Systematic Pathology, fifth ed. Churchill Livingstone, Edinburgh.

JBS 2: Joint British Societies' guidelines on prevention of cardiovascular disease in practice, 2005. Heart 91 (Suppl. V): v1–v52.

Levick, J.R., 2009. An Introduction to Cardiovascular Physiology, fifth ed. Arnold, London.

Marcia, G., Mark, A.L., 1983. Arterial baroreflexes in humans. In: Shepherd, J.T., Abboud, F.M. (Eds.) Handbook of Physiology. American Physiological Society, Bethesda.

Sagawa, K., 1983. Baroreflex control of systemic arterial pressure and vascular bed. In: Shepherd, J.T., Abboud, F.M. (Eds.) Handbook of Physiology. American Physiological Society, Bethesda.

Stevens, A., Lowe, J., 2000. Pathology, second ed. Mosby, Edinburgh.

Waller, D.G., Renwick, A.G., Hillier, K., 2009. Medical Pharmacology and Therapeutics, third ed. WB Saunders, Edinburgh.

Williams, B., Poulter, N.R., Brown, M.J., et al., 2004. British Hypertension Society guidelines for hypertension management 2004 (BHS-IV) summary. BMJ. 328, 634–640.

World Health Organization (WHO), 2003. International Society of Hypertension (ISH) statement on management of hypertension. J. Hypertens. 21, 1983–1992.

CAPILLARY FUNCTION AND THE LYMPHATIC SYSTEM

11

Chapter objectives

After studying this chapter you should be able to:

1. Describe the general structure of capillaries and identify the structural variations found in continuous, fenestrated and discontinuous capillaries.

2. Outline how the molecular size and lipid solubility of solutes influence the route by which they can cross capillary walls.

3. Explain the fundamental concepts behind the terms osmotic pressure, colloid osmotic pressure (oncotic pressure) and hydrostatic pressure.

4. Explain how hydrostatic and osmotic pressure gradients determine the distribution of water between the intracellular and extracellular compartments of the body.

5. Describe the physiological and clinical roles of macromolecules (colloids) in moving water from the interstitial fluid compartment into the circulation.

6. List the functions of the lymphatic system including its role as a tissue drainage pathway.

7. Discuss how disturbances of body water distribution, i.e. intracellular and extracellular oedema, can arise as a consequence of disease mechanisms.

Structure of capillaries

Aspects of the structure of capillaries are discussed, along with the other types of blood vessel, in Chapter 1. A diagram of a microcirculatory unit is shown in Figure 1.9. A capillary is a tube made up of a single layer of endothelial cells surrounded by a basement membrane. Capillaries have a lumen diameter in the range of 3–8 μm. As red cells have a diameter of about 8 μm they must deform to pass through capillaries. During passage along the 0.5–1.0 mm length of a capillary there is a volume of trapped plasma in between successive red cells. This flow pattern is known as bolus flow. Between adjacent endothelial cells there are gaps (pores or clefts) of varying size which contribute substantially to the permeability characteristics of the capillary wall. However, capillary structures are not all identical and three main types have been identified. These are designated continuous, fenestrated and discontinuous capillaries. It must be remembered that there are discrete variations in structure and function even within these three broad types of capillary.

Interesting facts

With the development of early microscopes in the 17th century, the Italian Malpighi was able to see capillary blood vessels for the first time.

Continuous capillaries (Fig. 11.1) are the least permeable group and they are found in skin, muscle, lungs, adipose tissue and the nervous system. They are the most widely distributed type of capillary. They have tight junctions in between adjacent endothelial cells which only allow the passage of relatively small molecules (Mr < 10 000). Larger molecules are thought to cross endothelial cells via the extensive invaginations (caveolae) which cover both surfaces of endothelial cells. Caveolae are linked to the formation of vesicles which can cross the cells transporting larger molecules. An intact basement membrane, which consists mainly of collagen, surrounds the endothelial tube. Pericytes partially surround the capillary and provide support. In some circumstances they are contractile and may be relaxed by nitric oxide generated in the endothelial cells (Chapter 9). Even within the classification of 'continuous' capillary endothelia there are considerable variations in structure and function. The least leaky capillaries are found in the brain (see p. 109).

Fenestrated capillaries (Fig. 11.2A) are much more permeable to water than continuous endothelia and they are found in tissues that have a high transcapillary water flux. These include the glomerulus of the kidney, intestinal villi and the choroid plexus of the brain (the site of cerebrospinal fluid formation). There are fenestrae (round holes) in the endothelial cells which have a diameter of 50–60 nm. The fenestrae are not generally completely open holes but are covered by a very thin diaphragm which is derived from the glycocalyx. Viewed from the

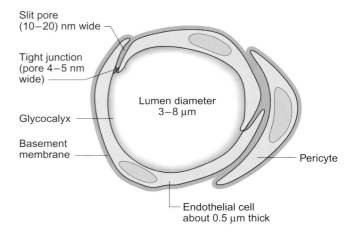

Fig. 11.1 Structure of a continuous capillary. Tight junctions between cells determine capillary permeability. Pericytes surround part of the capillary wall and provide support.

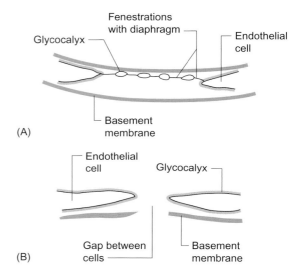

Fig. 11.2 Structure of junctions between adjacent endothelial cells. (A) Fenestrated capillary wall. In the fenestrae there is a thin diaphragm configured like a miniature cartwheel. The basement membrane is intact. (B) Discontinuous capillary wall. These have relatively large gaps in between cells (c. 100 nm) and an incomplete basement membrane.

blood side of the capillary, these diaphragms are said to resemble a cartwheel-like structure with 14 wedge-shaped gaps. As with continuous capillaries, fenestrated capillaries have an intact basement membrane.

Discontinuous capillaries (Fig. 11.2B) are found in tissues such as bone marrow, liver and spleen where there is a need for red blood cells to enter or leave the circulation. There are gaps, which may be over 100 nm in diameter, in between adjacent endothelial cells and an incomplete basement membrane which also has gaps in it. Red cells have a diameter of about 8000 nm (8 μm) but they can deform to pass through quite small holes.

Interesting facts

Capillary diameter is approximately 3–8 μm and red cell diameter is about 8 μm. The red cells deform to pass through the effectively rigid blood vessels.

Movement of substances across capillary walls

Capillary walls act as a 'semipermeable' membrane. Electrolytes and small lipophilic molecules cross the wall much more easily than plasma proteins. Solute transfer mechanisms can be divided into three broad groups on the basis of the physical characteristics of the solute.

1. Small lipid-soluble molecules, a group which includes oxygen, carbon dioxide and some drugs such as anaesthetic agents, can diffuse through the lipid bilayer which forms the plasma membrane of the endothelial cells. They can therefore cross almost the entire surface area of a capillary.

2. Small lipid-insoluble ions and molecules cannot easily cross cell membranes and so passage across capillary walls is confined to water-filled channels in between or through cells. There is a layer of negatively charged macromolecules (the glycocalyx) which covers the endothelial cells and lines the water filled channels. This also contributes to the permeability characteristics of the capillary wall. Small charged species (Na^+, K^+, Cl^-, etc.) may cross capillary walls in this way but, in addition, larger hydrophilic compounds such as glucose, amino acids and many drugs also use this route.

3. Large lipid-insoluble molecules will be particularly affected by the structure of capillaries outlined above. In continuous endothelia for instance passage of these molecules will be very limited under normal conditions. In other tissues some plasma protein can leak out of the circulation and the concentration of protein in the interstitial space may be 20–70% of the plasma concentration. Many physiologically important compounds circulate bound to proteins. These include lipids, many hormones, some vitamins and micronutrients such as iron and copper. Delivery of these compounds to cells is dependent on transcapillary wall passage of their unbound form and this also applies to many drugs. A further mechanism by which proteins can cross capillary walls is via endocytotic vesicle formation.

Water movement across capillary walls

Water can cross capillary walls via open channels between or through cells or by transcellular movement. In the latter case water must cross the plasma membrane

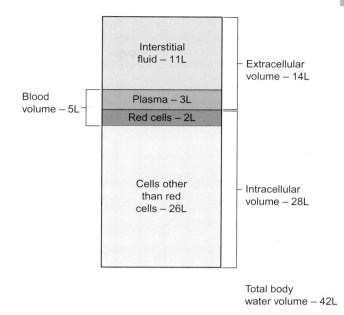

Fig. 11.3 Body water volume distribution. Typical distribution of total body water volume of 42 L into compartments in the 'textbook person'.

on each side of the endothelial cells. The mechanisms involved are of particular importance to whole body homeostasis.

The textbook person (male, 70 kg body weight, aged 20–25 years) contains about 42 L of body water, i.e. 60% of body weight. Distribution of this water is typically about one third (14 L) in the extracellular compartment and two thirds (28 L) in the intracellular compartment (Fig. 11.3). The 14 L of extracellular fluid comprise 3 L of blood plasma and 11 L of interstitial fluid. The 2 L of red blood cells are included in the intracellular compartment. These compartments should not be regarded as 'water-tight' and there is a continuous flux of water between them. This process aids the distribution of nutrients around the body. Calculations based on typical values for cardiac output, and the fact that about 60% of blood volume is plasma, show that approximately 4000 L of plasma pass through the microcirculation of an adult in the course of a day (Fig. 11.4). In this period there is a net outflow of approximately 8 L of water passing across capillary walls and into the interstitial fluid. Correspondingly, 8 L of interstitial fluid drain into the lymphatic system and eventually return to the circulation by this route. Of the 8 L of fluid entering the lymph capillaries, about half is reabsorbed during passage through the lymph nodes and the other half will re-enter the circulation at the subclavian veins (see p. 132). Failure to maintain the correct distribution of body water leads to the excessive accumulation of interstitial fluid—oedema.

The mechanisms behind these fluid movements are now discussed and a case history of a patient with oedema is introduced in Case 11.1:1.

CAPILLARY FUNCTION AND THE LYMPHATIC SYSTEM

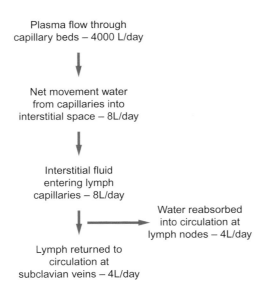

Fig. 11.4 Water movement through the lymphatic system. Typical values for the normal movement of water through the lymphatic system during each day.

Case 11.1 Capillary function and the lymphatic system: 1

A minor problem?

Peter is a 9-year-old boy who had generally been well apart from being troubled by mild eczema. A few days after a cold with a runny nose he found that his face and ankles had become swollen. If he pressed with a finger on the swollen ankles it left an indentation which only gradually disappeared (pitting oedema). His body weight had recently increased by 5 pounds (about 2.5 kg).

Peter's mother took him to their GP who checked his blood pressure (normal) and found nothing abnormal during chest ausculation or during examination of the jugular venous pulse. However, a dipstick test on a urine sample showed the presence of substantial amounts of protein. Peter was immediately referred to the local hospital where he came under the care of a paediatric nephrologist.

This case history raises the following questions:

1. What are the forces across blood capillary walls which determine the distribution of water between the intravascular and interstitial compartments?
2. What are the major pathophysiological mechanisms leading to the development of oedema? Which of these appear to be ruled out by the GP's examination?
3. What is the link between loss of protein in the urine and the development of oedema?

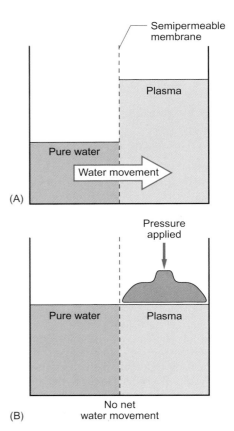

Fig. 11.5 Osmotic pressure of blood plasma. Model illustrating the concept of the osmotic pressure of blood plasma. The two compartments in each of the containers are separated by a semipermeable membrane. In each case the water and plasma were at the same level initially. In the top diagram the water moves by osmosis from the pure water compartment to the plasma. In the lower diagram a pressure is applied to the plasma which will just stop any water movement. By definition this is equivalent to the osmotic pressure of plasma, typically about 7.6 atmospheres or 5800 mm Hg. If a solution was placed in the right hand compartment in which the only dissolved solutes were the plasma proteins then the osmotic pressure would typically be about 21–29 mm Hg. Most of the osmotic pressure of plasma is contributed by the small solutes, particularly Na^+ and Cl^-.

Osmotic pressure of body fluids

Water moves by osmosis from an area of low osmotic pressure (dilute solution) to an area of high osmotic pressure (strong solution). Osmotic pressure depends on the number of solute particles rather than their size or chemical identity. The total osmotic pressure exerted by the components of blood plasma is about 7.6 atmospheres (5800 mm Hg). In the simple model shown in Figure 11.5 this would be the pressure that would need to be exerted on top of the plasma compartment in order to just stop water moving by osmosis. Most of the osmotic pressure of plasma is generated by the small particles which have the highest concentrations in plasma, especially sodium and chloride. Capillary walls are quite freely permeable to the small particles and so the concentrations of sodium and chloride in plasma and in interstitial fluid are similar and there is no significant osmotic pressure gradient generated by the small particles. The concentrations of the small cations (Na^+, K^+) and the small anions (Cl^-, HCO_3^-) each summate to approximately 150 mmol/L which means the osmolarity of plasma is approaching 300 mosmol/L. The normal range of plasma osmolarity is actually 275–290 mosmol/L. The fact that this is slightly less than 300 mosmol is partly due to electrostatic attraction between some anions and cations such as Na^+ and Cl^- so that a proportion are behaving as a single particle rather than two separate ones.

Colloids are large molecules which do not readily diffuse. Diffusion is discussed as a topic in Chapter 1. In plasma the natural colloids are the plasma proteins which, in most normal situations are too large to cross the capillary wall easily. Although their molar concentration in plasma is low, about 1 mmol/L, the concentration difference between plasma and interstitial fluid means there is a colloid osmotic pressure gradient of 21–29 mm Hg which will tend to move fluid from the interstitial compartment to the plasma compartment. The terms colloid osmotic pressure (COP) and oncotic pressure are used synonymously. The colloid osmotic pressure of plasma is attributable particularly to the albumin component. Albumin typically forms just over half of the total plasma protein concentration by weight (35–59 g/L out of a total of 70–78 g/L) but, in addition, albumin ($Mr = 69\,000$) is much smaller than the globulin family of plasma proteins. The number of osmotically active particles per gram of albumin protein is therefore much higher than for the other proteins.

It must be stressed that the proportion of the total osmotic pressure of plasma (5800 mm Hg) contributed by the plasma proteins (21–29 mm Hg) is very small. Sometimes there is a clinical need to increase the colloid osmotic pressure of blood plasma. This can be achieved with administration of either human serum albumin or synthetic colloids such as the polyfructose polysaccharides called dextrans. These substances may be referred to as 'plasma expanders' in clinical practice because they osmotically draw fluid from the interstitial space. These strategies are used in the clinical management of circulatory shock (see Chapter 14).

The Starling hypothesis

Starling published his ideas on capillary function in 1896 and they still form the basis of our understanding of capillary function today. Starling recognized that capillary walls are leaky to water but would retain the plasma protein. There is a gradient of hydrostatic pressure (capillary blood pressure—interstitial fluid pressure) which moves water out of capillaries and a gradient of colloid osmotic pressure (COP plasma—COP interstitial fluid) which would tend to move water back into capillaries (Fig. 11.6).

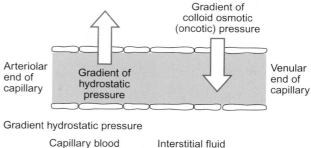

Gradient hydrostatic pressure

| Capillary blood pressure | — | Interstitial fluid pressure |

Gradient colloid osmotic pressure (COP)

| COP plasma | — | COP Interstitial fluid |

Fig. 11.6 The 'Starling hypothesis' of capillary function. The original hypothesis (1896) has been modified in the light of more recent research findings (see text).

Until recently it was thought that water moved out of capillaries at the arterial end and moved back into capillaries at the venous end of a capillary. However the osmotic pressure gradient in the Starling equation (see below) is now thought to be rather smaller than previously estimated. There is a relatively small net movement of water out of capillaries (which enters the lymphatic system) but large scale movement of water is not now thought to occur. The gradient of colloid osmotic pressure should be viewed as a force opposing the capillary blood pressure hydrostatic force and therefore reducing its impact. Nevertheless the balance of Starling forces is an important concept and is central to an understanding of the mechanisms of oedema (see p. 132).

The Starling forces can be expressed in a mathematical format using standard notation as follows:

$$J_v = K_f((P_c - P_i)) - \sigma(\pi_p - \pi_i)$$

where J_v = rate of fluid movement across the capillary wall, K_f = filtration coefficient (a measure of capillary water (hydraulic) permeability), P_c = capillary hydrostatic pressure, P_i = interstitial fluid hydrostatic pressure, π_p = colloid osmotic pressure of plasma, π_i = colloid osmotic pressure of interstitial fluid, σ = colloid osmotic reflection coefficient.

Typical values for the component 'Starling forces'

Capillary hydrostatic pressure is not constant along the length of the capillary. The existence of blood flow from the arterial to the venous end means that there must be a drop in pressure along a capillary. Absolute values for capillary blood pressure will depend partly on the state of constriction of the vessels at either end of the capillary. Thus, arteriolar constriction will impose a high resistance to flow and therefore there will be a big pressure drop across this segment and the pressure at the start of a capillary will be relatively low. Correspondingly arteriolar vasodilatation, as occurs in inflammatory reactions, leads to an increase in capillary pressure. Constriction of the venule would also tend to increase capillary pressure. Typical numerical values in a well perfused capillary might be:

capillary hydrostatic pressure: arteriolar end = 30–40 mm Hg
capillary hydrostatic pressure: venule end = 10–15 mm Hg
mean capillary hydrostatic pressure = 25 mm Hg

Speculation about the hydrostatic pressure in the interstitial space has aroused controversy. The interstitial fluid is not water which is normally free to move. The interstitial space contains macromolecules such as the protein collagen (types I and III), hyaluronates and proteoglycans. They effectively immobilize the water in a similar way to water trapped between the fibres of a sponge. Under normal circumstances this prevents the textbook person's 11 L of interstitial fluid from draining to their feet under the effects of gravity.

Pressure in the interstitial space is negative, i.e. subatmospheric. A typical pressure in a normally hydrated person might be about −2 mm Hg. When, in oedema, the interstitial fluid volume increases the interstitial fluid pressure rises and eventually becomes positive. The shape of the oedematous structure changes and the surface becomes hard, smooth and rounded—inflated by a positive pressure underneath the skin. When substantial oedema fluid accumulates it drains to the lowest point of the body, the ankles in someone still mobile and over the sacrum in someone who is bed-bound. The capacity of the macromolecules in the interstitial space to immobilize water has been exceeded. Interstitial fluid pressure in this case is of the order of +1 to +2 mm Hg.

A typical value for the colloid osmotic pressure in plasma is about 28 mm Hg and for interstitial fluid it is of the order of 8 mm Hg. The latter value varies considerably between tissues depending primarily on the capillary permeability. It is an interesting point to remember that, as the interstitial fluid volume is nearly four times plasma volume and the interstitial fluid protein concentration is about a quarter of the concentration in plasma, the total amounts of plasma protein distributed inside and outside the circulatory system (interstitial space) are roughly equivalent. The colloid osmotic reflection coefficient (σ) is an index of the molecular size selectivity of the capillary wall. Thus, if the structure of the wall was such that it was totally impossible for a given protein to cross it then σ = 1. This would be the case if the size of a protein was relatively large compared to the size of the pores in between or through cells. If however there was effectively no obstruction to the movement of the protein across the capillary wall then σ = 0.

The 'typical' figures for the 'Starling forces' quoted above do not all apply to the pulmonary circuit. Although capillary blood pressure in the lung is low, which reduces the tendency for water to leave the lung capillaries, the capillary walls are rather leaky (i.e. σ is relatively low) and so the protein content of the lung interstitial fluid is correspondingly high. This of course reduces the gradient of colloid osmotic pressure across the capillary wall. It is commonly supposed that we normally avoid the development of oedema in the lungs because pulmonary capillary blood pressure is low. In fact, because of the reduced colloid osmotic pressure gradient, it is the efficiency of the lung lymphatic drainage system which primarily protects us against pulmonary oedema.

Interesting facts

The total amount of blood vessel in a 20 to 25-year-old 70 kg male 'textbook person' would stretch three times round the world. Most of this tubing consists of capillary vessels rather than the major arteries and veins.

The lymphatic system

Although the two sets of 'Starling forces' almost balance, there is a net outflow of water from the circulation each day of about 8 L (Fig. 11.4). This volume is returned to the circulatory system via the lymphatic system. About half of the water component, but not the protein, is reabsorbed in lymph nodes. The remaining half of the volume and all the protein re-enters the circulation via ducts entering the venous drainage of the arms (see p. 131).

The functions of the lymphatic system can therefore be summarized as follows:

- tissue drainage system which helps to maintain appropriate body water distribution

Case 11.1 Capillary function and the lymphatic system: 2

Peter's proteinuria

The paediatric nephrologist examining Peter initiated a series of tests. Plasma [creatinine], a marker for glomerular filtration rate, was normal. A 24-hour urine collection showed that the proteinuria was heavy at 9 g/day. Further analysis of plasma proteins showed that plasma [albumin] was low but the [globulin] was slightly raised. Albumin has a comparatively low relative molecular mass. Normally only very small amounts pass through the glomerular filter and these are mainly reabsorbed in the proximal tubule of the nephron. Albumin excretion is therefore normally negligible but any change in glomerular permeability may result in amounts of albumin crossing the filter which exceed tubular reabsorptive capacity and hence lead to proteinuria. Globulins are larger molecules which would need very substantial changes in the permeability of the glomerular filter before they could appear in the urine. A modest increase in plasma [globulin] may however suggest an immune system basis to the glomerular disease.

A form of glomerulonephritis, probably minimal change disease, was suspected and so a treatment regimen based on steroids and diuretics was initiated.

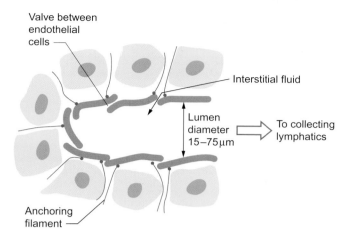

Fig. 11.7 Lymph capillary. Diagram of blind-ending tube of endothelial cells which constitutes a lymph capillary. It is held open by anchoring filaments. Interstitial fluid drains through the valve-like structures where the endothelial cells overlap to enter the lymph capillary. This occurs when interstitial fluid pressure exceeds intralymphatic pressure (see text).

- return of plasma proteins which have leaked out into the interstitial space back to the circulation
- absorption of digested fat in the form of chylomicrons into the lacteals (lymph capillaries) of the gut
- defence function at lymph nodes mediated by phagocytic cells and by lymphocytes.

Structure and function of lymph capillaries

Lymph capillaries, like blood capillaries, consist of a single layer of endothelial cells but they are blind-ending tubes. The cells sit on an incomplete basement membrane. Adjacent endothelial cells overlap and so fluid entering a lymph capillary has to pass through a valve-like structure. This is aided by the presence of anchoring filaments which radiate out into the surrounding tissue and oppose the collapse of the lymph capillary especially when interstitial fluid pressure rises (Fig. 11.7).

If pressure in the interstitial space is higher than pressure inside the lymph capillary water will be squeezed between overlapping endothelial cells into the lymph capillary. If fluid pressure within the lymph capillary is higher than in the surrounding interstitial fluid, the endothelial cells will be pushed together and the valve will be closed, hence preventing movement of water back out from the lymphatic into the interstitial space.

Factors which cause a change in the balance of the Starling forces may increase local interstitial fluid pressure and hence increase the volume of water entering a lymph capillary. These factors include an increase in capillary blood pressure (as in exercise or in heart failure), decreased plasma colloid osmotic pressure (as in malnutrition and renal or liver disease) and increased

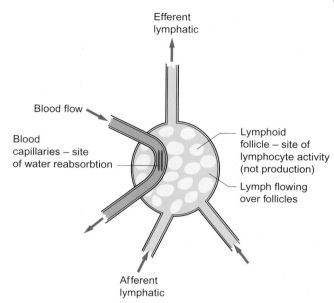

Fig. 11.8 Lymph node. Lymph enters the node and flows over the lymphoid follicles and is exposed to phagocytic cells and lymphocytes with antigen recognition sites and other functions in the immune system. Lymphocytes are produced in primary lymphoid tissues, the bone marrow and thymus. Water is reabsorbed in the lymph node back into blood capillaries. About half of the lymph formed is reabsorbed in this way.

permeability of capillaries (as in inflammatory reactions). Also, acutely, compression of the interstitial space by moving tissues, e.g. muscles, will transiently increase local interstitial fluid pressure and force fluid into the lymph capillary. This is thought to be an important mechanism in helping to maintain a negative interstitial fluid pressure. A further factor is the peristaltic movement in the walls of large lymphatics and the presence of valves in these vessels. This helps to move the lymph away from the interstitial compartment and so also contributes to maintaining negative interstitial fluid pressure.

Large lymphatic vessels

Lymph capillaries join together to form collecting lymphatics. Semilunar valves exist along all the lymphatic vessels in order to prevent backflow. As with the venous system, the lymphatics drain into progressively larger and larger lymphatics which have surrounding smooth muscle after the collecting lymphatics. The largest lymphatics are referred to as afferent lymph trunks. Peristaltic movements of the lymphatic wall help to propel fluid through the lymphatic system. This lymphatic pump can generate pressures in large lymphatics which approach the diastolic pressure in blood vessels.

At intervals along the lymph trunks there are lymph nodes (Fig. 11.8). These cavernous structures contain phagocytic cells and lymphocytes. The lymph nodes are also an important site for reabsorption of the water

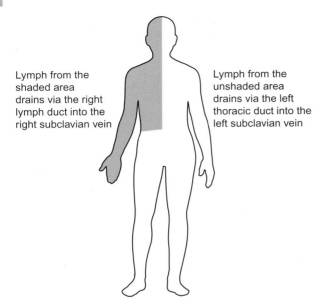

Lymph from the shaded area drains via the right lymph duct into the right subclavian vein

Lymph from the unshaded area drains via the left thoracic duct into the left subclavian vein

Fig. 11.9 Return of lymph to the systemic circulation. For most of the body the lymph drainage is via the left thoracic duct which enters the left subclavian vein. A smaller right lymphatic duct enters the right subclavian vein and drains the regions shown by the shaded area on this diagram.

Table 11.1	Typical concentrations of Na^+ and K^+ in the intracellular and extracellular fluid compartments	
	Intracellular fluid	*Extracellular fluid*
[Na^+]	10–20 mmol/L	140 mmol/L
[K^+]	150 mmol/L	4 mmol/L

basis for enlarged lymph nodes which may be either localized or widespread can be classified as follows:

- Primary tumours of the lymph node (lymphomas) which include the groups of diseases known as Hodgkin's lymphomas, non-Hodgkin's lymphomas and chronic lymphocytic leukaemia.

- Secondary neoplasm in the lymph nodes arising as a result of metastasis from a tumour elsewhere.

- Specific infections of lymph nodes such as tuberculosis, infectious mononucleosis (glandular fever) or local infections.

- Inflammatory reactions which cause lymph node hyperplasia.

Oedema

Oedema is excess accumulation of water in body fluid compartments. It often occurs as an expansion of the interstitial fluid compartment following a disturbance of the Starling forces. The mechanisms of interstitial oedema are discussed below but intracellular oedema will first be considered.

Typical concentrations of Na^+ and K^+ in the intracellular and extracellular fluid compartments are shown in Table 11.1. There is therefore a concentration gradient for Na^+ to leak into cells and Na^+ is also attracted by the net negative charge, mainly held on proteins, on the inside of cells. Correspondingly there is a gradient for K^+ to leak out of cells. Intracellular:extracellular ion gradients are maintained by the Na^+/K^+-ATPase (sodium pump) in the plasma membrane of cells. This expels $3Na^+$ to the extracellular compartment and returns $2K^+$ to the intracellular compartment. Each cycle of the pump requires the hydrolysis of an ATP molecule to provide energy. Some cell membranes contain as many as 1 million sodium pumps which may work at a rate of about 30 times per second and consume an ATP molecule each time they pump $3Na^+$ out of the cell. As the textbook person has about 10^{14} cells this is obviously a major energy cost. Keeping the sodium pump running accounts for about 30–40% of our total energy consumption. The consequence of failing to expel the excess Na^+ is osmotic swelling of cells, i.e. expansion of the intracellular fluid volume. This will occur in ischaemic tissues with inadequate ATP production which can swell to two to three times normal volume. This usually leads on

component of lymph back into the circulation. About half of the fluid which enters lymph capillaries will return to the circulation by this route. Several incoming (afferent) lymphatics drain into a series of sinuses within each lymph node. Bacteria and other foreign particulate matter are phagocytosed and antigens in the lymph trigger lymphoid tissues to increase the number of lymphocytes released into the lymph. Some of these will become antibody-producing cells.

After the filtering process the lymph emerges in an efferent lymphatic. The lymphatic drainage from the lower limbs and the abdominal viscera enters a large lymphatic trunk on the posterior abdominal wall. This continues to collect tributaries including the lymphatic drainage from the left arm and the left side of the head until the largest lymphatic in the body, the left thoracic duct, enters the left subclavian vein. This vessel carries the lymph formed in most of the structures of the body except the 'top right-hand corner'. The lymphatic drainage for the right arm, right side of the chest and the right side of the head enters the right subclavian vein via a smaller right lymphatic duct (Fig. 11.9). About half (3–4 L) of the lymph formed in the periphery returns to the circulation via the subclavian veins.

Lymph node enlargement (lymphadenopathy) is an important clinical sign and is a component of clinical examination. In addition to the location of enlarged lymph nodes, other characteristics of palpable nodes should be recorded. These include whether they are hard or soft, tender or non-tender, their size and whether they are mobile and discrete or matted together. The pathological

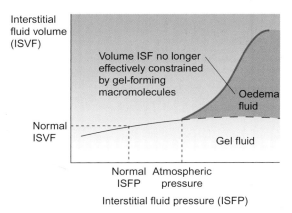

Fig. 11.10 Relationship between interstitial fluid volume and interstitial fluid pressure. For an explanation of this graph see the text.

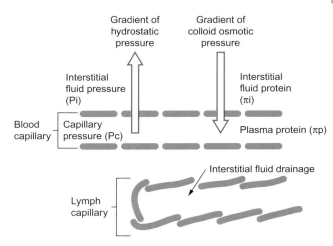

Fig. 11.11 Capillary function. Model of capillary function showing the forces which may contribute to the development of extracellular oedema.

to tissue death (see Chapter 1). Intracellular oedema can also occur as part of inflammatory reactions in which there is an increase in cellular sodium permeability.

Extracellular oedema

Key features of the interstitial compartment which are central to understanding the mechanisms of oedema are:

- interstitial fluid pressure is normally slightly negative, i.e. less than atmospheric pressure
- interstitial fluid is effectively immobilized in a gel form by protein and carbohydrate macromolecules.

Any change in the Starling forces across capillary walls which tends to expand the interstitial fluid volume (ISFV) will lead to an increase in interstitial fluid pressure (ISFP). Initially, this will oppose further movement of fluid out of the capillary by reducing the gradient of hydrostatic pressure. If the amount of water entering the interstitial compartment is sufficient to force the macromolecules apart the ISFV will be able to expand more easily without a substantial change in ISFP. This is illustrated in Figure 11.10 which shows the relationship between ISFV and ISFP. Normal ISFP is about $-2\,\text{mmHg}$. When ISFP becomes the same as atmospheric pressure the interstitial fluid is no longer adequately constrained by the interstitial macromolecules and so expansion of ISFV occurs. Eventually, further expansion of the ISFV is limited by the restraining influence of the skin. This is why the top of the graph in Figure 11.10 flattens. Once the water is no longer adequately constrained by the macromolecules it is able to move under the influence of gravity and will accumulate in the lower limbs if the subject is mobile or over the sacrum if the subject is in bed.

The fundamental mechanisms of extracellular oedema can be illustrated by reference to Figure 11.11 which summarizes the Starling forces. The common disturbances of these forces which can lead to oedema are:

- an increase in capillary blood pressure (P_c)
- a decrease in plasma colloid osmotic pressure (π_p)

- blockage of the lymphatic drainage
- an increase in capillary wall permeability (a change in K_f or σ).

Each of these mechanisms is now briefly discussed in relation to likely clinical scenarios.

Increase in capillary blood pressure

A common cause of oedema by this mechanism is in right sided heart failure. The compensatory response to ventricular failure is an increase in preload in order to raise stroke volume. This means an increase in the filling pressure of the right ventricle (right atrial pressure) mainly achieved by an increase in blood volume (see Chapter 6). The increase in right atrial pressure means that the pressure in the vessels preceding the atrium must be increased, i.e. in the vena cava, venules and capillaries if blood is to continue to flow back towards the heart. The rise in capillary pressure leads to extracellular oedema.

Hypertension per se does not lead to oedema. Blood pressure is usually high because of raised resistance to flow (Chapter 10). The main resistance vessels are the arterioles, which are pre-capillary vessels. Pressure in capillaries may therefore be normal as the high pressure in the arteries is dissipated moving the blood through the constricted arteriolar segment. It is only when hypertension leads to heart failure, due to the increased afterload effect, that people with high arterial blood pressure become oedematous.

Decrease in colloid osmotic pressure

Recognized causes of decreased plasma protein concentration include malnutrition (reduced amino acid availability to synthesize protein), liver disease (damage at the site of plasma protein synthesis), kidney disease (loss of protein in urine as a result of glomerular damage—the nephrotic syndrome) or in patients with extensive burns (a plasma protein-rich serous exudate covers the burned area and the water then evaporates leaving a dry protein coat). The case history in this chapter describes a patient with oedema secondary to renal disease.

Substantial generalized oedema occurs when the plasma albumin concentration falls below 25 g/L (normal range 35–50 g/L). There is however an interesting syndrome associated with a genetically determined failure to synthesize plasma albumin. Strangely this group of patients who have no albumin are not necessarily oedematous. This is incompletely understood.

Lymphatic blockage

The large lymphatic vessels may become occluded by tumours affecting lymph nodes or by breast tumours and their subsequent surgical clearance. It is important to remember the anatomy, the left thoracic duct enters the subclavian vein close to the left axilla.

Other causes of lymphatic insufficiency include congenital structural abnormalities, fibrosis following radiotherapy and infection. The tropical disease elephantiasis is associated with a filarial worm infection which blocks the lymphatic system. It is becoming recognized that failure of the lymphatic pump mechanism is an important component in the development of lymphoedema.

Increase in capillary wall permeability

This occurs due to the release of inflammatory mediators such as histamine, bradykinin, serotonin and various cytokines. The main site of action for these mediators is the post-capillary venules and they lead to an increase in the size of pores between endothelial cells. This not only increases the water permeability but may also lead to a significant loss of plasma protein into the interstitial space and, consequently, a reduction in the colloid osmotic pressure gradient, across the blood vessel wall.

In many cases the increase in capillary permeability occurs locally and generates local oedema (swelling), as for example at the site of a skin lesion. Evidence has more

Case 11.1 Capillary function and the lymphatic system: 3

Resolution of Peter's problems

Peter's glomerulonephritis responded well to treatment with steroids and glomerular permeability returned to normal. In children this problem typically follows an upper respiratory tract infection and is more likely to occur in atopic individuals who have a history of hay fever, asthma or allergic eczema. The excess fluid load, represented by the oedema and the increase in body weight, was cleared with the aid of the diuretics. A normal body fluid distribution was eventually re-established when the plasma [protein] returned to normal. This was delayed by the need for increased hepatic protein synthesis to replace that lost in the urine.

recently emerged that oedema formation can occur rapidly during acute inflammatory responses as a result of primary changes in interstitial fluid pressure (P_i). This follows interactions between dermal cells and the macromolecules in the interstitial space which are mediated by the cell adhesion molecules, the β_1-integrins (see Berg et al. 2001).

Further reading

Aukland, K., Reed, R.K., 1993. Interstitial–lymphatic mechanisms in the control of extracellular fluid volume. Physiol. Rev. 73, 1–78.

Berg, A., Rubin, K., Reed, R.K., 2001. Cytochalasin D induces oedema formation and lowering of interstitial fluid pressure in rat dermis. Am. J. Physiol. 281, H7–H13.

Browse, N., Burnand, K.G., Mortimer, P.S., 2003. Diseases of the Lymphatics. Hodder Arnold, London.

Levick, J.R., 2009. Cardiovascular Physiology, fifth ed. Arnold, London.

Michel, C.C., 1977. Starling: the formulation of his hypothesis of microvascular fluid exchange and its significance after 100 years. Exp. Physiol. 82, 1–30.

Michel, C.C., Curry, F.E., 1999. Microvascular permeability. Physiol. Rev. 79, 703–761.

Mortimer, P.S., Levick, J.R., 2004. Chronic peripheral oedema: the critical role of the lymphatic system. Clin. Med. 4, 448–453.

FETAL CARDIOVASCULAR SYSTEM AND CONGENITAL HEART DISEASE

12

Chapter objectives

After studying this chapter you should be able to:

1. Explain how the structure of the fetal heart and circulation differs from that in the adult.

2. Describe the structural changes at birth and during the neonatal period associated with the transition from the fetal to adult form of circulation.

3. Outline the changes in the functional characteristics of the circulation such as heart rate and blood pressure which occur during the growth of a child into an adult.

4. Describe some of the common differences in the pattern of ECG traces between children and adults.

5. Understand some of the common genetic and functional bases for congenital heart malformations.

6. Explain the clinical basis for the presentation, investigation and diagnosis of congenital heart defects.

7. Discuss the rationale for medical and surgical approaches to the correction of some congenital heart defects.

Introduction

Though the main functions of the fetal cardiovascular system are the same as in the adult, i.e. the distribution of oxygen and nutrients to the body and the transfer of carbon dioxide and waste products to the organ of excretion, there are some fundamental differences. Before birth the lungs are collapsed and filled with fluid and the organ of oxygenation, nutrient delivery and waste excretion is the placenta. The fetus is essentially a parasite and must extract oxygen and nutrients from the maternal circulation. Despite adaptations, such as an increased affinity of fetal haemoglobin (HbF) for oxygen compared with adult haemoglobin (HbA), the fetus exists in a state of relative hypoxia. Haemoglobin in the blood returning from the placenta is generally around 80% saturated with oxygen compared to above 98% in the pulmonary venous blood of a child or adult (see Chapter 1). Carbon dioxide levels are correspondingly elevated in the fetus. It is important to remember that the fetus is adapted to tolerate these conditions and aspects of this adaptation initially persist after birth.

The placenta consists of a system of villi inserted into lacunae containing maternal blood. The fetal blood vessels are contained within the villi which are bathed in maternal blood but there is no direct communication between fetal and maternal blood supplies. There is however only a short distance for diffusion of oxygen, carbon dioxide and nutrients between mother and fetus. The placenta is not simply an organ of passive diffusion, it also has synthetic and catabolic functions and provides active transport mechanisms for nutrients.

Some aspects of the evolution of the circulatory system from infant to adult help us to understand the fetal circulation. In the fetus the fluid-filled lungs pose a high resistance to blood flow and, as they are not involved in gas exchange, there is little value in directing blood flow to them.

As in adult life the brain, after the heart, is the dominant oxygen demanding organ. In contrast to the adult, in the fetus the oxygen supply comes from the placenta and so the most highly oxygenated blood arrives at the heart in the inferior vena cava rather than in the pulmonary veins. This blood is partially desaturated at around 80% despite the high affinity of HbF for oxygen. In order to ensure optimum supply of oxygen to the brain the fetal circulation has two major structural differences compared to that in the adult, the ductus arteriosus and the foramen ovale. Figure 12.1 summarizes the fetal circulation.

The foramen ovale, in conjunction with the Eustachian valve, directs most of the maximally oxygenated blood entering the right side of the heart directly into the left atrium. From here it passes via the left ventricle into the aorta and predominantly supplies the head. The Eustachian valve is essentially a fetal structure, though its remnants can be seen on an echocardiogram in up to 5% of adults. The valve maintains a separation between

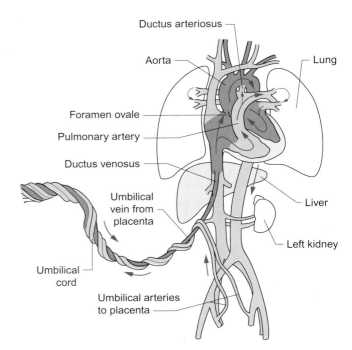

Fig. 12.1 The fetal circulation.

the inferior and superior vena caval flows in the fetus and thus preserves the relatively high saturation of blood passing into the left atrium and to the brain. Normal growth of the brain is a high priority for the fetus. This is illustrated by the preservation of head growth under conditions of stress such as placental insufficiency. This leads to asymmetric intrauterine growth retardation with the head being large with respect to the body.

Desaturated blood returning in the superior vena cava is streamed preferentially through the tricuspid valve into the right ventricle. It then passes out into the pulmonary artery where it is divided on the basis of flow resistance with the majority (approximately two thirds) passing through the ductus arteriosus and into the descending aorta. Roughly 2/3rds of the blood in the aorta supplies the abdominal organs and lower limbs and the remaining 1/3rd passes to the placenta. The key point regarding the placenta is that it has a low resistance to blood flow and so takes a high proportion of the aortic blood flow. Overall the peripheral resistance to flow is low. The collapsed lungs have a high resistance to flow in utero but this will change in the baby after birth.

The division of blood flow at the level of the right atrium has an important impact on the flow of blood around the aortic arch. Since the major recipient of the relatively well oxygenated blood is the brain, only a small proportion (about 10%) of the left ventricular output passes through the section of the aortic arch between the origin of the left subclavian artery and the opening of the ductus arteriosus.

Table 12.1 Main features of the fetal circulation compared with the adult circulation

Fetus	Adult
Newly oxygenated, but still partially desaturated, blood leaves the placenta and arrives at the right atrium in the inferior vena cava	Blood which is nearly fully saturated with oxygen arrives at the left atrium via the pulmonary veins
Pressure in right atrium is higher than that in the left atrium	Left atrial pressure is higher than that in the right atrium
Right-to-left shunting of blood occurs across the foramen ovale	There is no shunt at atrial level
The right ventricle supplies blood to the systemic circulation	The right ventricle only supplies blood to the pulmonary circulation
The right ventricle output predominantly passes through the ductus arteriosus into the aorta	The right ventricle output passes to the lungs
Resistance to blood flow is low in the placenta and this leads to a low peripheral resistance overall	Peripheral resistance to blood flow is high
Stiff, fluid-filled, lungs have high resistance to flow	Expanded, air-filled, lungs, have low resistance to blood flow

A further important feature of the fetal circulation is the flow of blood from the right ventricle into the systemic circulation via the ductus arteriosus. In the fetus the duct is comparable with the arch of the aorta. This can be visualized in fetal echocardiography where the 'ductal arch' must be distinguished from the aortic arch. In the fetus the two ventricles eject blood in parallel rather than in series, as in the adult.

To re-cap, the main features of the fetal circulation compared with the adult circulation are as shown in Table 12.1.

Sometimes transition from fetal to adult circulation at birth is incomplete, leading to so-called persistent fetal circulation. An example of a case history is shown in Case 12.1:1.

Interesting facts

Reptilian and amphibian hearts have three chambers with separation of oxygenated and deoxygenated blood by ridges within the ventricles. However the crocodile has a fully septated four chamber heart. In order to allow it to sustain dives for long periods it has a mechanical valve which diverts pulmonary blood flow to the systemic circulation whilst it is submerged.

How does the transition from fetal to adult circulation occur?

Changes at birth

On taking its first breath, the newborn infant instigates several simultaneous changes which will completely alter its circulation. Though most of these changes occur within minutes, they will take weeks to become fully complete.

The precise stimulus for the initiation of air breathing is not well understood. In utero the fetus makes some respiration-like movements but the process of birth drives the true onset of independent breathing. The clamping of the cord isolates the baby from the placenta. The associated increase in blood P_{CO_2} and decrease in P_{O_2} appear to be important in triggering the respiratory drive. The first few breaths are crucial, they must open the airways and complete the process of fluid clearance from the lung. Surfactant, a mixture of lipid, phospholipid and protein which lines the alveoli, is key to the reduction in surface tension necessary to allow the small airways to open. Anything which inhibits this fluid clearance can lead to failure to convert from the fetal to the neonatal pattern of circulation.

The first breath opens the airways and allows gas exchange across the alveolar membrane. The lungs expand and blood vessels open. This initiates a drop in the pulmonary vascular resistance (see Figure 12.5). Combined with the sudden rise in peripheral resistance resulting from the loss of the low-resistance placenta, there is a profound alteration in haemodynamics in the newborn infant. The blood leaving the right ventricle is preferentially directed through the now low-resistance lungs and returns to the left atrium. This increase in venous flow into the left atrium raises the left atrial pressure. At the same time there is a fall in right atrial pressure because venous return to this chamber has been reduced following the loss of the placental circulation. As left atrial pressure is now higher than right atrial pressure the foramen ovale, a flap valve, closes. Thus, in the newborn any detectable flow across the atrial septum is predominantly left to right. With the changes in pressures and the establishment of lung ventilation there is a sharp increase in blood oxygen content. This improved tissue oxygenation reduces the acidaemia to which the fetus has been adapted. Rising pH and $P_{a O_2}$ inhibit the synthesis of prostaglandins in the ductus arteriosus. This leads to closure of the ductus arteriosus separating the pulmonary circulation from the systemic circulation. Though generally the duct has closed within 24 hours of birth, early echocardiography demonstrates that a small left to right ductal shunt persists in a large minority of newborns for some days or even weeks. However this shunt is not usually of clinical significance.

| Case 12.1 | Fetal cardiovascular system and congenital heart disease: 1 |

A blue child

A newborn baby was noted to be cyanosed at 24-hour review. The respiratory rate was slightly increased at 60–70 breaths per minute but there was no respiratory distress. On auscultation there were no murmurs, the chest was clear and femoral arteries were easily palpable. A blood oxygen saturation check showed saturations of 78–82%. The baby was transferred to the special care baby unit (SCBU) and a hyperoxia test (increased inspired oxygen concentration) was performed. Arterial blood gases breathing room air showed $pH = 7.37$, $Po_2 = 3.5\,kPa$, $Pco_2 = 5.0\,kPa$, $[HCO_3] = 19\,mmol/L$, base excess $= -2.3\,mmol/L$ (see Chapter 1). When given 100% O_2 for 5 minutes arterial blood gas data were $pH = 7.36$, $Po_2 = 9.5\,kPa$, $Pco_2 = 5.5\,kPa$, $[HCO_3] = 19\,mmol/L$, base excess $= -2.2\,mmol/L$. A diagnosis of congenital cyanotic heart disease was made and after discussion with the regional paediatric cardiology unit dinoprostone infusion (a synthetic prostaglandin) was commenced and arrangements were made for transfer to the regional specialist centre.

On arrival echocardiography confirmed the putative diagnosis of transposition of the great arteries (TGA). The child was prepared for immediate balloon septostomy and was taken to the catheter laboratory.

Septostomy involves transvenous insertion of a catheter with a balloon at the end via the right atrium and patent foramen ovale into the left atrium. The balloon is then inflated and pulled back into the right atrium sharply in order to tear the interatrial septum. Care must be taken to avoid damaging the mitral valve or the inferior vena cava/right atrium junction.

The procedure was performed without complications. Post septostomy, oxygen saturations rose to 85–90%. The child was transferred back to the ward and after a few hours normal feeding was instituted.

Questions for consideration include:

1. What do the initial blood gas measurements tell us about the cardiopulmonary problems in this child?
2. What clinical signs help distinguish cardiac problems from a respiratory cause for cyanosis?
3. What is the rationale for the dinoprostone infusion?
4. How does blood flow around the circulation in a case of TGA?
5. How does septostomy affect the oxygen saturation of haemoglobin in this case?

Answers to these questions are discussed in the text of this chapter and in Case 12.1:2.

Over the first few days of life the process of adjustment proceeds with a continued fall in pulmonary artery pressure. This single physiological process accounts for many of the clinical features of congenital heart disease and cardiovascular problems in children.

Longer term changes in the heart during childhood and adulthood

Typically the pressure in the pulmonary artery will fall from the comparatively high level in the fetus to a normal adult level (25/5, mean = 10 mm Hg) over a period of a few weeks. The lower working pressure in the right ventricle means that during childhood it becomes increasingly dominated by the left ventricle in terms of muscle mass.

Apart from the fall in pulmonary pressure with time there are a number of physiological changes with maturation. Heart rate (HR) and blood pressure (BP) both vary with age and an appropriate normal range must be used in clinical practice. An adult with a heart rate of 120 bpm and a systolic BP of 85 mm Hg might be in the early stages of hypovolaemic shock but these would be perfectly normal values for a 1 year old. It is critically important to know the normal changes in physiological variables when assessing children, as they do not conform to textbook adult values.

Table 12.2 Heart rate and BP variations with age

Age (yr)	HR (bpm)	Systolic BP (mm Hg)
<1	110–160	70–90
1–2	100–150	80–95
2–5	95–140	80–100
5–12	80–120	90–110
>12	60–100	100–120

Table 12.2 summarizes the normal variation of HR and BP with age. An estimate of the normal systolic BP, for a given age in children, can be made from the formula: systolic BP = 80 + (2 × age in years).

The variation in heart rate reflects the relatively small size of the infant heart compared with its body mass and the relatively low compliance (increased stiffness) of the ventricles. The stiff ventricles mean that the stroke volume of the heart responds less dramatically to increasing venous return (preload effects) compared to an adult (see Chapter 4). In order to meet the demand for increased cardiac output the newborn heart rate must rise substantially, even at rest. Thus it is not unusual to see heart rates in newborns varying from 90 bpm when deeply asleep to 160 bpm when only slightly active. In the sick newborn under stress heart rates over 200 bpm may be seen with the heart still in sinus rhythm.

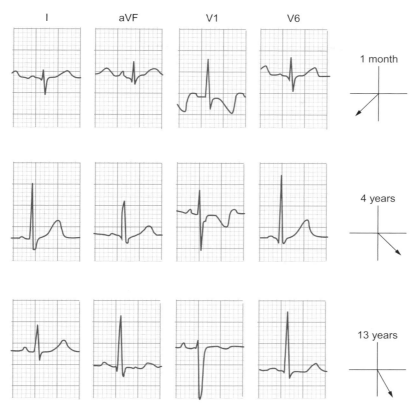

Fig. 12.2 ECG pattern—variation with age.

The normal ECG in childhood

Broadly speaking the ECG of the child has the same components as that of the adult, i.e. P waves, QRS complexes and T waves (see Chapter 7). However the relative contribution of the right and left ventricles to the shape of the ECG trace is different in children compared to adults. There is therefore a progressive change in the pattern of the ECG through childhood which reflects the declining contribution of the muscle mass of the right ventricle compared to the left ventricle. The large muscle mass of the newborn right ventricle affects the axis of the QRS complex in the frontal plane. The axis of the frontal QRS vector in the infant may be well past the upper limit of normal for the adult with the normal range being as high as +180°. Again, with time and the involution of the right ventricle, the axis 'swings' leftwards until it reaches the normal range for adults −30° to +90° (see Chapter 7). This change over time means that the acceptable axis for children in the frontal plane is very wide ranging. Broadly speaking, the axis should be inferior, i.e. between 0° and 180°. Deviation above the horizontal axis should be considered abnormal in the absence of evidence to the contrary. In the presence of physical evidence to support it a rightwards axis more extreme than usual may be suggestive of a residual load on the right ventricle. Put simply if the QRS vector is positive (i.e. pen deflection is upwards) in lead aVF then the vertical plane axis of the heart is probably normal.

The chest leads are particularly informative. In V_1 the QRS complexes are initially dominantly positive with a dominant R wave reflecting depolarization in the relatively hypertrophied septum. T waves in V_1 may be positive in the first 2 weeks of life but then become negative and remain inverted up until late childhood. The initial solely, or dominantly, positive deflection in V_1 slowly becomes equiphasic and by adulthood will be purely negative in the majority of normal ECGs. Figure 12.2 shows the typical variation.

Persistence of infantile ECG patterns may reflect a failure in the decline of RV pressures, as for example in the case of significant obstruction to the right ventricular outflow caused by pulmonary stenosis. Other causes of persistence of high pulmonary pressure (pulmonary hypertension) are a large ventricular septal defect (VSD), a patent ductus arteriosus (PDA) or, more rarely, primary pulmonary hypertension. Atrial septal defects (ASD) rarely cause pulmonary hypertension even though there may be a substantial left to right shunt. The persistence of infantile ECG patterns a month after birth should prompt urgent discussion with a specialist paediatric cardiology centre particularly in the presence of symptoms or signs supporting a diagnosis of congenital heart disease.

Broadly, the normal range for the intervals between successive components of the ECG for children are shorter than for adults and generally the younger the child the shorter the interval. This largely reflects the physical size of the heart, as a wave of electrical activity spreading through a smaller heart has a shorter distance to travel and so takes less time. This generalization applies for everything but the index referred to as the corrected QT interval (QTc). This is defined as the QT interval/square root (preceding R–R interval). Generally this falls with increasing age. Identification of the QTc has become clinically more important with increasing understanding of the role that abnormal repolarization plays in sudden death in young people. This may be evident in prolongation of the QTc above the normal range for an adult on the resting ECG.

Congenital heart disease

Congenital heart disease (CHD) affects around 1% of all children. The degree to which the heart can be distorted yet remain capable of supporting life is remarkable. One of the most frequently asked questions by parents is 'Why did it happen?' The frequently given answer is that, for the most part, we do not know.

It seems likely that with the wide variation of pathologies, largely sporadic in nature, a multifactorial aetiology is involved, possibly with a mix of genetic and environmental factors. Maternal factors such as diabetes and periconception infections such as rubella are strongly associated with congenital heart disease. Also congenital heart disease is strongly associated with other apparently unrelated structural defects, suggesting either a common environmental insult or a common genetic defect whose relationship affects tissues in the early embryo such that apparently unrelated organs are affected. Therapeutic and recreational drugs are associated with CHD, though whether the effects are direct or simply association is not clear. For example sodium valproate, an antiepileptic drug, inhibits folate metabolism. Its association with CHD may be by way of its interference with folate metabolism. Individuals using recreational drugs frequently live chaotic lives with poor nutritional status so that they are at risk of conditions associated with vitamin deficiency, which may be the fundamental cause of pathology and not the drugs per se.

Clearly 'genetic programming' is crucial to certain forms of congenital heart disease. As genetic knowledge advances more and more syndromes are linked with specific genetic lesions. For example, complete atrioventricular septal defect (AVSD) accounts for around 4% of all cardiac defects in the general population. However in children with Down syndrome (trisomy 21) it accounts for around 40% of the heart defects which are relatively common in this condition. About 40% of children with Down's syndrome have some form of congenital heart disease. Tetralogy of Fallot (see p. 146) and some related cardiac defects (pulmonary atresia with ventricular septal defect, truncus arteriosus, interrupted aortic arch) are associated with deletion in the q11 region of chromosome

22. However not all children with tetralogy of Fallot have the 22q11 deletion and usually those children with this deletion have substantial non-cardiac problems in addition to their cardiac defects. These include cleft palate, speech and learning difficulties, hypocalcaemia and immunological problems. However the q11 region of chromosome 22 contains several hundred genes and research is underway to see if some specific genes account for the cardiac problems associated with the large DNA deletion. One candidate is the TBX-1 ('TBOX-1') gene. In mice in which TBX-1 has been blocked or disabled cardiac defects similar to those found in 22q11 deletion syndromes in humans are found.

Conditions such as Marfan's syndrome and Williams' syndrome are associated with specific structural cardiovascular anomalies but not generally abnormalities in the connections of the heart. Marfan's syndrome is now known to be caused by defects in the gene for fibrillin located on chromosome 15q21. Defective protein leads to weakness in the connective tissues including those of the heart causing mitral valve prolapse due to dysfunction of the subvalvar apparatus and, more importantly, aortic root dilatation with risk of dissection which can be fatal if untreated. Preventive treatment is by replacement of the aortic root and ascending aorta with synthetic substitutes. Williams' syndrome is caused by a deletion of the elastin gene on chromosome 7q11. Typically this is associated with supravalvar aortic stenosis or peripheral pulmonary stenosis. Pulmonary valvar stenosis and atrial or ventricular septal defects are also recognized cardiac anomalies. Outside the heart renal artery stenosis and stenosis of other major fibrous vessels is also documented. Though all these defects may seem to arise logically from a defect of a structural protein, it is far from obvious why this condition should be associated with developmental delay and many other problems. As yet we understand far too little about the subtle interaction of structure and function in the developing embryo.

Not all congenital heart problems can be explained on a genetic basis however, as overall there is only a weak familial link with congenital heart disease. For siblings of an affected child, or children of affected parents, the overall incidence of congenital heart disease is only mildly increased from about 1% to 3–4%. Thus there must be other factors affecting the development of the fetal heart.

A second important element in the pathogenesis of congenital heart disease is how the growth of structures is dependent on the way they function during fetal development. Thus for vascular structures to grow appropriately they must have a blood flow which encourages them to develop correctly. For example, obstruction on the left side of the heart is frequently associated with problems at multiple levels. This may explain the association between stenosis of the aortic valve and coarctation of the aorta (narrowing of the aorta adjacent to the insertion of the ductus arteriosus into the aorta). As described earlier in this chapter, in the fetus only about 10% of the cardiac output traverses the isthmus—that part of the aortic arch between the origin of the left subclavian artery and the insertion of the duct. If stenosis of the aortic valve reduces the output from the left side of the heart—possibly only marginally—then flow across this critical region of blood vessel may be significantly reduced and normal development of the aorta discouraged.

In the condition called Shone's syndrome obstruction can occur at many levels on the left side of the heart. Mitral stenosis is often accompanied by aortic stenosis, aortic arch hypoplasia and coarctation of the aorta. It is proposed that impaired development of the mitral valve leads to decreased flow into the left ventricle, through the aortic valve and around the aortic arch. This reduced flow results in impaired development of these structures. At its most extreme it may be seen as hypoplastic left heart syndrome (HLHS) in which the left ventricle is completely underdeveloped, the aortic valve is severely stenotic or even atretic and the ascending aorta and aortic arch are hypoplastic. In the classical HLHS the ascending aorta is simply a functional extension of the coronary arteries and the blood supply to the head and neck vessels is completely retrograde around the arch and fed from the ductus arteriosus. The shunt at atrial level is completely reversed in the fetus and the right ventricle must support the whole circulation.

That the development of cardiovascular structures is dependent on the functional demand placed upon them is elegantly demonstrated by the findings from fetal echocardiography. Fetuses with very poorly developed ventricles at 16–20 weeks of gestation may have undergone complete involution by birth with only a tiny or even undetectable ventricular cavity on a postnatal echocardiograph. The two hypotheses for the genesis of congenital heart disease are not of course mutually exclusive. Subtle errors in the genetic code may be amplified by the interaction between development and function in utero. It is probable that a large proportion of congenital heart disease occurs due to disruption of normal development early in pregnancy, which is then amplified by the effect of changes in function.

Presentation of congenital heart disease

Murmurs

Murmurs are extra sounds caused by turbulent flow of blood during the cardiac cycle (see Chapter 8). Murmurs can initially be divided on the basis of cause; innocent or functional murmurs have no underlying structural cause whereas pathological murmurs result from specific abnormalities of cardiac structures.

Innocent murmurs are generally characterized by:

- low intensity (quiet)
- lack of radiation (can only be heard at one point)
- frequently vary with body position or state, e.g. only audible when sitting, when ill or after exercise
- lack of associated symptoms
- normal ECG findings.

Typical examples of innocent murmurs are:

- flow murmur—ejection murmur typically heard in the pulmonary area when the cardiac output is high
- vibratory (Still's) murmur—systolic murmur with buzzing musical quality localized to left sternal edge
- venous hum—continuous murmur heard at the base of the neck; typically abolished by lying down or pressing on the jugular vein
- carotid bruit—audible in the neck and thought to arise from blood flow into the brachiocephalic artery.

The intensity of a pathological murmur is largely dependent on the size of the hole through which blood must pass and the pressure gradient across the narrowest point. These are the factors which determine the velocity of flow and hence the likelihood of turbulence occurring (see Chapter 8). Thus with stenotic valves where the whole of the cardiac output must pass through the valve the intensity and length of the murmur increase with the degree of stenosis. However, for ventricular septal defects (VSD) the relationship between size and flow is complex as larger defects have a greater flow but a lower pressure gradient. Thus there is a peaked relationship between the intensity of the murmur and the size of the defect with very large defects generating little or no murmur and very small defects usually quieter murmurs because the flow is low despite maximal pressure difference. As the defect becomes vanishingly small the murmur disappears.

The time course of a murmur is very important in assessing its origin. Murmurs arise from jets of blood passing between chambers or vessels. The timing of the start and finish of the pressure gradient which generates the jet helps define its quality. For example, in the case of a VSD there is no pressure gradient during diastole as both ventricles fill. However almost immediately after the start of systole when the pressure in both ventricles has risen to the point where the atrioventricular valves have closed, i.e. immediately after the first heart sound, the pressure in the left ventricle is greater than that in the right. Thus the flow of blood through the VSD commences at the first heart sound and continues through into early diastole when the semilunar valves are heard to shut, i.e. the second heart sound. Thus the typical VSD murmur occurs throughout systole and is described as being pan- or holo-systolic (Fig. 12.3A). This may be compared with the murmur of aortic valve stenosis. Initially the pressure in the left ventricle is lower than in the aorta so there is a period between the first heart sound (closure of the mitral valve) and the opening of the aortic valve in which there is no blood flow out of the ventricle. The pressure in the ventricle rises to a peak during early systole at which time the volume of blood ejected from the ventricle is maximal and so the murmur reaches its maximum intensity. Then there is a period of reduced ejection of blood during which the pressure in the ventricle begins to fall. The intensity of the murmur falls to zero at the time the semilunar valves close. A recording of

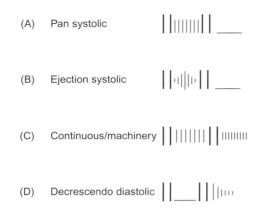

(A) Pan systolic

(B) Ejection systolic

(C) Continuous/machinery

(D) Decrescendo diastolic

Fig. 12.3 Audible patterns of typical murmurs. The pairs of vertical double lines represent the timing of the first and second heart sounds.

heart sounds, a phonocardiogram, has a typical diamond-shaped pattern for ejection systolic murmurs (Fig 12.3B).

Continuous murmurs can only occur where there is a persistent pressure difference between two vessels throughout the cardiac cycle. Apart from the innocent venous hum the commonest cause of continuous murmur is a patent ductus arteriosus (PDA). Since the aorta is always at a higher pressure than the pulmonary vasculature, even in diastole, the murmur occurs both in systole and diastole. However, since the pressure difference is greater in systole the quality of the sound varies between systole and diastole. Thus the murmur is continuous with two phases—it is often described as a machinery murmur (Fig. 12.3C). Large arteriovenous malformations are another cause of continuous murmurs.

Diastolic murmurs are often more difficult to hear because the pressure gradients are less than for systolic murmurs. The loudest diastolic murmurs tend to be caused by leakage (incompetence) in the semilunar valves. These typically occur in early diastole and are decrescendo in character. The typical decrescendo intensity profile reflects the fact that extracardiac vascular pressures fall during diastole whilst intraventricular pressures rise during diastole (Fig. 12.3D). Diastolic murmurs may also occur where there is stenosis of the atrioventricular (AV) valves, though these are likely to be difficult to hear. Classically described as 'rumbling' in quality the murmur has a low pitch rather different to high pressure murmurs. Increased flow through the AV valves may cause a murmur because of a functional stenosis.

A common mistake is to ascribe the murmur associated with a large atrial septal defect (ASD) to flow across the atrial septum. This would be a diastolic murmur but in fact the typical murmur is a systolic ejection murmur loudest over the pulmonary area and radiating to the back. This is actually generated by flow through the pulmonary valve which is functionally stenosed because of the increased flow rather than the valve being narrow. It may be possible to hear a diastolic murmur across the tricuspid valve which is also secondary to the increased flow through the right side of the heart.

Radiation

The term radiation is used to describe the spatial distribution of a murmur. It specifically applies to the direction in which a murmur is maximally audible away from the site of maximum intensity. Radiation is a key feature in identifying the cause of murmurs. For example innocent murmurs are typically localized without radiation. In order to interpret radiation as a clinical sign it is necessary to understand the normal anatomical relations of the heart.

The heart lies in an oblique orientation to the body, the apex being anterior and lateral with the base being posterior and medial. The aorta arises in parallel with this axis and turns upwards into the neck. The atrioventricular valves (tricuspid and mitral) lie in a plane perpendicular to this axis and slightly offset from each other. The pulmonary artery arises from the anterosuperior surface of the right ventricle but turns directly posterior before bifurcating into left and right pulmonary arteries. The ventricular septum falls in a plane which extends from apex to base but angles from left inferoposterior to right superoanterior. So what does this tell us about the radiation of murmurs?

It is easy to see how the jet of blood caused by aortic stenosis directs sound towards the right shoulder and neck. Pulmonary stenosis tends to be heard loudest over the left infraclavicular area, but because the artery points backwards the murmur can be heard over the left chest posteriorly. Branch pulmonary artery stenosis may be easily audible in the ipsilateral chest. Typically, the murmur of a VSD is loudest over the praecordium at the left sternal edge reflecting the posterior/anterior relation of the left and right ventricles (jet is from posterior to anterior).

Shunts

The normal ex utero circulation places the right and left ventricles in series with the pulmonary and systemic vascular beds between them (Fig. 12.4A). Though both pumps are combined in a single organ, the heart, they could be separate organs. This would make controlling the balanced output of each ventricle more difficult but not impossible. When blood passes from one side of the heart to the other bypassing the relevant end organs this is known as a shunt. Shunts may be intracardiac (e.g. VSD (Fig. 12.4B) or ASD (Fig. 12.4C)) or extracardiac (e.g. PDA (Fig. 12.4D) or arteriovenous malformation (Fig. 12.4E)). The main effect of a shunt is to volume load one or other side of the heart. Persistently high pulmonary blood flows associated with high driving pressure will eventually produce irreversible pulmonary hypertension. In the extreme case, systemic to pulmonary shunts may reverse, producing a flow of desaturated blood from right to left with consequent peripheral desaturation. This is known as Eisenmenger's syndrome.

The presence of a shunt will affect cardiac performance. For example a PDA will generally cause blood to pass from the aorta into the pulmonary circulation which

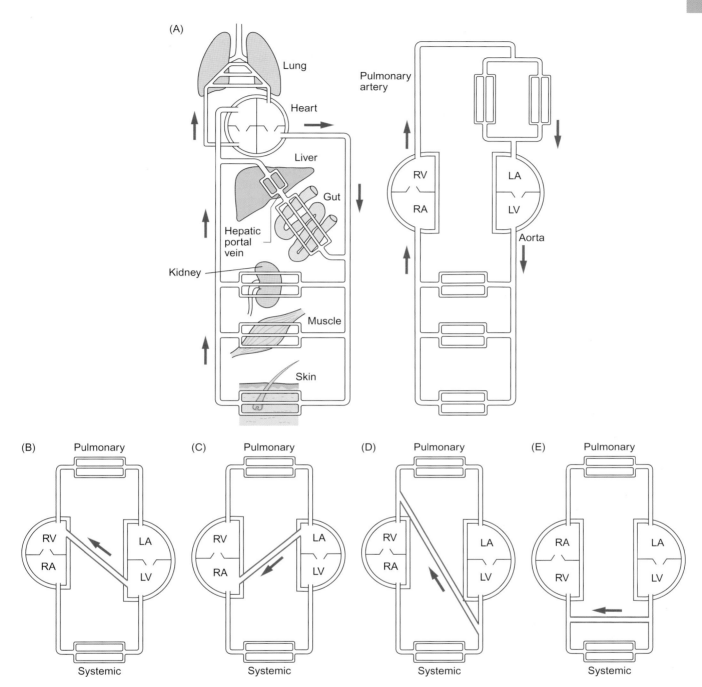

Fig. 12.4 Blood circulation and shunts. (A) Schematic diagram of circulation and various shunts. (B) Ventricular septal defect. (C) Atrial septal defect. (D) Patent ductus arteriosus. (E) Systemic arteriovenous malformation.

is at lower pressure. This extra blood, the shunt flow (S), is added to the flow already passing through the lungs from the right ventricle. Since the amount of blood returning to the right ventricle is equal to the amount passing through the systemic organs, the cardiac output (CO), the flow through the lungs is CO + S. The venous return to the left side of the heart from the lungs is equal to CO + S and may be considerably greater than the

resting systemic requirement. This produces volume loading of the left side of the heart with a dilated left atrium and ventricle and is associated with exercise limitation. Although the left ventricle has the capacity in a normal adult to increase its output to about five times resting levels (see Chapter 4), in the presence of a substantial shunt it may already be preloaded by several times the resting cardiac output at rest. Thus, during exercise, the left ventricle soon reaches its maximum output and the individual becomes exercise limited. In children this is frequently seen as having to stop for a rest before any of their playmates. Babies may become out of breath whilst feeding and have to stop to 'catch their breath'. In the case of premature infants the volume load on the left heart and high pulmonary blood flow may mean that they are unable to cope without mechanical ventilatory support.

Arteriovenous malformations may occur in either systemic or pulmonary circulation. These abnormal connections have a low resistance to flow and so increase flow through the circuit. This leads to volume loading of both sides of the heart. In extreme cases they may cause high output cardiac failure. The distinction between arteriovenous malformations and shunts connecting opposite sides of the heart is that the latter lead to volume loading of only one side of the heart.

Calculating shunts

Simple shunt ratios may be calculated using the Fick principle. In practice this is based on the fact that uptake of oxygen in the lungs must be equal to oxygen extraction (consumption) in the systemic circulation. A precise estimate of the flow in either the systemic or the pulmonary vascular bed can only be achieved with accurate measurement of absolute oxygen consumption, a measurement fraught with difficulty. However the ratio of the two flows may be calculated on the basis that oxygen uptake = oxygen extraction. If Q_p is the pulmonary blood flow and Q_s the systemic blood flow, then the following holds true if we ignore the small amount of dissolved oxygen (valid for inhaled O_2 concentrations <30%):

$$\text{pulmonary uptake of oxygen} = Q_p \times [\text{Hb}] \times 1.34 \times$$
$$\text{(pulmonary arteriovenous saturation difference)}$$

$$\text{systemic extraction of oxygen} = Q_s \times [\text{Hb}] \times 1.34 \times$$
$$\text{(systemic arteriovenous saturation difference)}$$

where [Hb] represents the concentration of haemoglobin in the blood in g/L and 1.34 is the volume (mL/gHb) of oxygen carried by a gram of haemoglobin when saturated (see Chapter 1). Since, at equilibrium, pulmonary uptake must equal systemic extraction then it follows that:

$$Q_p \times [\text{Hb}] \times 1.34 \times \text{(pulmonary}$$
$$\text{arteriovenous saturation difference)}$$
$$= Q_s \times [\text{Hb}] \times 1.34 \times \text{(systemic}$$
$$\text{arteriovenous saturation difference)}$$

and therefore

$$\frac{Q_p}{Q_s} = \frac{\text{aortic saturation} - \text{systemic mixed venous saturation}}{\text{pulmonary venous saturation} - \text{pulmonary artery saturation}}$$

Where the size of a VSD is small the amount of blood passing through it adds little to the workload of the left ventricle and so is of little significance. However left to right shunts in which the pulmonary blood flow is above twice the systemic flow may be sufficient to produce symptoms. As flow becomes relatively greater so do symptoms. Initially, the most telling sign of a large shunt in a baby is breathlessness, particularly when feeding, their most energy demanding activity. The other major energy demand after homeostasis is growth. Feeding behaviour and weight gain are important markers of cardiac function in the infant. Babies with large shunts feed slowly, become more breathless during feeding and often need calorie supplements or mechanical feeding support such as nasogastric feeds. Tissue oedema leads to relative tissue hypoxia because of impaired diffusion of oxygen. This reduces the efficiency with which nutritional calories can be utilized. Pulmonary oedema occurs because the high blood flow and high blood pressure lead to fluid outflow from the pulmonary capillaries at a rate greater than the lung lymphatics can cope with (see Chapter 11). Oedematous lungs are both stiff and less efficient for gas transfer. Thus the work of breathing is greatly increased due to decreased compliance of the lungs. This increase in energy demand also contributes to the poor weight gain.

Cyanosis

The third common presentation of congenital heart disease is cyanosis which may occur in the newborn for several reasons. Peripheral cyanosis, caused by poor perfusion of tissues with blood, must be differentiated from central cyanosis, caused by reduced oxygenation of blood in the central arterial tree (see Chapter 1). Central cyanosis can be viewed as having two major causes, 'respiratory', in which the cyanosis is secondary to lung disease with impaired gas transfer, and 'cardiac' in which the cyanosis is due to the mixing of partially desaturated (venous) and normally saturated (arterial) blood (see Case 12.1:2).

The single major distinguishing feature between the pulmonary and cardiac causes of cyanosis is the lack of response to increasing the inhaled oxygen concentration. If cyanosis is due to impaired gas transfer then increasing P_{O_2} in the inhaled gas mixture and hence increasing the concentration of O_2 within the alveolus should improve the transfer of oxygen into the blood. However in the case of cyanotic heart disease the blood passing through alveolar capillaries is already nearly fully oxygenated and so little change results from increasing the oxygen content of inhaled gas. The cyanosis is due to mixing of this oxygenated sample with blood which has not been exposed to oxygen in the pulmonary vascular bed. The lack of respiratory distress is suggestive of a cardiac cause for cyanosis, as is the presence of a murmur or other physical sign linked with cardiac disease. However these are not 100% predictive as respiratory distress may occur secondary to the effects of heart failure or hypoxia whilst murmurs are frequently not present in cyanotic lesions particularly in the newborn period.

The key to understanding cyanosis is analysis of the routes which saturated and desaturated blood take through the circulation. Cyanosis will occur where desaturated blood is able to enter the systemic circulation. Many different possibilities occur and frequently they are clinically indistinguishable. Cyanosis must occur where there is loss of some part of the standard circuit, e.g. pulmonary or tricuspid atresia, where systemic and pulmonary venous returns must be joined before re-dividing to supply systemic and pulmonary vascular beds. In other cases the mixing may not be obligatory, but functional, resulting from a combination of lack of a divider between the systemic and pulmonary circulations and haemodynamic conditions within the heart. An ASD, normally not a cyanotic lesion, may produce cyanosis if the right heart pressures rise above those of the left such as when an infant cries—producing transient cyanosis as desaturated blood passes from right atrium to left atrium.

Ultimately management of cyanotic heart disease relies on surgical repair. This may be definitive, in which a normal circulation with two separate ventricles is achieved, or palliative in which stable saturations are achieved even though a normal circulation cannot be produced (see Blalock–Taussig shunt and Fontan circulation described on p. 147). Medical therapy may be important in stabilizing the child prior to surgery, e.g. the use of exogenous prostaglandin to maintain ductal patency prior to the insertion of a synthetic shunt to give a stable pulmonary blood flow (see Case 12.1:1).

Change from in utero to ex utero physiology: impact on physical signs

The change from in utero to ex utero physiology also has a profound influence on the presentation of congenital heart disease. Left-to-right shunts may be clinically undetectable at birth because of the high pulmonary pressure. As the right ventricular pressure falls (Fig. 12.5) VSD murmurs will become louder as the degree of left-to-right shunting increases. Parents frequently question the quality of newborn examination when significant defects are missed at the routine examination. However the paediatrician may take comfort in the fact that some murmurs may not be present in the first few days of life. This is a key feature differentiating obstructive lesions such as pulmonary stenosis or aortic stenosis from shunting lesions such as VSDs. In the former, since the cardiac output must pass through these valves at all times, a murmur will be audible from birth whereas the latter will depend upon the relative pressures between right and left ventricles which changes in the first few days of life. Initially, with right and left ventricular pressures equal, shunts from one side of the heart to the other will be minimal and in fact a mild degree of de-saturation may be observed reflecting right-to-left shunting.

The volume of left-to-right shunt with a VSD demonstrates a similar variation over time as the murmur. Initially a newborn baby may tolerate a large VSD because the high pulmonary pressure associated with fetal life restricts the amount of blood passing from the

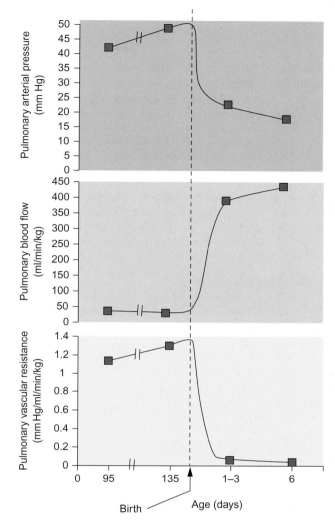

Fig. 12.5 Changes in pulmonary artery pressure, pulmonary blood flow and pulmonary vascular resistance at birth.

left to the right ventricle and back through the pulmonary circulation. Commonly infants become more breathless over the first few weeks of life as the flow through the shunt increases and the volume load on the left ventricle increases. Babies may develop significant cardiac failure. Unless steps are taken to restrict the pulmonary blood flow then permanent damage may occur in the pulmonary vascular bed with the development of pulmonary hypertension. Clinically this is indicated by an improvement in the heart failure, a worrying sign. For some children the pulmonary vascular resistance never falls and they never show signs of heart failure.

By contrast, the residual presence of prenatal structures may obscure complex underlying lesions. For example it is common in transposition of the great arteries (TGA) for children to present at a few days of age with profound cyanosis or collapse. The underlying lesion in TGA is a complex failure of septation in which the aorta arises from the right ventricle and the pulmonary artery arises from

Case
12.1
Fetal cardiovascular system and congenital heart disease: 2

Causes of cyanosis (see questions posed in Case 12.1, Box 1)

1. It is important to distinguish cardiac from respiratory causes of cyanosis. The hyperoxia test (increasing inspired Po_2) is a classic way to do this, and is often more helpful in the child with some breathing difficulties. The basic principle lies in the distinction between a problem with gas transfer and one of circulation. Cardiac cyanosis is not responsive to increasing the inspired oxygen to any great extent. An increase in arterial Po_2 of only 5.5 kPa in this case is strong evidence in favour of cardiac disease.

2. Clinically respiratory disease is usually associated with increased work of breathing which is described as respiratory distress. Respiratory distress is an overall term for signs such as subcostal recession, tracheal tug, nasal flaring and grunting. Cardiac cyanosis may be effortless— certainly in older children. In general babies are tolerant of cyanosis because of the hypoxaemia present in the fetal environment.

3. Dinoprostone is a synthetic prostaglandin (PGE_2). Prostaglandins are important in the natural closure of the ductus arteriosus. Prostaglandins inhibit closure of the duct. Exogenous prostaglandin is given in many types of congenital heart disease where flow through the duct is critical to maintaining pulmonary blood flow or peripheral perfusion. In the case of TGA it is important to maintain high circulating volume in the pulmonary circuit as this promotes shunting of oxygenated blood back into the systemic circulation across the atrial septum.

4. In the normal circulation deoxygenated blood is carried in the systemic veins to the right atrium. From the right atrium it passes through the tricuspid valve into the right ventricle from which it is pumped across the pulmonary valve into the pulmonary artery and thence to the pulmonary capillary bed. Oxygenated blood returns to the heart in the pulmonary veins to the left atrium. Blood crosses the mitral valve into the left ventricle from whence it is pumped via the aortic valve into the aorta and around the body. Eventually it passes through the systemic capillary bed and is collected in venules which drain into the venous system.

5. In the case of TGA the systemic venous return is to the right atrium and then to the right ventricle. However the right ventricle is connected to the aorta and hence pumps de-oxygenated blood back around the body. The pulmonary venous return is to the left atrium and thence to the left ventricle. However the left ventricle is connected to the pulmonary artery and thus directly back to the lung. Fully oxygenated blood is circulated back to the pulmonary circulation.

6. The function of balloon septostomy is to open up the atrial communication thereby improving mixing of systemic venous return (desaturated) and pulmonary venous return (saturated) and thus increasing the systemic saturation of haemoglobin with oxygen.

the left ventricle. Thus there are essentially two separate circulations. Venous blood returns from the body to the right atrium, passes into the right ventricle and is pumped out round the body again. Fully saturated oxygenated blood returns from the lungs to the left atrium, passes into the left ventricle and is then pumped back to the lungs via the pulmonary artery. Clearly in a completely separate circulation oxygen would be extracted until the point where tissues would become hypoxic and die. In order to be compatible with life there must be some mixing of oxygenated and deoxygenated blood. This can occur if the foramen ovale remains open and is of a good size and if the ductus arteriosus remains patent. Mixing only occurs at the foramen ovale but the ductus arteriosus is crucial for maintaining left atrial pressure by filling the pulmonary circulation. As in the normal circulation the pulmonary pressure is lower than systemic pressure and so shunting at the duct is always left to right (systemic to pulmonary).

Initially the child may appear well as the duct remains patent and there is a good flow of blood to the lungs. It should be noted that TGA is frequently not associated with a murmur. Clinical cyanosis may be difficult to identify in the first 48 hours of life because of facial congestion following delivery and a relatively high saturation (85–90%). Infants may behave quite normally leading to routine discharge. However as the ductus arteriosus closes over the subsequent few days the child may become increasingly cyanosed and breathless with increasing hypoxia and acidaemia. The child commonly presents to the emergency department in a collapsed or near collapsed state.

A single anatomical abnormality may vary sufficiently to present with completely different clinical pictures. Take for example the anatomical variability of Fallot's tetralogy. This is the combination of a large subaortic VSD which does not provide any obstruction to flow (not 'restrictive'), and an overriding of the aorta across the ventricular septum, subpulmonary and pulmonary stenosis and right ventricular hypertrophy. At one end of the spectrum the pulmonary obstruction is mild and the pulmonary blood flow is high—remember the VSD is not restrictive. A murmur of pulmonary stenosis may be noted in the newborn period (the VSD is not restrictive and therefore does not produce a murmur). However saturations will be near normal with predominantly left-to-right shunt across the VSD though some mixing at the ventricular level will occur. As the pulmonary vascular resistance falls the left-to-right shunt may increase and the child may become breathless but systemic blood will remain almost fully saturated with oxygen. By comparison, where the pulmonary obstruction is severe, resistance to blood flow to the lungs is greater than that to the body and so desaturated blood preferentially enters the systemic circulation and the child may present with a murmur and cyanosis in the newborn period.

Early and late management of congenital heart disease

Management of congenital heart disease can be divided into three main categories. Firstly there is medical versus surgical management. Thereafter the surgical management may be considered as curative or palliative, i.e. whether the surgeon is able to produce a normal circulation with two ventricles pumping blood separately or whether the best that can be achieved is stabilization and minimization of exercise restriction with surgical reconstruction which does not achieve a normal circulation.

One of the major success stories in modern neonatal medicine has been the medical management of ductus arteriosus patency. Since the key role of E-series prostaglandins in maintaining ductal patency was identified in 1975, two opposing management strategies have had a major impact on the physician's ability to stabilize neonates. Prostaglandins act to maintain ductal patency. A synthetic prostaglandin infusion can be used to re-open and maintain ductal patency in conditions such as pulmonary atresia, TGA or hypoplastic left heart syndrome in which the circulation is critically dependent on ductal patency. Many infants with life threatening congenital heart disease can be stabilized with the use of relatively simple and safe prostaglandin therapy until definitive surgical management is arranged. Conversely in the preterm neonate the PDA can be a troublesome problem causing heart failure and high flow pulmonary oedema resulting in dependency on mechanical ventilation. Treatment with indometacin, a non-steroidal anti-inflammatory drug which inhibits production of prostaglandins, induces ductal closure. The use of indometacin has greatly reduced the number of preterm infants requiring surgical ligation of the duct.

In the infant with a high left-to-right shunt the high output cardiac failure may be managed with diuretics in order to offload excess pulmonary fluid. As with adults a combination of loop (furosemide (frusemide)) and potassium sparing (amiloride, spironolactone) diuretics are used to avoid inducing electrolyte imbalance. In some instances angiotensin converting enzyme (ACE) inhibitors are used to try and reduce pulmonary blood flow by lowering systemic vascular resistance and thereby increasing systemic cardiac output at the expense of pulmonary blood flow. The introduction of ACE inhibitors should only be made with extreme caution in infants, as they frequently have inadequate cardiac reserve to meet the increased demand.

It is almost axiomatic that any congenital heart lesion which requires medical management in early life requires definitive surgical intervention. Advances in surgical and anaesthetic techniques, including cardiopulmonary bypass, have allowed the surgical management of more and more complex lesions with low mortality. Average surgical mortality for all congenital heart disease is now around 2%.

Interesting facts

With the huge improvement in the techniques used, average surgical mortality for all congenital heart disease is now around only 2%.

Though the primary aim of surgical intervention is to reconstruct a circulation which is as close to normal as possible with a single operation this is not always feasible. Some hearts cannot be reconstructed with two ventricles whilst the constraints of surgical technique mean that in other conditions for which two ventricle repair is technically feasible the limitations of early repair mean that initial palliation with later definitive repair is the optimum strategy.

The first intervention which may be performed is a balloon septostomy. This palliative, interventional technique involves the passage of a balloon-tipped catheter from the systemic veins via the right atrium and foramen ovale into the left atrium. The balloon is then inflated and forcibly withdrawn from left to right atrium, tearing the atrial septum and improving atrial mixing. First performed by William Rashkind in 1966, this procedure is most frequently used in TGA to improve spillover of saturated blood from the left atrium to the right atrium whence it can then be circulated to the body. It is one of the earliest interventions a newborn is likely to receive and can be life saving, preventing a terminal hypoxic spiral and relieving the dependence on prostaglandin to maintain ductal patency.

Palliative techniques such as Blalock–Taussig (BT) shunts (connection of the subclavian artery to the pulmonary artery, originally directly but now usually with a Gore-Tex tube) allow the maintenance of pulmonary blood flow in circumstances where this may be restricted such as in tetralogy of Fallot or pulmonary atresia. This stabilizes systemic saturation and encourages growth of the pulmonary arteries whilst protecting the lung vasculature from damage by high pressures and flows. The construction of the shunt is such that it provides a significant resistance between the systemic and pulmonary circulations, balancing adequate blood flow against damage to the pulmonary vasculature. Initially performed in 1944, this was one of the first palliative repairs for cyanotic heart diseases though now definitive repair is more common. Other forms of artificial shunt exist from the aorta to the pulmonary artery, though it is technically more difficult to obtain controlled results. More recent practice has involved the introduction of conduits from the right or, more rarely, left ventricle to pulmonary

Case 12.1 Fetal cardiovascular system and congenital heart disease: 3

Corrective surgery

The child described in Case 12.1:1 proceeded to corrective surgery on day 7 of life. This involved switching the pulmonary artery and aorta with coronary transfer and re-implantation using cardiopulmonary bypass to provide a circulation to the rest of the body during surgery. The operation was uneventful and after 3 days of mechanical ventilation the baby was transferred back to the ward on the fourth postoperative day. The postoperative recovery was otherwise uneventful and the infant was discharged on the tenth postoperative day with normal feeding established.

What is the effect of the corrective operation on the circulation?

The arterial switch operation reconnects the appropriate great arteries to the appropriate ventricles, i.e. pulmonary artery to right ventricle and aorta to left ventricle. Apart from suture lines the only residual abnormalities are that the pulmonary valve remains in the aortic position and the aortic valve lies between the right ventricle and the pulmonary artery. The normal crossover relation of the aorta and pulmonary artery are also disrupted with the pulmonary artery generally lying anterior to the aorta.

artery, the Sanno procedure. This was originally developed to avoid the problem of a reduction in coronary circulation during diastole which may occur with BT shunts. Since the pulmonary artery pressure is lower than systemic at all points of the cardiac cycle, diastolic steal can occur in which coronary perfusion is compromised by preferential flow into the pulmonary system during diastole. Remember that coronary perfusion occurs primarily during diastole (see Chapter 5).

Where there is unrestricted pulmonary blood flow the aim is to reduce the pressure and flow in the lungs. This may be achieved by pulmonary artery banding, the application of a tight ligature around the pulmonary artery, thereby creating an artificial stenosis. This is used in patients who have large VSDs whose anatomy is not favourable for primary closure. For example multiple muscular VSDs may allow high pulmonary blood flow and be easily identifiable on echocardiogram. However they are often difficult to see once the heart is opened and emptied of blood, particularly as the trabeculations in the right ventricle obscure the orifices. Pulmonary artery banding reduces pulmonary blood flow and the pressure in the pulmonary arterial bed, thereby preventing long term damage to the lung vasculature whilst the child grows. With luck the muscular septum will hypertrophy and close the defects spontaneously, or some form of surgical intervention can be attempted later once the child is larger. Once the VSDs have been closed the band may be

removed and the circulation functions normally. Pulmonary artery banding is also used to protect the pulmonary vascular bed in lesions with a single ventricle and unobstructed pulmonary flow. This is particularly important in cases with only one ventricle, as the long-term plan can only be palliative and the quality of palliation is critically dependent on the pressure in the pulmonary arterial tree (see Fontan circulation below). Pulmonary artery banding, whilst an apparently simple procedure, is far from uncomplicated. The operation is a move from one stable state to another – akin to changing canoes in midstream. The potential for catastrophic loss of cardiac output is significant.

In some conditions there is inadequate development of one or other of the ventricles and so two ventricle repair is not possible. Traditionally this was palliated with a repair involving either restricting pulmonary blood flow with pulmonary artery banding or augmenting it with some form of shunt, e.g. Blalock–Taussig. This left the child with an inadequate saturation of their blood with oxygen and a permanent left to right shunt and subsequent volume loading of the single ventricle. However in the late 1960s Francis Fontan demonstrated that with favourable pulmonary artery pressure it was possible to make a direct connection of the systemic venous system to the pulmonary artery. The resulting circulation has no active pumping of blood into the lungs (normally the function of the right ventricle) but relies on passive filling augmented by the negative intrathoracic pressure generated by respiration to promote flow into the lungs. Key to the success of this strategy is the similar value of mean central venous pressure (5–7 mm Hg) and mean pulmonary artery pressure (around 10 mm Hg). Whilst not providing as efficient a system as a two ventricle repair, the Fontan circulation provides a long-term palliation well into early adulthood. Beyond this, longer term outlook is poor however, with the likely need for a transplant at around 30 years of age.

Interesting facts

Gore-Tex is a material widely used in waterproof jackets and boots. It is also a material used to repair and replace damaged major blood vessels.

The construction of a Fontan circulation is staged to allow for the changing haemodynamics of the pulmonary vasculature. Initially the pulmonary vasculature needs to be protected and pulmonary blood flow maintained. In situations such as tricuspid atresia and VSD with hypoplastic right ventricle this may require banding of the pulmonary artery to restrict pulmonary blood flow and lessen damage to the pulmonary vascular bed. It is critical to avoid long-term damage to the pulmonary vascular bed as elevated pulmonary artery pressures will prevent completion of the Fontan circulation. Alternatively, where there is inadequate pulmonary blood flow the creation of a shunt to augment the blood flow may be necessary. Between 4 months and 1 year of age, depending on the lesion and progress of the child, the next stage may be completed with connection of the superior vena cava (SVC) to the right pulmonary artery. Usually any arterial shunt is tied off at this time. Then, between 2 and 6 years of age, the venous connections may be completed with connection of the inferior vena cava (IVC) to the pulmonary arteries. Prior to the completion of the venopulmonary connections the blood of the child will be poorly saturated with oxygen. However, after completion of the surgery the systemic blood saturation with oxygen will generally be in the mid to high 90+% range. Various residual shunts, e.g. the venous drainage from the cardiac muscle itself which returns via the coronary sinus to the right atrium, will generally mean that full saturation can never be achieved.

Further reading

Allen, H.D., Gutgesell, H.P., Clark, E.B., Driscoll, D.J., 2000. Moss and Adams Heart Disease in Infants, Children, Adolescents and Young Adult, sixth ed. Lippincott/Williams & Wilkins, Philadelphia.

Anderson, R.H., Baker, E.J., Macartney, F.J., Rigby, M.L., Shinebourne, E.A., Tynan, M., 2009. Paediatric Cardiology, third ed. Churchill Livingstone, Edinburgh.

Behrman, R.E., Kliegman, R.M., Jenson, H.B., 2007. Nelson Textbook of Pediatrics, eighteenth ed. WB Saunders, Philadelphia.

Campbell, A.G.M., McIntosh, N., 1998. Forfar and Arneils Textbook of Pediatrics, fifth ed. Churchill Livingstone, Edinburgh.

Park, M.K., 2002. The Paediatric Cardiology Handbook, third ed. Mosby, St Louis.

Tulzer, G., 2000. Fetal cardiology. Curr. Opin. Pediatr. 12, 492–496.

EXERCISE AND THE CARDIOVASCULAR SYSTEM

13

Chapter objectives

After studying this chapter, you should be able to:

1. Explain the essential differences between dynamic and static forms of exercise.

2. Describe the background to the changes in cardiac output which support the metabolic needs of muscles during dynamic exercise.

3. Discuss the mechanisms which ensure an appropriate distribution of blood flow during dynamic exercise.

4. Understand the concept of an exercise induced 'oxygen debt'.

5. Describe the problems posed for the cardiovascular system by static forms of exercise.

6. Evaluate the potential benefits associated with different types of training regimens.

7. Explain the use of exercise testing as a way of monitoring the functional capacity of the heart in patients with cardiovascular disease.

Physiological responses to exercise

In broad terms, there are two types of exercise, dynamic and static. Dynamic (isotonic) exercise encompasses activities such as running, cycling, swimming in which large numbers of muscles are involved in rhythmic contraction and relaxation. Static (isometric) exercise is of the sustained straining type, perhaps illustrated by a weightlifter or someone trying to move a heavy object. Muscles are maintained in a contracted state during static exercise. Some forms of exercise, such as rowing, have components of both static and dynamic exercise. In each type there are metabolic demands which must be met by the circulatory system. The functional capacity of the circulatory system is frequently the main limiting factor determining performance. Unless there is some form of lung disease, respiratory function is not normally a limiting factor for exercise performance.

Understanding exercise physiology is not just important in a sporting context. Clinically, exercise testing is used to evaluate the cardiopulmonary performance of patients with a range of circulatory or respiratory disorders. The form of exercise used in this case is normally dynamic exercise performed on a treadmill or exercise bicycle so that physiological recordings including ECG, arterial blood pressure, arterial blood oxygenation and O_2 consumption rate, can be made. Exercise stress testing provides information about the functional exercise capacity of an individual and may be used to monitor progress after therapeutic interventions. It also facilitates investigation of exercise-induced symptoms, such as angina, and uncovers 'silent' changes in the ECG, for example, which may only occur during exercise. Exercise testing must, of course, only be undertaken with due regard for patient safety.

The two basic types of exercise are now discussed separately.

Interesting facts

At rest, the average red blood cell does a complete circuit of the circulatory system, including the lungs, in about 1 minute. In very vigorous dynamic exercise this time may be reduced to only about 12 seconds.

Dynamic (isotonic) exercise

In dynamic exercise there is a linear relationship between exercise intensity and oxygen consumption. After cessation of exercise there is a gradual decrease in oxygen consumption as the 'oxygen debt' is cleared. These events are discussed later in this chapter.

The key cardiovascular changes which support the metabolic needs of contracting muscles in dynamic exercise are:

- an increase in heart rate
- an increase in stroke volume of the heart

Case 13.1 Exercise and the cardiovascular system: 1

Developing exercise intolerance

Peter Jones is a 63-year-old man who, in his younger days, was a professional soccer player. With the training regimens that this involved he maintained a high level of physical fitness. For many years after his retirement as a football player he had kept himself active, particularly with regular games of golf. Recently he had found that this made him very tired. This was especially noticeable on the uphill sections of the course. He had also noticed that he became breathless when climbing the stairs in his house. This worried him because his father had died following a heart attack aged 58 years.

Peter knew that his father had smoked heavily from his teenage years and in his latter years had suffered considerably with angina. Apart from a very occasional cigarette Peter had effectively been a non-smoker and had not experienced episodes of angina. Nevertheless, he was concerned about the decline in his physical capacity which he felt could not just be attributed to advancing years. Peter, therefore, made an appointment to see his family doctor.

This scenario gives rise to the following questions:

1. What are the normal cardiovascular responses to exercise?
2. How can exercise capacity be improved by training?
3. What factors limit exercise ability with increasing age?

- a modest increase in mean arterial blood pressure
- changes in the distribution of blood flow to support exercising muscles.

Increased extraction of oxygen from arterial blood (see Chapter 1) in exercising muscles will also contribute to the increase in oxygen delivery.

Initiation of the cardiovascular responses to exercise

Identification of the key physiological events at the initiation of dynamic exercise has long been contentious and is still the subject of debate, despite the existence of theoretical models for more than 100 years. Reflex control of the circulation normally relies on sensory information provided from baroreceptors and chemoreceptors (see Chapter 10). These same reflexes function during ongoing exercise, but mean arterial BP, P_{O_2} and P_{CO_2} do not change significantly at the start of exercise. The changes in cardiac function during exercise therefore occur too rapidly to be explained by activation of baroreceptor and chemoreceptor reflexes.

The most popular hypothesis used to explain the initiation of cardiovascular responses to exercise is the feedforward' or 'central command' theory. This suggests that the areas of the brain which drive muscle contraction at the start of exercise also produce the drive to increase heart rate and lung ventilation. This theory was first proposed in 1913 and numerous modifications have been suggested since then. The parts of the brain particularly involved in 'central command' are thought to be the motor cortex and the hypothalamus. The cerebellum, which has the major role in the coordination of muscle movement, is also involved in coordinating the cardiovascular response to exercise.

Areas within the medulla control the sympathetic and parasympathetic nerves which normally regulate heart rate and cardiac contractility as part of the baroreceptor reflex (see Chapter 10). At the start of exercise, the influence of central command over the medullary centres is to decrease vagal tone and to increase sympathetic drive, thus increasing heart rate. Part of this response may be an alteration in the operation of the baroreceptor reflex (see Chapter 10). Under normal conditions, this reflex keeps blood pressure relatively constant at a 'set point'. During exercise, central command induced changes in this set point have the same effect as a blood pressure which is too low, hence leading to an increase in heart rate.

Reflex activation of the sympathetic nervous system also leads to peripheral vasoconstriction (see Chapter 9). This occurs particularly in the splanchnic and kidney circulations and in the vessels of non-contracting muscles. This helps to divert blood flow to active muscles. The central command mechanism is probably complemented by feedback from metabolite concentrations, particularly [K^+], detected by chemoreceptors in contracting muscles and information from mechanoreceptors within moving joints and muscles.

Cardiovascular changes in sustained exercise

Cardiac output is a function of both heart rate and stroke volume. Figure 13.1 shows the effect of different intensities of dynamic exercise on cardiac output, heart rate and stroke volume in healthy young individuals. Intense exercise in trained athletes may require a fivefold increase in cardiac output. Changes in stroke volume reach maximum levels at a moderate exercise intensity (see below). Beyond this level, further increases in cardiac output are provided solely by increases in heart rate. Increased oxygen delivery to tissues is also achieved by increasing the extraction of oxygen from arterial blood (see Chapter 1). Thus, the arterial–venous oxygen content difference widens with increasing exercise intensity.

Maximum heart rate in intense exercise in a physically fit 20 year old 'textbook person' is 180–195 bpm. This figure changes with age so that maximum heart rate in a 10-year-old may be 210 bpm (see Chapter 12), whereas in a person aged 65 it is only about 165 bpm. Central command dominates heart rate control in mild exercise but, in more intense forms of exercise, autonomic reflexes (see Chapter 10) and the indirect effects of metabolites

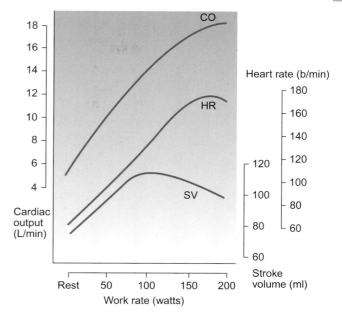

Fig. 13.1 Responses to sustained dynamic exercise. Typical plateau responses of heart rate, stroke volume and cardiac output to different intensities of sustained dynamic exercise in a fit young individual.

(see Chapter 9) generated in contracting muscles become increasingly important. Secretion of adrenaline (epinephrine) and noradrenaline (norepinephrine) from the adrenal medulla, and their effect on the sinoatrial node, also contributes to the increase in heart rate.

Stroke volume of the heart increases during dynamic exercise but reaches a maximum level at an exercise intensity of about half maximum O_2 consumption (Fig. 13.1). The extent of changes in stroke volume appears to vary with the type of dynamic exercise and the physical fitness of the individual. In trained individuals there may be relatively greater changes in stroke volume at lower workloads. In Chapter 4 the factors determining the stroke volume of the heart are identified as:

- preload effects (Frank–Starling mechanism)
- contractility effects
- afterload effects.

Increased filling of the right ventricle (increased preload) occurs as a result of increased contraction of limb muscles and therefore increased venous return to the heart. A simple, but often neglected, concept is that increases in cardiac output can only be achieved if there is an equivalent increase in venous return of blood to the heart, you can't get out what you don't put in! Sympathetic nervous system activation during dynamic exercise will lead to venoconstriction which also increases preload on the heart. When resting in a supine position, because there is less effect of gravity on venous return from the lower part of the body, stroke volume is already higher than in an upright posture. The cardiac output increases which occur during exercise in a supine position

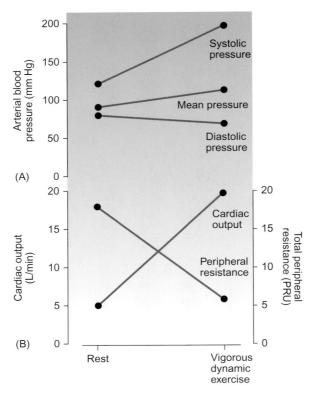

Fig. 13.2 Effects of vigorous dynamic exercise. Typical effect of vigorous dynamic exercise on cardiac output, total peripheral resistance and arterial blood pressure shown as systolic, diastolic and mean pressures. Note: the units for expressing total peripheral resistance (PRU) are derived from the formula:

$$\text{Total peripheral resistance} = \frac{\text{Mean arterial pressure}}{\text{Cardiac output}}$$

Thus:

$$PRU = \frac{mm\,Hg \cdot min}{litre}$$

Compare the responses to dynamic exercise shown in this figure with those for static exercise (Fig. 13.5).

(e.g. swimming) are achieved almost entirely as a result of an increase in heart rate because stroke volume is already approaching maximum levels at the start of exercise.

Contractility increases in the heart are associated with an increase in myocyte intracellular [Ca^{++}] and lead to an increased force of ventricular contraction (see Chapter 4). Sympathetic nervous system activation in exercise and the release of adrenal medulla catecholamines will lead to increased contractility via activation of β-adrenoceptors. The modest increase in mean arterial blood pressure (Fig. 13.2) which normally occurs in dynamic exercise will impose an increased afterload on the heart and hence tend to moderate the preload and contractility induced increases in stroke volume outlined above.

Changes in arterial blood pressure during dynamic exercise are summarized in Figure 13.2. The increase in

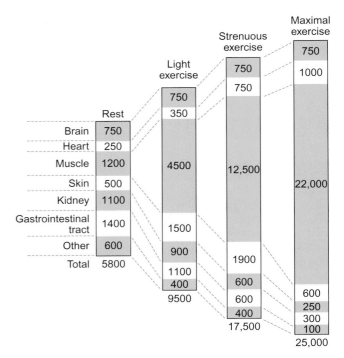

Fig. 13.3 Distribution of cardiac output at different levels of exercise. (From Richardson DR, Randall, DC and Speck DF 1998 Cardiopulmonary system. Fence Creek Publishing, Madison, CT, with permission; data was originally adapted from Chapman CB, Mitchell JH 1965 The physiology of exercise. Scientific American 212:91.)

systolic pressure reflects the increased force of ventricular contraction during exercise. Diastolic pressure reflects a combination of changes in resistance to blood flow, particularly through the dilated blood vessels in exercising muscles, and the increase in heart rate. This point needs some further explanation. Metabolite-induced vasodilatation in exercising muscles leads to a decrease in the resistance to blood flow (Fig. 13.2). During diastole, therefore, blood will flow out of the aorta more easily and so the phase of the arterial pressure curve which corresponds to diastole will become steeper. Diastole is terminated at the next time the aortic valve opens. As heart rate increases in exercise this point will be reached more quickly and the pressure fall during diastole will be ended when the next heart beat starts. Overall, mean arterial blood pressure is still mainly regulated by the baroreceptor reflex.

Distribution of blood flow in exercise

The distribution of blood flow during dynamic exercise is summarized in Figure 13.3. At rest, 20–25% of resting cardiac output is distributed to the muscles, a flow rate of the order of 1 L/min. During maximal exercise about 90% of the increased cardiac output goes to the muscles, a muscle blood flow rate of perhaps 22 L/min. The changes in cardiac output during exercise are discussed above but it must also be remembered that the total peripheral resistance during maximum dynamic exercise is of the order of one third of the resting resistance (Fig. 13.2). Two opposing mechanisms produce a redistribution of blood flow during exercise. In exercising muscles the increased metabolic rate leads to metabolite-induced vasodilatation (see Chapter 9). There is also activation of the sympathetic nervous system during exercise which causes α-receptor-mediated vasoconstriction. In exercising muscles the metabolite vasodilatation overwhelms the effect of the sympathetic vasoconstriction response leading overall to vasodilatation. In circuits such as the kidneys and splanchnic circulation, where there is no exercise-induced metabolite vasodilatation, sympathetically driven vasoconstriction dominates and blood flow is lower than resting levels (Fig. 13.3).

Plasma renin activity, and therefore generation of the vasoconstrictor angiotensin II (see Chapter 9), also increases during exercise and is thought to contribute to the changes in blood flow in the abdominal viscera. However, studies using angiotensin converting enzyme inhibitor drugs, which block the formation of angiotensin II, have shown no effect on maximum oxygen uptake or on exercise performance, suggesting that activation of the renin-angiotensin system is not a critical factor in exercise responses.

Blood vessels in the brain have little α-adrenoceptor-linked vasoconstrictor tone and so brain blood flow does not change during exercise. The myocardium also has little neural vasoconstrictor tone and so metabolite-induced vasodilatation predominates in the heart. Coronary blood flow therefore relates directly to work done by the cardiac muscle. Redistribution of blood flow during exercise throughout the body is also aided by the vasodilator effects of nitric oxide produced by vascular endothelial cells (see Chapter 9). Increased blood flow along a blood vessel leads to increased shear stress between the blood and the endothelial cells. This is a trigger for the release of the vasodilator nitric oxide produced by constitutive enzymes in the endothelium.

The skin has a particular role to play in thermoregulation. Heat generated in exercise is dissipated through increased skin blood flow (see Chapter 9). In moderate exercise, skin blood flow increases three to four fold. In intense exercise, cutaneous vasoconstriction occurs (Fig. 13.3). This has the effect of diverting more blood to exercising muscles but the corollary is that body temperature must rise.

The net effect of all these changes is that muscle blood flow can increase 20 fold during intense exercise (Fig. 13.3).

Oxygen debt and the recovery from exercise

As there is a short lag period between the onset of exercise and the development of the full cardiorespiratory response to that level of exercise, an 'oxygen debt' occurs

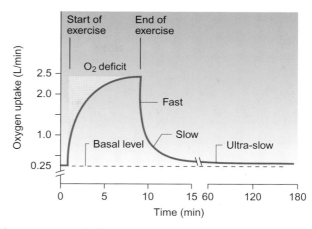

Fig. 13.4 Oxygen deficit. Development of an oxygen deficit (debt) at the start of exercise because the rate of oxygen uptake does not initially match the intensity of exercise. Recovery from the oxygen deficit occurs in three phases once the exercise has finished. (From Astrand P-O, Rodahl K 1986. Textbook of work physiology. McGraw Hill Publishing, New York, with permission.)

(Fig. 13.4). This oxygen debt has three chemically identifiable components:

1. A decrease in cellular [ATP] as it is used to drive muscle movement.

2. Depletion of creatine-phosphate stored within cells as an immediate mechanism for rephosphorylating ADP to ATP (muscle cells contain about four to five times as much creatine-phosphate as ATP).

3. Accumulation of lactic acid in muscles. It has been produced anaerobically and cannot be converted back to pyruvate so that it can enter mitochondria and be metabolized aerobically until sufficient supplies of oxygen are available.

Recovery from exercise has three phases. The 'fast' phase (Fig. 13.4) represents the rephosphorylation of ADP and creatine stores within the muscle. Following vigorous exercise the half-life for this phase is about 30 seconds. During the 'slow' phase, which has a half-life of about 15 min, lactate is resynthesized into glucose and then glycogen. The ultra-slow phase of recovery from exercise lasts for several hours. It is caused by a rise in body temperature during exercise which produces an increased metabolic rate and hence an increase in oxygen consumption. The extent of the oxygen debt in any given individual will of course reflect the intensity of exercise and how well the cardiovascular and respiratory systems function.

Interesting facts

The differences between the work done during maximum dynamic exercise and maximum static exercise can be observed whilst watching major events such as the Olympic Games on television. Runners are gasping for breath at the end of a race but a world record setting weightlifter is hardly out of breath at all.

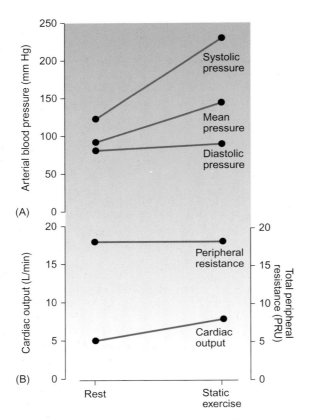

Fig. 13.5 Effects of vigorous static exercise. Typical effect of vigorous static exercise on cardiac output, total peripheral resistance and arterial blood pressure shown as systolic, diastolic and mean pressures. The units for total peripheral resistance (PRU) are defined in the legend to Figure 13.2. Compare the responses to dynamic exercise (Fig. 13.2) to those for static exercise shown in this figure.

Cardiovascular responses to static exercise

Static exercise involves the sustained development of muscle tension. In maximum static exercise the energy expenditure (oxygen consumption) is relatively small compared to maximum dynamic exercise. This is illustrated by the fact that a weightlifter, unlike a runner, is not very obviously breathless after completing a lift. There are however considerable effects of static exercise on the cardiovascular system. The changes in heart rate are less marked than in dynamic exercise but there is a reflexly induced increase in diastolic as well as systolic blood pressure. An increase in cardiac output, driven by 'central command', is not matched by the extensive metabolite induced vasodilatation found in dynamic exercise so diastolic blood pressure increases (Fig. 13.5).

Two factors limit the increase in stroke volume during static exercise. Any whole body straining exercise associated with breath holding and closure of the glottis will result in an increase in intrathoracic pressure. This will tend to compress the inferior vena cava and reduce venous return to the heart. Such a series of changes in

| Case 13.1 | Exercise and the cardiovascular system: 2 |

Exercise testing

The doctor examined Peter and found that his blood pressure was 160/95 and said that if it was still the same next week he would suggest that Peter should start taking a thiazide diuretic. An ECG recorded in the surgery failed to show any obvious abnormality but the doctor was still concerned about Peter's description of tiredness on moderate exercise. He therefore referred Peter for investigation in the exercise stress testing laboratory in the local hospital.

Pulmonary function tests were performed by spirometry. Measurements of forced expiratory volume in 1 second (FEV_1) and forced vital capacity (FVC) were made and the results were found to be within the normal range for a person of Peter's height, age and gender.

Peter was then exercised on a treadmill whilst a 12 lead ECG was recorded. At the slowest treadmill speeds, 1.7 and 3 miles per hour (mph) on a gradient of 10° Peter felt reasonably comfortable with the level of exercise but at 3 mph there were initial signs of S-T segment depression in leads I, aVL, V_5 and V_6 on the ECG. When the treadmill speed was increased to 4 mph Peter started to feel uncomfortably breathless halfway through the planned 3 minute test. At the same time the S-T segment depression reached a level which made the laboratory staff stop the test. A diagnosis of myocardial ischaemia in the lateral wall of the left ventricle was proposed. Peter was referred to the cardiologists for an angiogram investigation. This subsequently provided evidence of narrowing of three main coronary arteries probably as a result of atheroma.

This history raises the following questions:

1. What are the main risk factors for development of atheroma and which are relevant for consideration of the case of Peter?
2. Why did Peter become breathless on exertion?
3. What further laboratory/clinical data would be useful in helping to understand this case?

the cardiovascular system are known as the Valsalva manoeuvre (described on p. 157). Flow of blood through exercising muscles is also limited by the sustained muscle contraction. The second factor limiting stroke volume in static exercise is the increase in arterial blood pressure (Fig. 13.5) which will impose an afterload on the heart (see Chapter 4). Very substantial increases in mean arterial pressure occur during maximal isometric exercise. These occur particularly with arm exercise and so are not just related to changes in venous return. Chemoreceptor reflexes originating within the arm muscles are thought to be important in this event.

Interesting facts

The list of people who have died from cardiovascular collapse following a rise in intra-abdominal and intrathoracic pressure whilst sitting on the toilet includes Elvis Presley, George III and Catherine the Great.

Valsalva manoeuvre

This is a series of cardiovascular events associated with static exercise such as weightlifting but they also occur in any form of straining movement including defaecation. Indeed the associated increase in heart rate may have catastrophic consequences for patients with already compromised cardiac function.

The key event of the Valsalva manoeuvre is a rise in intrathoracic pressure produced by contraction of the abdominal and thoracic wall muscles and hence attempted expiration against a closed glottis. The manoeuvre was first described in 1707 by the Italian anatomist Valsalva. The cardiovascular responses are frequently divided into four phases.

Phase I: a sudden rise in arterial pressure associated with the increased intrathoracic pressure. A small decrease in heart rate occurs.

Phase II: the sustained high intrathoracic pressure compresses the vena cava hence leading to reduced venous return and a fall in cardiac output. Arterial pressure starts to fall. The baroreceptor reflex therefore produces a tachycardia.

Phase III: when the straining response ends and intrathoracic pressure decreases there is, transiently, a further small rise in heart rate.

Phase IV: as venous return is no longer impeded, venous blood, which has been pooled in the lower part of the body, surges back to the heart resulting in a rise in cardiac output and arterial blood pressure. The consequence is a reflex bradycardia before the circulatory control mechanisms return to their normal resting state.

The series of changes in heart rate during the Valsalva manoeuvre are dependent on an intact autonomic nervous system. This provides the basis for a non-invasive test for the functional competence of the autonomic nervous system. It can be used, for example, in patients with long-standing poorly controlled Type I diabetes mellitus in whom autonomic nervous system dysfunction is a common problem.

Training effects of exercise

Epidemiological studies have shown that there is a genetic component to endurance exercise performance. The actual genetically determined factors are quite difficult to unravel but seem to include aspects which determine maximum oxygen uptake and the level of exercise at which lactate accumulation occurs. However, within any one individual, maximum oxygen uptake and exercise performance may be improved by training.

Training effects are an increase in physical performance as a response to repeated exercise. Such benefits do not come easily and a typical regimen to improve performance might be exercise to the level of 60% of maximum oxygen consumption, carried out for 20–30 minutes, at a frequency of two or three times a week for at least 8–10 weeks.

The nature of training effects achieved depends on the type of training undertaken. This might be based on a dynamic exercise programme (also called isotonic, aerobic or endurance training) or a static exercise schedule (isometric, strength or power training). With dynamic exercise training there is an increase in the size of the chambers of the heart and an increase in both resting stroke volume and ejection fraction (see Chapter 4). Static exercise training leads to an increase in the thickness of the left ventricle wall and, as a consequence, a decrease in stroke volume and ejection fraction. This form of training therefore brings few benefits in cardiovascular performance.

The athlete who bases a training programme on dynamic exercise is likely to achieve a greater maximum oxygen consumption as a result of an increased cardiac output. For any given workload, the trained athlete is likely to have a lower heart rate than an unfit person. However the maximum heart rate that can be achieved does not change with training. Recovery back to resting heart rate after exercise is quicker in a trained individual.

A lower peripheral resistance in the trained athlete will tend to reduce arterial blood pressure and hence decrease cardiac afterload. A sustained reduction in arterial blood pressure means that there has been a resetting of the baroreceptor reflex (see Chapter 10). The site where this change occurs is thought to be the cardiovascular control centres in the caudal hypothalamus.

Cardiovascular health benefits of exercise

Below the level of the changes brought about by training regimens, there is evidence that individuals who indulge in regular physical activity have a reduced incidence of myocardial infarction and reduced mortality from cardiovascular disease. The type of exercise considered to be beneficial is the dynamic type characterized by walking, swimming and cycling. Static (isometric) exercise regimens do not appear to be beneficial in this context. Exercise programmes are also thought to contribute to the rehabilitation of patients following a myocardial infarction.

The mechanisms behind these beneficial effects of exercise are not entirely clear but they probably include a decrease in atherogenesis (see Chapter 8) or an improvement in the heart's ability to tolerate the consequences of ischaemia. This may be manifested by a decrease in thrombotic or arrhythmic events in the heart. After a period of exercise, blood pressure in hypertensive subjects is reduced for several hours. This appears to be associated with a resetting of the baroreceptor reflex.

Clinical uses of exercise testing

Oxygen consumption is directly proportional to the work performed and is the best single measurement of exercise intensity. Correspondingly maximal oxygen consumption ($V_{O_{2}max}$), which depends on a combination of the maximum achievable cardiac output and the oxygen extraction from the blood in the periphery, provides an index of the functional capacity of the entire circulatory system. This is the basis for the now widespread use of exercise stress testing in cardiovascular medicine. Although $V_{O_{2}max}$ is not routinely measured directly, it is inferred from the maximum exercise capacity. Compared to some

other ways of assessing cardiac performance such as coronary angiography an exercise test has the advantage that it is non-invasive. The main uses are to evaluate chest pain and arrhythmias, to screen for coronary artery disease and to determine the functional capacity of an individual.

The patient exercises on either a treadmill or stationary exercise bicycle. The exercise level is progressively increased through a series of standardized stages until a level is reached at which the test is terminated. One widely used protocol based on a treadmill test is the Bruce test. The workload is increased every 3 minutes. Table 13.1 summarizes the different stages of the test. The lowest level of exercise (functional class III) is set at a level of oxygen consumption which is about three times resting levels whereas the highest level of the test is about 13 times normal resting oxygen consumption. A patient with a maximum work capacity of only 17 mL O_2/min/kg b.w. (functional class II) would have a reduced exercise tolerance for normal daily activities. During the test the patient is continually observed and questioned about developing symptoms of angina and breathlessness. Arterial blood pressure is regularly recorded together with ECG and heart rate.

Observations which provide markers for the presence and severity of coronary artery disease include the following:

- duration and extent of exercise capability

- extent of upward or downward deflection of the ST segment of the ECG—these changes are usually myocardial ischaemia related

- a fall in blood pressure during exercise

- development of arrhythmias.

As exercise testing is a potentially hazardous procedure detailed guidelines (Box 13.1) have been published which stipulate contraindications for starting an exercise test and for terminating a test. The examples shown in these two tables have been selected from the much more extensive guidelines published in 2002 by an American

---

Case 13.1

Exercise and the cardiovascular system: 3

Treatment and outcome of case

Further tests by the cardiology team showed that Peter's myocardium was reasonably healthy. He was considered to be a good candidate for coronary artery bypass graft surgery and was referred to the cardiac surgeons.

Postsurgery recovery was uneventful and after a period of several weeks had elapsed Peter found that his exercise tolerance had improved markedly. He was once again able to climb the stairs in his house without discomfort and to complete a round of golf. He was advised to exercise every day with a walk of 3–5 miles.

Table 13.1 Modified Bruce treadmill exercise test

Functional class	Typical patient status	Treadmill		Oxygen consumption (mL/min/kg b.w.)
		Speed (mph)	Gradient (%)	
I	Normal healthy active	4.2	16	46
I	Normal healthy sedentary	3.4	14	35
I	Borderline	3.0	13	28
II	Symptomatic	1.7	10	17
III	Symptomatic (e.g. post MI or elderly)	1.5	8	10

Note: resting oxygen consumption by the textbook 70 kg person is 250 mL/min based on 3.6 mL/min/kg b.w.

Box 13.1 Detailed guidelines for beginning and terminating an exercise stress test

Contraindications for beginning exercise testing

Acute myocardial infarction up to 2 days previously
Unstable angina which is not adequately controlled
Symptomatic cardiac arrhythmias
Severe aortic stenosis
Acute pulmonary embolus
Severe arterial hypertension
High degree atrioventricular block

Criteria for terminating exercise testing

Moderate to severe angina
Drop in blood pressure of more than 10 mm Hg
Signs of poor tissue perfusion such as cyanosis or pallor
Dizziness or near syncope (fainting)
Subjects wish to stop
ECG changes develop which are characteristic of significant myocardial ischaemia
Sustained ventricular tachycardia
Significant arrhythmias

College of Cardiology and American Heart Association (ACC/AHA) task force.

Exercise testing is not foolproof and the sensitivity of the test for detecting coronary heart disease is overall only 66%. Not surprisingly testing does predict severe disease more accurately than mild disease. In addition to false negatives the test will also throw up false positives. For unexplained reasons false positives are six to eight times more common in females than in males. Despite these problems exercise testing remains a very important way of evaluating patients, particularly those with ischaemic heart disease.

Further reading

Astrand, P.-O., Rodahl, K., Dahl, H.A., Strømme, S.B., 2003. Textbook of Work Physiology, fourth ed. Human Kinetics, Champaign, IL.

Gibbons, R.J., Balady, G.J., Bricker, J.T., et al., 2002. ACC/AHA 2002. Guideline update for exercise testing: summary article. Circulation 106, 1883–1892.

Herd, J.A., 1991. Cardiovascular response to stress. Physiol. Rev. 71, 305–326.

Jones, J.H., Linstedt, S.L., 1993. Limits to maximal performance. Annu. Rev. Physiol. 55, 547–569.

McArdle, W.D., Katch, F.I., Katch, V.L., 2006. Exercise Physiology: Energy, Nutrition and Human Performance, sixth ed. Lippincott/Williams and Wilkins, Baltimore.

Robergs, R.A., Keteyian, S.J., 2003. Exercise Physiology, second ed. McGraw-Hill, New York.

Waldrop, T.G., Eldridge, F.L., Iwamoto, G.A., Mitchell, J.H., 1996. Central Neural Control of Respiration and Circulation During Exercise, American Handbook of Physiology Section 12: Exercise: Regulation and Integration of Multiple Systems. American Physiological Society, Bethesda, MD.

Wilmore, J.H., Costill, D.L., Kenny, W.L., 2007. Physiology of Sport and Exercise, fourth ed. Human Kinetics, Champaign, IL.

HAEMORRHAGE AND CIRCULATORY SHOCK

14

Chapter objectives

After studying this chapter you should be able to:

1. Explain the importance of changes in arterial blood pressure following haemorrhagic shock both in relation to the perfusion of tissues and the role of a fall in blood pressure in triggering compensatory responses.

2. Describe the immediate physiological responses to haemorrhage which help to sustain arterial blood pressure.

3. Understand how a change in the balance of the 'Starling forces' across capillary walls leads to the 'internal transfusion', a movement of interstitial fluid into the circulation.

4. Explain how changes in kidney function, plasma protein synthesis in the liver and red blood cell production in the bone marrow eventually lead to the replacement of lost blood volume.

5. Discuss the concept of decompensated or irreversible shock and outline the pathophysiological mechanisms involved.

6. List the four main types of mechanism behind circulatory shock responses.

7. Outline the basis for using blood, crystalloid and colloid solutions as replacement body fluids.

Introduction

Blood volume in the textbook subject is of the order of 5 L (see Chapter 1) and at any one time about 65% of this volume is in the venous compartment of the circulation. A reduction in blood volume may occur in many ways. Loss of whole blood through blood vessel trauma either directly out of the subject or into other tissues such as the lumen of the stomach or a thigh muscle is referred to as haemorrhage. However, excessive vasodilatation of peripheral blood vessels will induce similar physiological responses to loss of blood volume. These processes increase the 'volume' of the circulatory system whilst the volume of blood it contains remains unchanged leading to a relative hypovolaemia.

Normal physiological compensatory responses will usually cope with low levels of blood loss (up to 10% blood volume) without problem. This happens frequently on a voluntary basis with people who lose 500 mL blood while attending a blood donor session. The fundamentals of these physiological responses are firstly short-term maintenance of arterial blood pressure so that tissue perfusion is sustained and, secondly, over a longer time course, the lost blood volume is replaced. These mechanisms, which link together many of the individual topics covered in greater detail earlier in this book, will now be reviewed. Severe insults to the circulatory system lead to the syndrome of circulatory shock. This topic is discussed at the end of this chapter. A case history of a patient who has suffered a haemorrhage is shown in Case 14.1:1.

Interesting facts

Approximately two thirds of the blood volume is in the small and large veins. Loss of blood volume mainly affects the volume of blood in the venous compartment rather than the rest of the circulation.

Arterial blood pressure changes in response to haemorrhage

Rapid (time course in minutes) blood volume losses of the order of 5–10% in someone with normally functioning circulatory reflexes produce little if any change in mean arterial pressure. A rapid 15–20% haemorrhage will cause a modest reduction in mean arterial pressure from a normal textbook value of about 93 mm Hg (see Chapter 9) to about 80–90 mm Hg. Recovery from such a haemorrhage using normal physiological mechanisms should be uneventful. A 20–30% blood volume loss might typically result in a drop in mean arterial blood pressure to 60–80 mm Hg and generate some indications of shock responses but such a haemorrhage would not normally be fatal. A blood volume loss of 30–40% however would lead to a substantial reduction of mean arterial blood pressure to 50–70 mm Hg with serious shock responses which may become irreversible. Blood volume loss beyond 50% would normally be fatal.

Case 14.1 Haemorrhage and circulatory shock: 1

Gastrointestinal bleed

Linda Hamilton is 50 years old and has suffered from mild rheumatoid arthritis for 8 years. Her symptoms are managed with diclofenac 50 mg twice a day (an NSAID with analgesic and anti-inflammatory actions). She has not been troubled with major joint disruption. Over the last 3 weeks she has noted an occasional darkening of her stools. One morning she woke feeling normal but after breakfast became quite light headed. She then suffered some abdominal discomfort and felt slightly anxious. During the late morning she developed a violent abdominal cramp and had an intense urge to defaecate. The stools she passed were dark and extremely offensive.

She called her GP for advice and she immediately advised Mrs Hamilton to call an ambulance and go to A&E. The GP explained that Mrs Hamilton may be bleeding into her gut from an ulcer. (This is a well recognized side effect of NSAIDs.)

Whilst waiting for the ambulance to arrive Mrs Hamilton began to feel more unwell. She became nauseous and, whilst in the ambulance, vomited a considerable amount of altered blood. The paramedics checked her pulse and blood pressure. Her heart rate was 115 bpm and her blood pressure 128/85 mm Hg. Her peripheries were cool and capillary refill time was 4 seconds. The paramedics inserted a large bore cannula into a vein in her arm and gave her 500 mL of Gelofusine. Her heart rate settled slightly to 95 bpm and she described feeling less unwell.

While she is still in the ambulance the following questions arise:

1. How is Linda's blood pressure being maintained at this time? What evidence is contained in the history to indicate the physiological mechanisms involved?
2. What is the rationale for the infusion of a colloid solution (Gelofusine)?

The fundamental links between blood loss and hypotension are described in Chapter 4 and are summarized in Figure 14.1. Decreased blood volume leads to decreased right atrial pressure and consequently decreased filling of the right ventricle. This leads to a decrease in stroke volume (Starling's law) and therefore to a reduction in cardiac output. A 20% reduction in blood volume would typically result in an initial reduction in resting cardiac output from about 5 L/min to about 3 L/min. As mean arterial pressure is the product of cardiac output and peripheral resistance there is a fall in blood pressure as identified above. An important first aid point is that it is inadvisable to prop up someone who has suffered a haemorrhage to a sitting position. This would only further reduce the preload effects on the heart.

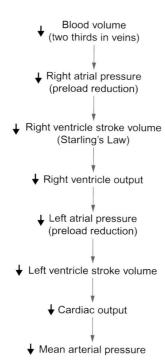

Blood volume
(two thirds in veins)

↓ Right atrial pressure
(preload reduction)

↓ Right ventricle stroke volume
(Starling's Law)

↓ Right ventricle output

↓ Left atrial pressure
(preload reduction)

↓ Left ventricle stroke volume

↓ Cardiac output

↓ Mean arterial pressure

Fig. 14.1 Link between haemorrhage and fall in arterial blood pressure.

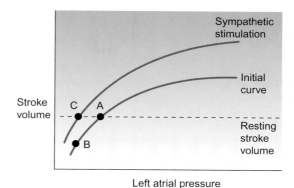

Fig. 14.2 Cardiac response to fast haemorrhage. Representation of cardiac function responses to moderate levels of fast haemorrhage. (A) Normal resting stroke volume. (B) Reduced stroke volume following a haemorrhage (decreased preload) if no compensatory responses occurred. (C) Restoration of stroke volume following activation of the sympathetic nervous system and, consequently, an increase in cardiac contractility. Preload, represented by left atrial pressure is still lower (C) than before the haemorrhage (A).

The compensatory responses which would help to restore blood pressure are triggered by the cardiovascular reflexes discussed in Chapter 10. Of prime importance is the carotid sinus baroreceptor reflex. The modified nerve endings which constitute the baroreceptor become less stretched as blood pressure falls. Fewer action potentials will therefore pass up the glossopharyngeal nerve and enter the brain at the level of the medulla. Following central processing of the baroreceptor input there will be activation of sympathetic outflow and inhibition of the parasympathetic nerve supply to the heart. The consequences are an increased heart rate (tachycardia) and an increase in cardiac contractility, both of which contribute to a raised cardiac output despite decreased preload effects on the heart (see Chapter 4). Re-establishment of a normal resting stroke volume as a result of a sympathetically induced increase in cardiac contractility is illustrated in Figure 14.2. In otherwise normal subjects, a significant tachycardia does not occur until the blood loss has exceeded 700–800 mL (10–15%).

Sympathetic nervous system activation also leads to α_1-receptor-mediated vasoconstriction (see Chapter 9). The regions of the circulation which are particularly affected by sympathetic vasoconstriction responses include the skin, gut, kidney and skeletal muscle. The brain and coronary circulations are relatively preserved especially during the sequel to a haemorrhage amounting to about 20% or less blood volume loss. Concurrent sympathetically mediated venoconstriction will help to maintain central venous pressure and hence limit the fall in preload on the right side of the heart. An unfortunate practical aspect of this venoconstriction is that it may hinder attempts to gain access to the circulation with a venous cannula so that infusion of blood or other replacement body fluids can commence.

The patient who has suffered a haemorrhage and has therefore activated these compensatory responses appears pallid due to cutaneous vasoconstriction, with cold clammy skin, possibly with peripheral cyanosis, and a weak rapid pulse. The responses to haemorrhage will vary considerably between individuals depending on factors such as age and gender, nutrition and fluid balance, season of the year and environmental temperature as well as less easily defined individual characteristics. The extent and speed of the haemorrhage will be important as well. When haemorrhage reaches levels of the order of 25–35% blood loss the sympathetic activation outlined above is succeeded by inhibition of sympathetic outflow and progression to circulatory shock as described later in this chapter. Peripheral cyanosis (see Chapter 1) is associated with a reduced local blood flow and hence greater than normal extraction of oxygen from the remaining blood. Sweating is regulated by the sympathetic nervous system and so is another manifestation of the baroreceptor reflex. Some of these autonomic nervous system mediated changes feature in the case history of Linda Hamilton outlined in Case 14.1:1. A simple but quite effective test of peripheral circulatory function is the nail capillary refill test. Pressure is applied to a finger nail bed until it has blanched. This indicates that blood has been forced away from the area. When pressure is removed the time taken for blood to return to the nail bed (indicated by a change in colour) is measured. Normally capillary refill time will be less than 2 seconds. A longer time indicates reduced tissue perfusion. This test is particularly useful in children as other signs of imminent circulatory collapse appear relatively late.

Short-term responses which help to restore lost blood volume

In Chapter 11 the 'Starling forces' which determine the movement of water across capillary walls are described. Fundamentally, the capillary blood pressure (hydrostatic pressure) tends to move water out of the capillary bed into the interstitial fluid. This is opposed by a gradient of colloid osmotic pressure which will tend to draw water from the interstitial compartment back into the capillary.

Following a haemorrhage, there may be a fall in mean arterial pressure but, in addition, a compensatory peripheral vasoconstrictor response occurs. As the main resistance vessels (see Chapter 9) are the arterioles, vessels which come immediately before the capillaries, there will be a fall in capillary blood pressure following a haemorrhage. This will alter the balance of the Starling forces and, as the colloid osmotic pressure of plasma is initially unchanged, this will result in a net movement of water from the interstitial space into the blood. This is illustrated in Figure 14.3. The rate and extent of this internal replacement of lost blood volume will depend on the rate and degree of blood loss. A rapid loss of 20% of blood volume (about a 1000 mL haemorrhage in the 'textbook person') will lead to perhaps 600 mL of interstitial fluid entering the blood over a period of around 10 minutes. This is sometimes referred to as an 'internal transfusion'. As skeletal muscle constitutes about 50% of body weight this tissue is a major source of the interstitial fluid for the internal transfusion.

A further factor which helps to maintain the internal transfusion is hormonally driven glycogen breakdown in the liver (Fig. 14.3). Sympathetic activation and an associated increase in adrenaline (epinephrine) secretion from the adrenal medulla lead to release of glucose from glycogen stores and, as a consequence, an increase in plasma and interstitial fluid osmolarity. More than half of total body water is held inside cells (see Chapter 11) and the rise in osmolarity draws fluid into the interstitial space from the intracellular compartment. It has been estimated that this fluid movement from the intracellular compartment contributes about half of the volume of the internal transfusion.

The colloid osmotic pressure of plasma will gradually fall as a result of dilution with interstitial fluid. At the same time, capillary blood pressure will gradually rise back towards normal levels as a result of the internal transfusion. Eventually a new equilibrium will be established between the Starling forces and so the internal transfusion will cease.

A consequence of the internal transfusion is haemodilution, a fall in haematocrit. Many patients who have suffered a haemorrhage will already have a low haematocrit by the time they reach hospital. While on the one hand

---

Case 14.1 Haemorrhage and circulatory shock: 2

A deterioration in Linda's condition

Just as the ambulance arrives at the hospital Mrs Hamilton vomited again. This time about 1.5 L of fresh blood was produced. Mrs Hamilton became agitated and the paramedics set-up another 500 mL of Gelofusine whilst rushing her into the Resuscitation Room. The A&E staff repeated Mrs Hamilton's observations; her pulse was now 136 bpm and weak. Blood pressure had fallen to 73/25 mmHg. She responded to commands but was not coherent. Her peripheries were cold and clammy. Her capillary refill time was greater than 6 seconds.

The resuscitation team inserted a second large bore cannula and continued to give IV fluid. O negative blood was given whilst the blood taken from the second cannula was sent for basic full blood count, biochemistry, clotting and cross-match of 5 units. Her initial [Hb] came back at 64 g/L (normal range for a woman: 115–160 g/L).

After 2 units of O negative blood and 2 L of 0.9% saline (normal saline) Mrs Hamilton was responsive. However she remained tachycardic (pulse 106 bpm beats per minute) and hypotensive (blood pressure 102/65). She was catheterized soon after arrival in the hospital and her urine output remained low at around 1 mL/kg/h.

The following questions arise concerning the status of Linda's circulatory system at this time.

1. What other, undetected, changes have been proceeding as a response to the gastrointestinal bleeding?
2. What information does the assessment of capillary refill time provide?
3. What physiological changes lead to the low urine flow rate?

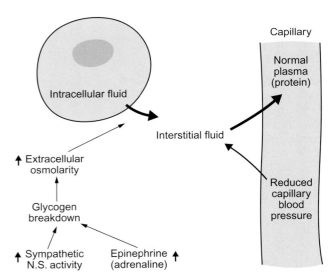

Fig. 14.3 'Internal transfusion'. Factors influencing 'internal transfusion', the net movement of water from the interstitial and intracellular compartments into the intravascular compartment following a haemorrhage.

this reduced haematocrit will lower blood viscosity (see Chapter 8) and make it easier for blood to flow round the body, the reduced viscosity also lowers the resistance to blood flow and potentially contributes to a further fall in blood pressure. The reduced oxygen carrying capacity of blood as a result of haemodilution will restrict oxygen delivery to already poorly perfused tissues.

Longer term responses which help to restore lost blood volume and electrolytes

Shifting water between the various fluid compartments in the body as a short-term measure still leaves the problem of replacing the overall water loss following a haemorrhage. This is achieved by a combination of changes in glomerular filtration rate in the kidneys and hormonally mediated changes in kidney tubular function (Fig. 14.4).

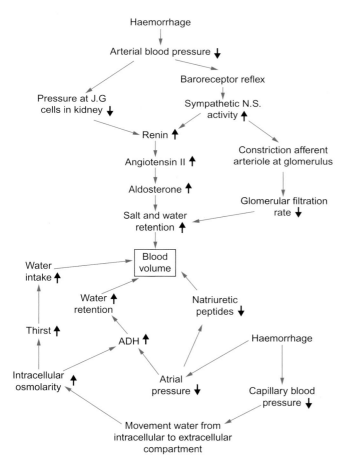

Fig. 14.4 Summary of the hormonal control of salt and water retention in the kidney. The events on the top half of this diagram are triggered by a fall in arterial blood pressure. The lower half represents events which are a consequence of changes in the venous and capillary segments of the circulation. After a moderate (e.g. 20%) haemorrhage these mechanisms will restore total body water and salt content to normal over about a 3 day period if salt and water intake are adequate.

Assuming an adequate oral salt and water intake, in the case of a 20% blood volume loss the body fluid volumes would be returned to normal over a period of about 3 days.

Sympathetic activation, as a result of the fall in blood pressure and the baroreceptor reflex, leads to intrarenal vasoconstriction. This particularly affects the afferent arterioles but also the efferent arterioles at the glomeruli. This leads to a reduction in glomerular filtration rate which helps to conserve water and electrolytes. The potential danger of prolonged intrarenal vasoconstriction is ischaemia leading to acute tubular necrosis (ATN). The nephron becomes blocked with swollen and necrotic tubular epithelial cells and the patient becomes oliguric (less than 100 mL urine per day). ATN is recoverable provided volume replacement is achieved and glomerular function is re-established within an adequate time course.

The main hormones involved in salt and water retention are described below.

Renin-angiotensin aldosterone system (see Chapter 9)

The main triggers for increased renin release following haemorrhage are firstly an increase in sympathetic nerve activity which, via a β-adrenoceptor mechanism on the juxtaglomerular (JG) cells, will increase renin secretion (Fig. 14.4). This increase in renin secretion is therefore linked to the fall in blood pressure at the carotid sinus baroreceptor. Secondly, the JG cells respond directly to a fall in renal artery blood pressure to increase renin secretion. An increase in renin secretion will increase the generation of angiotensin II (Ang II). This has two beneficial roles in the acute response to haemorrhage. The immediate vasoconstrictor effect of Ang II helps to maintain arterial blood pressure. Ang II is also the major stimulus to increased aldosterone synthesis in the zona glomerulosa of the adrenal cortex.

Aldosterone has a sodium retaining and potassium excreting action on the distal segments of the nephron. Water is absorbed osmotically along with the sodium retained. Ang II is also involved, by its action on the subfornical organ of the brain, in promoting thirst responses. A patient who had suffered an acute 20% haemorrhage and has had no fluid replacement therapy would experience an intense thirst within an hour or so. This is mainly due to changes in the environment of the thirst centre in the hypothalamus associated with the fluid shifts which generate the internal transfusion (see p. 164).

Natriuretic peptide hormones (ANP and BNP)

Release of these hormones, particularly from the atria of the heart, is an important aspect of normal blood volume regulation (Fig. 14.4). Expansion of blood volume with the consequent increase in central venous pressure and increased stretch of the right atrial wall is the normal trigger for release of natriuretic peptides. Actions of natriuretic peptides include inhibition of the action of aldosterone and a vasodilator action, especially within the kidney, which increases GFR. Following a haemorrhage, natriuretic peptide hormone levels will be suppressed as a consequence of the reduction in central venous pressure. The sodium and water losing effects of the peptides will be reduced thus contributing to maintaining the extracellular fluid volume.

Antidiuretic hormone (ADH)

This peptide hormone is synthesized in the hypothalamus and released into the circulation from the posterior pituitary (Fig. 14.4). The major physiological triggers for secretion are a fall in blood volume, detected by stretch receptors in the atria and great veins (see Chapter 10), or a rise in the osmolarity of blood passing through the hypothalamus. ADH secretion will therefore be increased following haemorrhage.

ADH was initially named vasopressin in recognition of the vasoconstrictor actions of the hormone. Following a haemorrhage high levels of the hormone will contribute to the rise in peripheral resistance, particularly in the cutaneous circulation of the face. These are minor effects compared to sympathetically mediated vasoconstriction however.

The antidiuretic actions of ADH result from an increase in the water permeability of the inner medullary collecting duct of kidney tubules. This allows increased osmotically driven water reabsorption in this segment of the nephron and therefore a reduction in urine volume. Patients who have suffered a haemorrhage have a reduced urine flow rate and are said to be oliguric if their urine flow rate is less than 400 mL/day. In an adult the term anuria is used if urine flow rate is less than 50 mL/day.

Replacement of the remaining components of the lost blood volume

Following the 'internal transfusion' and the activation of salt and water retention in the kidneys the remaining plasma proteins and red blood cells in the circulation are diluted. Plasma proteins are mainly synthesized in the liver and increased synthesis leads to replenishment within about 1 week of a moderate haemorrhage.

Red blood cell production occurs in the bone marrow under the control of the kidney hormone erythropoietin (Epo). The reduced red cell mass and hence reduced oxygen carriage after a haemorrhage is detected within the kidney and results in increased Epo production. The red cells lost during a 20% haemorrhage are replaced in about 4–6 weeks.

Interesting facts

Blood transfusion was attempted in the 17th century, sometimes successfully but often disastrously. The reasons for this did not become apparent until the discovery of blood groups in the early 20th century by the Austrian-born immunologist Landsteiner.

Case 14.1 Haemorrhage and circulatory shock: 3

A successful resolution of Linda's problems

Linda was transferred to a high dependency care unit where she underwent a further decompensation. She was resuscitated with 2 units of cross-matched blood and 1 L of normal saline. It was felt that her condition was not fully satisfactory and an urgent surgical consultation was requested. She was further stabilized and then taken for emergency laparotomy which resulted in the successful repair of a bleeding duodenal ulcer.

The following questions arise:

1. What is meant by decompensated shock?
2. What are the likely consequences of failing to manage circulatory shock adequately?

Decompensated or irreversible shock following haemorrhage

The events described above constitute the compensatory responses to haemorrhage. Most normal people can recover from the loss of up to about 25% of blood volume by purely physiological responses, although clinical intervention will accelerate recovery and minimize end-organ damage. If the blood loss exceeds about 30% of total blood volume and there is a delay of more than 3–4 hours before volume replacement therapy commences, the patient may enter the syndrome of decompensated or irreversible shock. Subsequent full restoration of blood volume may be to no avail.

An increase in sympathetic nervous system activity helping in various ways to sustain arterial blood pressure as described above is a key feature of the compensatory responses to haemorrhage. Decompensation is associated with a fall in arterial blood pressure as a consequence of substantial peripheral vasodilatation. This follows a reduction in sympathetic vasoconstrictor activity which originates in the central pathways in the brain which control sympathetic outflow. Circulating levels of vasoconstrictor hormones such as Ang II, vasopressin and catecholamines remain high but are unable to counter the fall in sympathetic activity. This phase is associated with bradycardia.

The decline in blood pressure has an adverse effect on cardiac function with reduced coronary perfusion. This results in a dangerous positive feedback loop as the fall in cardiac output will lead to further reduction in blood pressure and therefore further impaired coronary blood flow and hence further reduced cardiac performance. The poor tissue perfusion also has an adverse effect in peripheral tissues as it leads to local metabolic acidosis. Accumulation of tissue metabolites, such as H^+ (see Chapter 9), leads to vasodilatation and a further reduction in arterial blood pressure.

Decompensated shock represents a downward spiral of events which may be difficult to interrupt. The general principles of circulatory failure management are firstly to ensure adequate lung ventilation and provide extra oxygen, secondly to restore blood volume by infusion of blood or other fluids and thirdly to use interventions which improve cardiac performance. Experts in this area sometimes refer to the 'golden hour'. Optimal management of haemorrhage within this window of opportunity is crucial for minimizing morbidity and mortality. Correct recognition of the signs and symptoms of reversible shock helps to avoid the onset of catastrophic circulatory collapse.

Causes of shock

Physiological shock is the failure to provide end organs with adequate nutrients. Shock can be conveniently considered under four main headings:

1. hypovolaemic shock—reduction of blood volume
2. cardiogenic shock—pump failure
3. distributive shock—a fall in peripheral resistance and, consequently, decreased arterial blood pressure
4. obstructive shock—occlusion of a blood vessel.

In each case tissue perfusion is reduced and there is an inadequate supply of oxygen to the tissues.

Changes in the body which follow a haemorrhage (hypovolaemic shock) have been outlined above. It should be stressed that there is considerable variation in the responses between different individuals. The prognosis for individuals who suffered identical haemorrhages may be quite different.

In cardiogenic shock following events such as myocardial infarction (see Chapter 5) or serious arrhythmias there will be a fall in systemic arterial blood pressure as a result of the fall in cardiac output. In contrast to hypovolaemic shock, central venous pressure and pulmonary vein pressure are both likely to be increased. Poor left ventricular performance will lead to a rise in filling pressure on the left side of the heart and the possibility of pulmonary oedema. Fluid replacement therapy must therefore be very carefully managed. The changes in kidney function, which are primarily triggered by the fall in arterial blood pressure, will be broadly similar in haemorrhagic and cardiogenic shock.

Septic shock is a common cause of distributive shock and may be associated with bacterial, viral, fungal or protozoal infections. These infections may lead to the release of a wide range of toxic mediators which cause cell damage and cell death. Septic shock represents a complex series of events which may be collectively referred to as the systemic inflammatory response syndrome (SIRS). In the initial phases of septic shock, there is peripheral vasodilatation and a high cardiac output with excess peripheral perfusion and adequate urine flow rate. Later stages of septic shock are associated with vasoconstriction and a fall in cardiac output as a result of increased production of vasoconstrictor agents such as Ang II, catecholamines and thromboxanes. Treatment of the infection is a crucial part of management strategies.

Anaphylactic shock is another form of distributive shock. It represents an immediate hypersensitivity reaction which usually occurs within 30 minutes of exposure to an antigen such as a drug (e.g. penicillin), a specific protein (e.g. in a peanut) or an insect venom (e.g. a bee sting). It is mediated by immunoglobulin E (IgE) and leads to the release of mediators such as histamine which are stored in granules within mast cells. Vasodilatation and an increase in capillary permeability follow the release of histamine (see Chapter 11).

Fluid replacement therapy

The primary reason for fluid replacement therapy is to maintain tissue perfusion by ensuring an adequate cardiac output and a sufficiently high arterial blood pressure. Optimizing the preload effects on the heart in order to maintain cardiac output is an important aspect of fluid management. However care must be taken to avoid overload as this may lead to pulmonary oedema, especially if the patient is already in cardiac failure (see Chapter 6).

An extensive clinical analysis of fluid replacement therapy in a wide range of clinical conditions is outside the scope of this book but some general principles can be established. In relation to calculating the quantity of replacement body fluid the following points are relevant:

- estimate the amount of fluid already lost
- allow for future anticipated abnormal loss as for example in cases of excessive sweating or diarrhoea
- maintain normal daily fluid intake requirements (typically about 2500 mL/day).

Use of blood as a replacement fluid

In the case of haemorrhage blood transfusion is preferable as soon as appropriate cross-matched blood is available. This will improve the oxygen carrying capacity of the circulation but there are a number of potential problems with blood transfusion in addition to the fundamental difficulties of cost, availability, ethical/religious considerations and potential for transmission of infection.

- Cross-matching of blood does take some time which may be critical in an emergency situation. Even then adverse immunological reactions may take place.

- Transfusion which increases the haematocrit above an optimal level of 30–35% may increase the viscosity of blood (see Chapter 8) and hence the flow characteristics may change. Old stored red cells lose part of the flexibility which is essential for them to pass through capillaries (see Chapter 11). This may contribute to the obstruction of small vessels and cause local hypoxia.

- Stored blood loses platelets and is deficient in clotting factors. This may leave the patient with reduced ability to coagulate blood, a dangerous situation particularly during surgery. An effective clotting mechanism can be restored by administering clotting factors and extra platelets.

- Citrate is used as an anticoagulant for stored blood and, as this is metabolized, a metabolic alkalosis (see Chapter 1) will develop over the next 1–2 days.

- 2,3,DPG (see Chapter 1) which is generated inside red cells disappears during storage. This means that the affinity of haemoglobin to bind oxygen increases. The red cells pick up oxygen at the lungs without problem but fail to deliver it adequately in the tissues.

- Other potential sources of problems include a low $[Ca^{++}]$ and high $[K^+]$ in stored blood.

Use of crystalloid solutions as replacement fluids

The term crystalloid covers a range of replacement body fluids. The two simplest solutions are 0.9% saline (9 g sodium chloride/L) and 5% dextrose (50 g glucose/L). Combinations of these two solutes in different proportions (e.g. 0.45% NaCl + 2.5% glucose) together with solutions which more closely reflect the composition of plasma by the inclusion of other constituents (e.g. Hartmann's solution, Ringer-lacate solution) are all isotonic solutions. This means that they do not change the size of cells they come into contact with.

Hypertonic saline solutions (1.8% up to 10% saline) are available for use in special circumstances.

The characteristic of crystalloid solutions is that as the solutes are small they cross capillary walls. The volume of distribution is therefore at least all of the extracellular fluid compartment. The distribution of Na^+ and Cl^- in body fluids is predominantly extracellular and so saline infusion will mainly expand the extracellular space. Dextrose solutions are handled differently. Once infused into the circulation the glucose will be taken up into cells and either metabolized or stored as glycogen. Giving isotonic dextrose solution is therefore ultimately equivalent to an infusion of distilled water. The difference is that there is a sufficient time delay for the solution to become distributed around the body and mix with other body fluids before the glucose is removed. There is therefore dilution of body fluids but no osmotic lysis of cells. Some of the water will enter the intracellular compartment by moving down the osmotic gradient created by the dilution of the extracellular fluid. The volume of distribution of the water is therefore the same as for total body water, i.e. two thirds intracellular and one third extracellular (see Chapter 1).

Use of colloid solutions as replacement fluids

Colloids are large molecules which are initially distributed within the plasma compartment as they are too big to escape across many capillary walls in significant amounts. Colloids in common clinical use include albumin, polygelatins, starch derivatives and dextrans. They are used to raise the colloid osmotic pressure of plasma and therefore prevent or reverse the movement of water from the plasma into the interstitial fluid. The volume of colloid solution needed in order to increase the intravascular volume and therefore the preload on the heart by a given amount will be much smaller than for a crystalloid solution.

Human albumin (rmm = 69 000) is quantitatively the most important contributor to the colloid osmotic pressure of blood. It is normally held within the vascular compartment unless capillary permeability is increased (see Chapter 11). Infusion of an isotonic solution containing human albumin can be used to increase blood volume. However the half-life of albumin in plasma is relatively short, 10% of administered albumin leaves the circulation within 2 hours and 95% within 2 days. Human albumin is used for volume replacement in shock and in burned patients but is not recommended for routine volume replacement because supplies are limited and effective cheaper alternatives are available.

Polygelatin solutions are polypeptides which have commercial names including Haemaccel and Gelofusine (rmm = 35 000) and are isotonic with plasma. They can be given safely in large volumes but, as the cut-off for the size of molecule that can pass through the glomerular filter in the kidney is about 70 000, their half-life in the circulation is only about 4 hours. Large amounts of these polygelatines passing through the nephron may cause an osmotic diuresis and therefore increase urinary fluid loss. They are useful for acute resuscitation procedures but for longer term circulatory support longer half-life colloids need to be used.

Hydroxethyl starches (HES) are highly branched glucose polymers (rmm 70 000 or 200 000) with a circulatory half-life of approximately 17 days. Some disruptions of the clotting cascade are associated with the use of HES.

Dextrans are large polysaccharide molecules (rmm 40 000 or 70 000) with a circulatory half-life of 2–12 hours. They are very effective at increasing the colloid osmotic pressure of plasma but suffer from some side effects. They interfere with cross-matching of blood and a maximum recommended dose should not be exceeded because of the risk of renal failure developing. The clinical uses of dextrans are limited by the availability of alternatives. Up to 5% of patients may develop anaphylaxis.

Selection of suitable volume replacement therapy is a complex decision for which the volume and composition of the fluid lost is a prime consideration. It is also an area of considerable controversy. The relative merits of crystalloid or colloid solutions for fluid replacement during surgery and in resuscitation is a subject for heated debate.

Interesting facts

Medicines will be well used when the doctor understands their nature, what man is, what life is and what constitution and health are. Know these well and you will know their opposites; you will then know well how to devise a remedy.

Leonardo da Vinci (1452–1519)

Further reading

Chien, S., 1967. Role of the sympathetic nervous system in haemorrhage. Phys. Rev. 47, 214–288.

Länne, T., Lundvall, J., 1992. Mechanisms in man for rapid refill of the circulatory system in hypovolaemia. Acta Phys. Scand. 146, 299–306.

Schadt, J.C., Ludbrook, J., 1991. Haemodynamic and neurohumoral responses to acute hypovolemia in conscious mammals. Am. J. Phys. 260, H305–H318.

accessory pathway – second, abnormal, electrical connection between atria and ventricles.

adenosine – a nucleoside composed of the purine base adenine and the pentose sugar ribose. It has vasodilator actions in the peripheral circulation and a range of actions on the heart.

afterload – the force per unit cross-sectional area of muscle that opposes contraction. It depends on the arterial pressure, chamber radius and wall thickness. Arterial blood pressure is often used as a proxy for afterload but this is not rigorously correct. Aortic valve stenosis would, for example, increase the afterload on the left ventricle. Afterload can be thought of simply as the resistance to the outflow of blood from a ventricle.

alveolus – air sacs at the distal portion of the bronchial tree in which the majority of gas exchange takes place.

aneurysm – abnormal localized dilation of an artery wall.

angina pectoris – chest pain or discomfort arising from hypoxia of the myocardium.

angiogenesis – development of new blood vessels as sprouts from existing vessels.

angiography – radiological imaging of blood vessels after injection of radiographic contrast medium.

angioplasty – a technique used to expand a narrowed blood vessel. A catheter with a deflated balloon tip is passed through the narrowed vessel. The balloon is then inflated and pulled back through the narrowed segment of blood vessel.

anuria – either complete cessation of urine flow or a rate less than 50 mL/day.

aortic stenosis – narrowing of the aortic valve; may be supra-valvar if narrowing is in the ascending aorta or sub-valvar if there is obstruction in the left ventricular outflow tract.

apoptosis – a form of programmed individual cell death that occurs normally during embryological development. It also occurs in pathological processes such as atrophy and in neoplasms. It is an energy-dependent process, which is not associated with an inflammatory reaction.

arrhythmia – abnormal rhythm of cardiac muscle excitation and contraction. Arrhythmias may be normal and benign (e.g. sinus arrhythmia) or may indicate serious pathology. Arrhythmia is really a very unsatisfactory word as the word prefix 'a-' implies the complete absence of a rhythm. The term dysrhythmia is much more satisfactory but it is not in widespread use.

arteriolosclerosis – thickening and hardening of arterial walls. The term includes, but is not specific to, atherosclerosis.

ASD – atrial septal defect.

atherosclerosis – degenerative disease of large and medium-sized blood vessels (normally arteries) that are exposed to a high blood pressure.

atrioventricular node (AV node) – a group of cells with automaticity which normally provide the only connection between the atrial and ventricular myocardium. Key role is to delay ventricular contraction at the end of diastole to allow atrial contraction to 'top up' the ventricle with blood. Under certain circumstances the AV node may take over the control of heart rate when there is damage to the SA node.

auscultation – listening for sounds within the body such as cardiac murmurs, breath sounds or fetal heart sounds. Usually, but not necessarily, a stethoscope is used.

automaticity – the capacity to generate spontaneous depolarization and initiate contraction of cardiac muscle; applies to various elements of the conducting system of the heart.

autoregulation – mechanism which keeps blood flow through a tissue at a constant level despite changes in arterial perfusion pressure.

baroreceptor reflex – physiological control mechanism that helps to keep arterial blood pressure relatively constant. The major arterial baroreceptors are located in the carotid sinus and aortic arch. The efferent (output) side of the reflex is via the sympathetic and parasympathetic nerves, which regulate cardiac output and the sympathetic control of arteriolar tone.

bradycardia – a slower than normal heart rate.

breathlessness – awareness of breathing. May be physiological (as after exercise) or pathological (as a result of respiratory or cardiac disease mechanisms – then called dyspnoea).

cardiac output – volume of blood expelled per minute from each of the ventricles of the heart.

cardiomyopathy – a primary pathological problem of cardiac muscle.

cardio-thoracic ratio (CTR) – an assessment of heart size made from an anterior–posterior chest X-ray. The maximum width of the cardiac shadow (C) and the maximum width of the thorax (T) at the inside of the ribs are measured. CTR = C/T.

cardioversion – application of a direct current (DC) through the myocardium in order to simultaneously depolarize all cells. This allows the heart to recommence coordinated sinus rhythm. Used in emergencies in which a serious arrhythmia causes inadequate cardiac output or electively, with lower energy, to induce sinus rhythm in an otherwise haemodynamically stable arrhythmia.

catabolic – metabolic state in which larger molecules are broken down into smaller molecules, often excretory products such as carbon dioxide or urea.

colloid osmotic pressure (COP) – the component of the total osmotic pressure of a fluid (e.g. plasma) which is attributable to large molecules (e.g. proteins or artificial macromolecules) which cannot move between fluid compartments in the body.

compliance – a measure of the ease of inflation of a vessel; defined as the change of volume of an inflatable structure (such as a lung or blood vessel) per unit change in inflating pressure; analogous to the mechanical concept of elasticity (see also distensibility).

contractility – force of contraction at a given myocardial fibre length. Positive inotropes (such as β_1 adrenoceptor agonists) increase contractility. Contractility changes must be distinguished from preload effects which alter myocardial fibre length.

crepitations – a crackling sound which may be heard on auscultation of the chest. The quality of the sounds varies from fine, high pitched sounds produced in the distal air spaces to coarser low pitched sounds which originate more proximally in the lungs.

cyanosis – a blue colouration of the skin or mucous membranes produced by the presence of abnormal amounts of deoxygenated haemoglobin (Hb) in arterial blood. There is no internationally agreed quantitative definition but more than 50 g of deoxygenated Hb per litre of blood is a commonly used standard. Cyanosis may be central (poor oxygenation of arterial blood) or peripheral (stagnant local blood flow).

cytokines – a family of messenger proteins which stimulate the maturation or activation of a variety of cells including lymphocytes and macrophages. Originally known as lymphokines, when it was thought that they were only secreted by lymphocytes, cytokines have a wide variety of different physiological and pathological effects, including the maturation of haemopoietic stem cells.

diastole – filling phase of the ventricle in the cardiac cycle.

distensibility – a term which describes the elastic properties of an expandable structure, such as a blood vessel or the lungs. It is expressed as the change in volume of the structure divided by the change in the inflating pressure. The term distensibility is often used as if it is synonymous with the term compliance. Strictly, distensibility is the compliance divided by the original volume of the structure, i.e., the volume before the pressure inside was increased and the structure was inflated.

ductus arteriosus – embryological structure allowing blood to flow from pulmonary artery to descending aorta.

dysplasia – changes in the histological appearance of cells which suggest that they have become neoplastic. Usually applied to epithelia.

dyspnoea – awareness of abnormal difficulty in breathing.

dysrhythmia – see 'arrhythmia'.

ECG axis – the theoretical vector along which the wavefront of ventricular myocardial depolarization progresses. Usually this term applies to the average or net vector taken over the whole cardiac cycle. There can also be P-wave and T-wave axes.

echocardiography – a non-invasive method for observing the movement of the walls and valves of the heart using a beam of ultra-high frequency sound. Reflections of the sound beam are monitored and used to build a picture of the movement of cardiac structures.

electrocardiography (ECG) – the electrical events associated with the depolarization and repolarization of cardiac muscle are recorded using electrodes placed in standard positions on the surface of the skin.

embolus – mass of foreign material which is transported in the blood stream. Common embolic materials include thrombus, fat or air. Eventually the embolus lodges in a blood vessel which has a smaller lumen diameter than the embolus and thus blocks the vessel.

endocardium – the endothelial cells and associated connective tissue which line the cavities of the heart.

endocytosis – the physiological mechanism by which fluid is taken in small discrete amounts into the cell cytoplasm from the interstitial fluid.

epicardium – the layer of serous pericardium which covers the surface of the heart.

Eustachian valve – embryological structure which lies at the entry of the inferior vena cava into the right atrium and directs oxygenated blood towards the foramen ovale. Remnants can be seen in post-natal life; described as the Chiari apparatus.

fibrillation – completely discoordinated electrical activity of either atria or ventricles. Sustained ventricular fibrillation is not consistent with life. The name arises from the macroscopic appearance of the fibrillating chamber being full of threads or worms.

flutter – refers to very fast regular contractions of the atria (250–300 b/min).

foramen ovale – embryological structure allowing blood to flow from right to left atrium thereby by-passing the lungs in the fetus. More modern nomenclature is oval foramen.

gangrene – a characteristic 'blackening' of necrotic tissue. Produced by infection with anaerobic bacteria and tends to occur in tissues which have a resident bacterial flora, e.g. skin and large bowel.

glycocalyx – a layer of macromolecules which covers the surface of cells. An example is the layer of negatively charged molecules covering the endothelial cells which line the circulation.

hydrostatic pressure (HP) – the pressure in a fluid, i.e. the force per unit area acting on the walls of the structure containing the fluid. Physiologically/clinically can be expressed in units of mm mercury (mmHg), kilopascals (kPa) or cm water (cmH$_2$O).

hyperaemia – increased blood flow.

hyperplasia – the increase in the size of an organ or tissue as a result of an increase in the number of constituent cells. Can only occur in labile or stable tissues, i.e. tissues which can undergo mitotic division.

hypertension – a sustained period of raised arterial blood pressure.

hypertrophy – the enlargement of a tissue or organ resulting from an increase in the size of the constituent cells, *not* an increase in number. Examples include cardiac hypertrophy in hypertension and skeletal muscle in athletes.

hypoxia – a shortage of oxygen, but not an absolute lack (anoxia).

incompetence – a term used to describe valves in the heart which fail to prevent the backflow of blood (regurgitation) through the valve after valve closure.

infarct – an area of necrosis produced by an obstruction of the circulation.

inflammation – a mechanism by which the body reacts to many different forms of injury. Acute inflammation has both vascular and cellular components and usually lasts for days or a few weeks. In chronic inflammation, there is a mixed cellular response, including macrophages and cells derived from macrophages, and the process can last for months or years.

inotrope – neurotransmitter (e.g. norepinephrine/noradrenaline) or hormone (e.g. epinephrine/adrenaline) or a drug (e.g. digoxin) that alters contractility of the heart muscle. Positive inotropes increase contractility and negative inotropes decrease contractility.

ischaemia – shortage of blood flow, often a result of an obstruction to the circulation.

juxtaglomerular apparatus – it is composed of two groups of cells in the kidney. Modified smooth muscle cells in the wall of the afferent arteriole just before it enters the glomerulus are also known as 'granular cells'. The macula densa cells form part of the wall of the kidney tubule where the ascending limb of the loop of Henle becomes the distal tubule. The granular cells secrete renin probably partly in response to signals originating in the macula densa.

Korotkow sounds – Nicolai Korotkow was a Russian surgeon. In 1905 he described the use of ausculation of the turbulence noises produced when a blood vessel is partially occluded as the basis for the non-invasive measurement of arterial blood pressure.

lead (for ECG recording) – the combination of two electrodes which is used to define a specific direction for the ECG, e.g. lead I, lead II, etc.

leucocyte – white blood cell.

lymph – interstitial (tissue) fluid which enters the lymphatic system, effectively a tissue drainage system.

lymphocytes – all lymphocytes originate as stem cells in the bone marrow. Those which become T-lymphocytes mature in the thymus gland. Those which become B-lymphocytes mature in the bone marrow. Together they form the basis of the immune system.

macrophage – a mononuclear cell derived from blood monocytes with phagocytic properties. Prominent in the chronic inflammatory response.

metabolite – a term used to refer to mediators such as carbon dioxide, H^+ adenosine, K^+ and lactic acid. Accumulation of these mediators in a tissue leads to vasodilation and an increase in local blood flow. In this way the distribution of blood flow around the body is regulated.

murmur – a sound heard during auscultation of the heart or a blood vessel produced by turbulent blood flow.

myocardium – heart muscle.

necrosis – the changes which occur in organs or tissues after cell death in a living body. Often taken to include cell death.

oedema – the accumulation of abnormal amounts of interstitial fluid in a tissue. Occurs when the normal balance between the hydrostatic pressure of the circulation and the osmotic force of the plasma proteins is upset.

oliguria – a urine flow rate which is insufficient to excrete the daily production of nitrogenous waste material (urea). Less than 300 mL/day.

oncotic pressure – the component of the total osmotic pressure of a fluid (e.g. plasma) which is exerted by the large non-diffusible molecules such as plasma proteins or infused macromolecules used as plasma expanders. Oncotic pressure means the same as colloid osmotic pressure.

orthogonal – at right angles.

orthopnoea – breathlessness which develops when a non-upright posture is assumed.

pacemaker – the site of origin of electrical depolarization which leads to the contraction of cardiac muscle, normally the sino-atrial node.

pacing – regulation of the rate of cardiac contraction by the use of an artificial pacemaker.

palpitations – sensation described by a patient of the awareness of the heart beating.

PDA – patent ductus arteriosus; persistence of the ductus arteriosus into post-natal life. More modern nomenclature persistent arterial duct.

pericardium – a bag-like structure which surrounds the heart and the origins of the great vessels.

pericytes – elongated contractile cells which wrap around precapillary arterioles outside the basement membrane.

PFO – patent foramen ovale—persistence of the foramen ovale in the post-natal heart.

phosphodiesterase – enzymes which promote the breakdown of the cyclic nucleotides (cyclic AMP, cyclic GMP) which act as second messengers in cell signalling. Inhibition of phosphodiesterase enzymes by drugs increases the concentration of the second messenger within a cell and potentiates its actions.

precapillary sphincter – cuff of smooth muscle around the entrance to a capillary.

preload – the force acting to stretch the ventricular muscle fibres at the end of diastole and therefore determines the maximum resting length of the sarcomeres. Increased preload leads to increased force of ventricular contraction (Starling's Law). The end-diastolic volume and the filling pressure (atrial pressure) are often used as proxys for the preload of the heart although neither is rigorously correct.

prostaglandins – family of biological mediators which are derived from the metabolism of arachidonic acid through the cycloxygenase (COX) pathway.

pulmonary hypertension (PHT) – elevation of the pressure in the pulmonary vascular bed. Implies abnormality of the pulmonary arteriolar resistance vessels and does not apply to focal obstructions (which are stenoses).

pulmonary stenosis – narrowing of the pulmonary valve.

radiation (for heart murmurs) – abnormal heart sounds can sometimes be heard away from the heart in the direction of blood flow. Thus the murmur of aortic valve stenosis can radiate and be listened to over the carotid artery.

regurgitation – abnormal movement of blood back through a closed, but incompetent, heart valve.

remodelling – changes in the structure of the heart and/or blood vessels in response to cardiovascular diseases such as myocardial infarction or hypertension. These remodelling changes are often not advantageous and have become an important focus for drug therapy.

respiratory quotient –

$$RQ = \frac{\text{Carbon dioxide produced}}{\text{Oxygen consumed}}$$

A typical value for RQ for someone on a mixed diet is 0.8.

sarcomere – the contractile unit in striated muscle which is composed of parallel arrays of myosin and actin filaments. Each sarcomere is bounded by a Z line.

shock – a syndrome of altered circulatory and metabolic function as a result of inadequate perfusion of tissues with blood.

shunt – an abnormal flow of blood between two normally separated structures. The volume of the shunt determines its clinical significance.

sino-atrial node (SA node) – a group of cells in the right atrium adjacent to the superior vena cava, which have high automaticity and usually provide the control of heart rate. Also known as the primary pacemaker.

sphygmomanometer – device used in arterial blood pressure measurement consisting of an inflatable cuff to occlude a blood vessel and a gauge to record pressure inside the cuff.

stenosis – narrowing of a valve or vessel.

surfactant – a complex mixture of proteins and phospholipids crucial in reducing surface tension in the alveoli in the lungs.

syncope – a temporary loss of consciousness (a faint) due to inadequate blood flow to the brain.

systole – contraction phase of the ventricle in the cardiac cycle.

tachycardia – a faster than normal heart rate.

textbook person – a 70 kg male aged 20–25 years. 'Normal' values quoted in textbooks usually refer to such an individual.

thrombus – an aggregate of platelets and fibrin with enmeshed leucocytes formed in living vessels with flowing blood. Thrombi may fragment and embolize (thromboembolism).

Valsalva manoeuvre – series of changes in heart rate and arterial blood pressure which accompany raised intrathoracic pressure. This occurs during straining as, for example, when trying to lift a heavy weight. It forms the basis of a test for the competence of autonomic function.

vasculitis – an inflammatory disease of blood vessels.

vasoconstriction – contraction of smooth muscle in a blood vessel wall, and hence reduction of the lumen diameter. The term vasoconstriction should specifically apply to vessels on the arterial side of the circulation.

vasodilation – relaxation of a blood vessel wall, and hence an increase in lumen diameter on the arterial side of the circulation.

vasovagal attack – an event characterized by a transient reduction in arterial blood pressure, increase in heart rate, peripheral vasoconstriction and sweating. It may be accompanied by a temporary loss of consciousness (syncope) and is most commonly associated with the emotional stress accompanying fear or pain.

vegetation – an infected mass which appears on a heart valve. It may be said to have the gross appearance of a fungus. Composed of bacteria and thrombus, may embolise.

venoconstriction – constriction of blood vessels on the venous side of the circulation, i.e., venules and veins. The term vasoconstriction is used to apply to vessels on the arterial side.

venodilation – the opposite of venoconstriction.

VSD – ventricular septal defect.

Index